MASTER TECHNIQUES IN OTOLARYNGOLOGY—HEAD AND NECK SURGERY

Head and Neck Surgery

THYROID, PARATHYROID, SALIVARY GLANDS, PARANASAL SINUSES AND NASOPHARYNX

Series Editor

EUGENE N. MYERS, MD, FACS, FRCS EDIN (HON)

Volume Editors

Master Techniques in Otolaryngology—Head and Neck Surgery
Head and Neck Surgery: Larynx, Hypopharynx, Oropharynx, Oral Cavity and Neck
Volume 1
Robert L. Ferris, MD, PhD, FACS

Master Techniques in Otolaryngology—Head and Neck Surgery
Head and Neck Surgery: Thyroid, Parathyroid, Salivary Glands, Paranasal Sinuses and Nasopharynx
Volume 2
Robert L. Ferris, MD, PhD, FACS

Master Techniques in Otolaryngology—Head and Neck Surgery: Reconstructive Surgery
Eric Genden, MD

Master Techniques in Otolaryngology—Head and Neck Surgery: Skull Base Surgery
Carl H. Snyderman, MD
Paul Gardner, MD

Master Techniques in Otolaryngology—Head and Neck Surgery: Rhinology
David Kennedy, MD

Master Techniques in Otolaryngology—Head and Neck Surgery: Facial Plastic Surgery
Wayne Larrabee Jr, MD and James Ridgeway, MD

Master Techniques in Otolaryngology—Head and Neck Surgery: Otology and Lateral Skull Base Surgery
J. Thomas Roland, MD

Head and Neck Surgery

THYROID, PARATHYROID, SALIVARY GLANDS, PARANASAL SINUSES AND NASOPHARYNX

VOLUME 2

Series Editor

Eugene N. Myers, MD, FACS, FRCS Edin (Hon)

Distinguished Professor and Emeritus Chair
Department of Otolaryngology
University of Pittsburgh School of Medicine
Professor, Department of Oral Maxillofacial Surgery
University of Pittsburgh School of Dental Medicine
Pittsburgh, Pennsylvania

Editor

Robert L. Ferris, MD, PhD, FACS

UPMC Endowed Professor and Chief, Division of Head and Neck Surgery
Vice Chair for Clinical Affairs, Department of Otolaryngology
Associate Director for Translational Research
Co-Leader, Cancer Immunology Program
University of Pittsburgh Cancer Institute
Pittsburgh, Pennsylvania

Wolters Kluwer | Lippincott Williams & Wilkins
Health

Philadelphia · Baltimore · New York · London
Buenos Aires · Hong Kong · Sydney · Tokyo

Acquisions Editor: Ryan Shaw
Print Production Manager: Marian Bellus
Product Developmental Editor: Dave Murphy
Design Manager: Doug Smock
Manufacturing Manager: Beth Welsh
Marketing Manager: Daniel Dressler
Production Services: SPi Global

9 8 7 6 5 4 3 2 1

Printed in China

Library of Congress Cataloging-in-Publication Data
CIP data available from the publisher upon request.
ISBN 978-1-4511-4367-6

Care has been taken to confirm the accuracy of the information presented and to describe generally accepted practices. However, the author, editors, and publisher are not responsible for errors or omissions or for any consequences from application of the information in this book and make no warranty, expressed or implied, with respect to the currency, completeness, or accuracy of the contents of the publication. Application of this information in a particular situation remains the professional responsibility of the practitioner; the clinical treatments described and recommended may not be considered absolute and universal recommendations.

The author, editors, and publisher have exerted every effort to ensure that drug selection and dosage set forth in this text are in accordance with the current recommendations and practice at the time of publication. However, in view of ongoing research, changes in government regulations, and the constant flow of information relating to drug therapy and drug reactions, the reader is urged to check the package insert for each drug for any change in indications and dosage and for added warnings and precautions. This is particularly important when the recommended agent is a new or infrequently employed drug.

Some drugs and medical devices presented in this publication have Food and Drug Administration (FDA) clearance for limited use in restricted research settings. It is the responsibility of the health care provider to ascertain the FDA status of each drug or device planned for use in his or her clinical practice.

LWW.com

This series of books is dedicated to Barbara, my wife and best pal.

*Our daughter, Marjorie Fulbright, her husband Cary and their sons,
Alexander F. Fulbright and Charles J. Fulbright.*

*Our son, Jeffrey N. Myers, MD, PhD, his wife Lisa and their sons
Keith N. Myers, Brett A. Myers, and Blake D. Myers.*

All of whom I love and cherish.

Eugene N. Myers

The conception, development, and realization of a large new effort such as this requires much devotion and support from staff and loved ones. In particular, I would like to dedicate this book to my phenomenally supportive and successful wife, Laura, without whom I could not have accomplished very many things in my career. I also appreciate the close mentoring relationship and guidance I have enjoyed over many years from Dr. Eugene N. Myers (Series Editor), who continues to provide opportunities for my career growth and contributions to the field of head and neck surgery.

Robert L. Ferris

Ricardo L. Carrau, MD, FACS
Professor
Department of Otolaryngology–Head and
Neck Surgery
Director of the Comprehensive Skull Base
Surgery Program
The Ohio State University Medical Center
Columbus, Ohio

Francisco J. Civantos, MD, FACS
Associate Professor
Department of Otolaryngology
University of Miami Health System
Miami, Florida

Claudio R. Cernea, MD
Professor
Department of Head and Neck Surgery
University of São Paulo Medical School
Department of Head and Neck Surgery
Federal University of São Paulo
São Paulo, Brazil

Jimmy Yu-wai Chan, MD, MS, FRCS
Chief, Division of Head & Neck Surgery,
Division of Plastic & Reconstructive Surgery
Department of Surgery
Queen Mary Hospital
The University of Hong Kong
Hong Kong, Republic of China

Mu-Kuan Chen, MD, MS, PhD
Professor
Chung Shan Medical University
Chief Medical Director
Changhua Christian Hospital
President
Taiwan Head and Neck Society
Taichung City, Taiwan, Republic of China

Woong Youn Chung, MD
Chief, Division of Endocrine Surgery
Department of Surgery
Yonsei University College of Medicine
Seoul, South Korea

Gary L. Clayman, DMD, MD, FACS
Professor of Surgery and Director of Head
and Neck Cancer Program
Alando J. Ballantyne Distinguished Chair
of Head and Neck Surgery
Department of Head and Neck Surgery
The University of Texas MD Anderson
Cancer Center
Houston, Texas

Pavel Dulguerov, MD
Chief of Head and Neck Surgery
Department of Otorhinolaryngology Head
and Neck Surgery
Geneva University Hospital
Geneva, Switzerland

Umamaheswar Duvvuri, MD, PhD
Assistant Professor
Department of Otolaryngology
University of Pittsburgh Medical Center
VA Pittsburgh Health System
Pittsburgh, Pennsylvania

David W. Eisele, MD, FACS
Andelot Professor and Director
Department of Otolaryngology–Head and
Neck Surgery
Johns Hopkins University School of
Medicine
Baltimore, Maryland

Robert L. Ferris, MD, PhD, FACS
Editor
UPMC Endowed Professor and Chief,
Division of Head and Neck Surgery
Vice Chair for Clinical Affairs, Department
of Otolaryngology
Associate Director for Translational
Research and
Co-Leader, Cancer Immunology
Program
University of Pittsburgh Cancer Institute
Pittsburgh, Pennsylvania

Jeremy L. Freeman, MD, FRCSC, FACS
Professor of Otolaryngology–Head and
Neck Surgery
Professor of Surgery, University of
Toronto
Temmy Latner/Dynacare Chair in Head
and Neck Oncology
Mount Sinai Hospital
Toronto, Ontario, Canada

Sheng-Po Hao, MD, FACS
Professor and Chairman
Department of Otolaryngology–Head and
Neck Surgery
Shin Kong Wu-Ho-Su Memorial Hospital
School of Medicine
Fu Jen Catholic University
Taipei, Taiwan, Republic of China

Keith S. Heller, MD, FACS
Professor of Surgery
Chief
Division of Endocrine Surgery
Department of Surgery
NYU Langone Medical Center
New York, New York

Heinrich Iro, MD, PhD
Professor and Chairman
Department of Otorhinolaryngology–Head
and Neck Surgery
University of Erlangen-Nuremberg
Erlangen, Germany

Sang-Wook Kang, MD
Assistant Professor
Department of Surgery
Yonsei University College of Medicine
Seoul, South Korea

Seiji Kishimoto, MD
Professor and Chairman
Department of Head and Neck Surgery
Tokyo Medical and Dental University
Tokyo, Japan

Yoon Woo Koh, MD, PhD
Associate Professor
Department of Otorhinolaryngology
Yonsei Head and Neck Cancer Center
Yonsei University College of Medicine
Seoul, South Korea

Jesus Medina, MD, FACS
Professor
Department of Otolaryngology
University of Oklahoma, College of
Medicine
Oklahoma City, Oklahoma

**Eugene N. Myers, MD, FACS, FRCS
Edin (Hon)**
Series Editor
Distinguished Professor and Emeritus
Chair
Department of Otolaryngology
University of Pittsburgh School of
Medicine
Professor, Department of Oral
Maxillofacial Surgery
University of Pittsburgh School of Dental
Medicine
Pittsburgh, Pennsylvania

Jeffrey N. Myers, MD, PhD, FACS
Professor
Department of Head and Neck Surgery
The University of Texas MD Anderson
Cancer Center
Houston, Texas

James L. Netterville, MD, FACS
Mark C. Smith Professor
Director of Head and Neck Surgery
Bill Wilkerson Center for Communication
Sciences
Vanderbilt Medical Center
Nashville, Tennessee

Kerry D. Olsen, MD
Professor of Otolaryngology
Department of Otorhinolaryngology, Head
and Neck Surgery
Mayo Medical School and Mayo Clinic
Rochester, Minnesota

Mark S. Persky, MD
Professor and Chairman
Department of Otolaryngology–Head and
Neck Surgery
Beth Israel Medical Center
Physician-in-Chief
Continuum Otolaryngology Service Line
Professor of Clinical Otolaryngology
Albert Einstein College of Medicine
New York, New York

Gregory W. Randolph, MD, FACS
Director of the General Otolaryngology
Service
Director of the Thyroid and Parathyroid
Surgical Service
Massachusetts Eye and Ear Institute
Harvard Medical School
Boston, Massachusetts

K. Thomas Robbins, MD
Professor
Division of Otolaryngology–Head and
Neck Surgery
Southern Illinois University School of
Medicine
Executive Director
Simmons Cancer Institute at Southern
Illinois University
Simmons Cancer Institute Endowed Chair
of Excellence in Oncology
Springfield, Illinois

Ashok R. Shaha, MD, FACS
Professor of Surgery
Jatin P. Shah Chair in Head and Neck
Surgery
Cornell University Medical College
Memorial Sloan-Kettering Cancer Center
New York, New York

Alfred A. Simental, MD, FACS
Chairman, Division of Otolaryngology–
Head and Neck Surgery
Department of Otolaryngology–Head and
Neck Surgery
Loma Linda University School of
Medicine
Loma Linda, California

Brendan C. Stack Jr, MD, FACS, FACE
Professor
Department of Otolaryngology–Head and
Neck Surgery
University of Arkansas for Medical
Sciences
Little Rock, Arkansas

James Y. Suen, MD
Distinguished Professor and Chair
Department of Otolaryngology–Head and
Neck Surgery
University of Arkansas, College of
Medicine
Little Rock, Arkansas

David J. Terris, MD
Porubsky Distinguished Professor and
Chairman
Department of Otolaryngology
Georgia Regents University
Department of Otolaryngology–Head and
Neck Surgery
Medical College of Georgia
Augusta, Georgia

Ralph P. Tufano, MD, MBA, FACS
Professor
Department of Otolaryngology–Head and
Neck Surgery
Johns Hopkins University School of
Medicine
Director
Division of Head and Neck Endocrine
Surgery
The Johns Hopkins Hospital
Director, The Johns Hopkins Hospital
Multidisciplinary Thyroid Tumor Center
Baltimore, Maryland

Alexander C. Vlantis, FCSHK
Associate Professor
Department of Otorhinolaryngology–Head
and Neck Surgery
The Chinese University of Hong Kong
Consultant
Department of Otorhinolaryngology–Head
and Neck Surgery
Prince of Wales Hospital
Hong Kong, Republic of China

Randal S. Weber, MD
Professor and Chairman
Department of Head and Neck Surgery
The University of Texas MD Anderson
Cancer Center
Houston, Texas

**William Ignace Wei, MS, FRCS, FRCSE,
FRACS(Hon), FACS(Hon), FHKAM**
Director
Li Shu Pui ENT, Head & Neck Surgery
Center
Hong Kong Sanatorium & Hospital
Hong Kong, Republic of China

Master Techniques in Otolaryngology—Head and Neck Surgery occupies a unique place in the pantheon of outstanding textbooks in the field of head and neck surgery. The topics are highly technical approaches to the field of head and neck oncology dealing with an extensive variety of both benign and malignant pathologics. The description of the surgery is accompanied by outstanding illustrations. This text is unique because each chapter is authored by an individual acknowledged to be a thought leader in the field without the luxury of contributions made by residents or fellows.

The chapters are carefully edited to reflect the effective style of Dr. Eugene N. Myers. The result is a true compendium of expert advice on nearly every topic in head and neck oncology. This reference will be a valuable addition to the library of even the most experienced surgeon, as it offers an opportunity to compare and contrast your personal approach to the methodology currently being taught by international experts.

Jonas T. Johnson, MD, FACS
The Dr. Eugene N. Myers Professor and Chair of Otolaryngology
University of Pittsburgh School of Medicine

Series Preface

Since its inception in 1994, the *Master Techniques in Orthopedic Surgery* series has become the go to text for surgeons in training and in practice. The user-friendly style of providing and illustrating authoritative information on a broad spectrum of techniques of orthopaedic surgery obviously filled a need in orthopaedic educational materials. The format has become a standard against which others are compared, and there are now 13 volumes in the series with other volumes in the planning phase.

When I was approached to be the series editor, I already knew what a daunting task it would be from my previous experience with editing surgical texts, but I felt this unique approach could become a valuable fixture in the catalogue of literature on surgery in all the subspecialty fields of Otolaryngology. This first edition includes volumes on Head and Neck Oncology, Reconstructive Surgery of the Head and Neck, Cranial Base Surgery, Rhinology, Aesthetic Surgery, and Otology and Lateral Skull Base Surgery.

I have recruited real masters to be volume editors including Robert L. Ferris, Eric Genden, Carl H. Snyderman and Paul Gardner, David Kennedy, Wayne Larrabee and James Ridgeway, and J. Thomas Roland, respectively. Having a separate volume on Reconstructive Surgery of the Head and Neck as a separate companion piece for the volume on Head and Neck Oncology is somewhat nontraditional but enabled us to include more topics.

I do hope that you will find the *Master Techniques* to be a useful addition to your surgical armamentarium for the benefit of your patients.

Eugene N. Myers, MD
Series Editor

Learning surgical techniques, as well as particular operations, is a rite of passage during training and continues afterward. Often we learn from our mentors and colleagues their well thought-out technical approaches and rationale for each approach and surgical maneuver, ultimately creating a hybrid of preferences and surgical style unique to each individual surgeon. Nonetheless, surgical techniques have many aspects in common to different individuals, conjoined by the relevant anatomy and its distortion often by neoplastic pathology. Thus, we endeavor to provide a compilation of individual approaches to unique as well as common surgical procedures, articulated by a single author who is an acknowledged surgical leader, a "Master" of each technique. In this new and unique volume, we have endeavored to transmit, through an outstanding group of world-renowned surgeon-authors, the rational for a particular surgical procedure and the technical details.

Often a surgical atlas is a composite of techniques blended together and usually written primarily by younger, early-stage surgical trainees (fellow or resident) on behalf of the more senior authors. However, we set out with the express intent to bypass this traditional approach, and instead to create single-author chapters written by the master surgeon herself/himself. The effort associated with this was greater for each individual surgeon, since they had to spend more time than usual writing the technical details of their particular assigned surgical procedure. The product is an outstanding and unique compilation of technical material, rationale, preoperative, intraoperative, and postoperative pearls (accompanied by various pitfalls to avoid).

The reader benefits from these single-author contributions from world-renowned surgical scholars, the Masters themselves, many of whom designed, refined, or in fact created the surgical technique authored and promulgated in each chapter. They hand-selected or created color pictures, videos, and sketches made exclusively for this edition in the vast majority of cases. We consider this volume a unique contribution to the surgical field not only for residents and fellows but also for advanced trainees and for ongoing surgical practitioners familiar with a particular surgical approach in their own practices.

We are deeply appreciative of the efforts of our colleagues, the Masters, who agreed to such an unusual and protean task, to describe their assigned technique in the first person as a single-author chapter. Our appreciation will be exceeded, in our opinion, by the benefit of their contribution to the head and neck surgical community who receive the fruits of years of refinement and development of these surgical approaches. Ultimately our patients stand to reap the rewards of this new set of volumes, which will hopefully enrich our care of patients and the positive clinical outcomes they experience.

Robert L. Ferris, MD, PhD, FACS

I would like to acknowledge Jonas T. Johnson, MD, for providing me with the stimulus to take on the task of editing a new project—*Master Techniques in Otolaryngology—Head and Neck Surgery*. It has proved to be a daunting task but I believe in the positive impact this will have on those doing head and neck surgery and their patients.

I also acknowledge the dedicated assistance of Agnes C. Zachoszcz and Charmaine Wallace in the preparation of the book.

I also gratefully acknowledge Robert Hurley who recruited me into the project and Ryan Shaw, his successor, for his strong support. David Murphy Jr, who had the daunting task of supplying the technical backup and put the book together.

Contents

Video Content

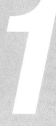

SENTINEL NODE BIOPSY IN CANCER OF THE ORAL CAVITY AND UPPER AERODIGESTIVE TRACT

Francisco J. Civantos

INTRODUCTION

The approach to the N0 neck in patients with early invasive squamous cell carcinoma of the upper aerodigestive tract remains controversial. A "watchful waiting" policy has traditionally been used in order to avoid the unnecessary morbidity in the majority of patients in whom neck metastases will never develop. Patients at risk have been identified by the characteristics of the primary lesion, such as thickness >4 mm, tumor size >2 cm, anatomic location, microinvasion, and perineural infiltration. However, none of these represent a fool proof means of defining the population at risk.

When an early, invasive primary cancer of the oral cavity is identified and no clinically or radiologically involved cervical lymph nodes (LNs) are present, we must still consider management of the LNs. The 20% to 30% risk of occult metastases must be weighed against the morbidity of dissecting necks that do not contain metastatic cancer. Sentinel node biopsy is appropriate for situations where the expected risk of metastases falls in the 5% to 15% range, which might be too high to feel comfortable with watchful waiting but too low to justify the potential morbidity of a selective neck dissection.

In order to validate this technique for cancer of the oral cavity, a trial funded by the National Cancer Institute was completed in North America under the auspices of the American College of Surgeons Oncology Group (ACOSOG). The results of the ACOSOG trial revealed, after central step sectioning and immunohistochemistry for cytokeratins, a negative predictive value (NPV) of 96% and false-negative rate of 9.8%. Interestingly, for T1 cancers in both groups of surgeons, in the setting of a 25% true-positive rate, the false-negative rate was 0% and NPV was 100%. Similarly, for the group of experienced surgeons, false-negative rate was 0% and NPV was 100%.

HISTORY

The typical patient who is a candidate for sentinel node biopsy presents with a visible and accessible cancer in the oral cavity. The patient will typically have seen or felt a lesion in the oral cavity, perhaps with the tongue, or at the time of brushing the teeth. The lesion is typically mildly uncomfortable. There may be a history of bleeding. The lesion may have been identified by the patient's dentist or physician as biopsy-proven squamous cell carcinoma.

PHYSICAL EXAMINATION

On physical examination, there is a lesion, which is ideally <2 or 3 cm in size and has some degree of thickness, which the examiner estimates to be several millimeters thick but not massively invasive. The lesion may be red or white and will generally be rough or irregular. It may be ulcerated. The patient has no movement abnormalities of the tongue or trismus. There is no palpable pathologic adenopathy.

INDICATIONS

The sentinel node biopsy procedure is best applied to T1-T2 cancers. Thus, oral cavity, oropharynx, and selected supraglottic laryngeal cancers, staged cT1N0 or cT2N0, should be considered for sentinel lymph node (SLN) biopsy. Appropriate clinical and radiographic evaluation should be used to stage these preoperatively. This might correspond to about 2 to 6 mm depth of invasion, but this is a hypothetical concept at this point, and greater experience and larger published clinical trials on sentinel node biopsy as the initial approach to the neck are needed to confirm this concept. The majority of patients on the ACOSOG validation trial were in this group. Extremely thin lesions, which might be mistaken for in situ or dysplastic lesions and subsequently turn out to be minimally invasive on biopsy, are not appropriate as the risk of metastases to the cervical lymphatics is negligible, at 2% or less. Lesions that feel mildly thick or gritty, or have some firmness, without massive invasion, are ideal. Some authors report SLN biopsy for cT3N0 tumors, but the size (>4 cm) reduces the accuracy of lymphatic mapping due to alternative drainage patterns, and thus, these are not recommended for SLN biopsy in my experience.

CONTRAINDICATIONS

In my opinion, lesions that extend deep into tongue muscle or deep into the buccal or palate region are better served with selective neck dissection. If a cancer is <3 cm in maximum diameter but has significant fixation of the tongue or other manifestation of deep invasion, then this lesion is truly a T4 lesion and results with sentinel node biopsy are unlikely to prove accurate and useful. Sentinel node biopsy has a low false-negative rate, but the NPV will be less if the population selected has a very high rate of metastases. In other words, a 4% rate of false negatives is acceptable if applied to a population with a 15% risk of metastases, but if applied to a population where most of the patients have micrometastases, the miss rate will be unacceptably high. Thus, deeply invasive lesions or lesions >4 cm are better served by either selective neck dissection or, if desired, sentinel node mapping and biopsy followed by immediate neck dissection. The latter approach can assist in making decisions about the contralateral side of the neck and provide improved identification of micrometastases, while eliminating the risk of false negatives leading to undertreatment of the patient. Patients with suspicious LNs on physical examination or imaging are also not candidates for this procedure. T3-T4 lesions, with trismus, bone invasion, tongue fixation, or other signs of massive deep invasion, are too deep to feel comfortable that the injection has fully mapped the drainage of the lesion, and such findings represent a contraindication to sentinel lymph node biopsy (SLNB).

PREOPERATIVE PLANNING

Imaging Studies

If the primary tumor meets criteria described above, the next issue is whether the neck is grossly involved. While the sentinel node technique is an excellent technique for detecting micrometastases, it is less useful for detecting nonpalpable but grossly involved LNs. This appears to be particularly true with squamous cell carcinoma. It is postulated that when a large percentage of the LN is replaced by cancer, physiologic obstruction occurs and alternative patterns of lymphatic drainage develop. It is important to detect the presence of such gross disease on preoperative imaging and avoid applying this technique to that group of patients, in order to avoid false positives. Generally contrast-enhanced computerized tomography (CT) and magnetic resonance imaging (MRI) (if iodine allergic) are the imaging modalities used. These should be strictly interpreted, and patients should be excluded if there are nodes >1.5 cm in size for levels I and II; >1.2 cm in size for levels III, IV, V, and VI; with central necrosis, irregular enhancement, or a poorly defined or irregular capsular border; or with groups of three or more asymmetrically located LNs, with a minimal axial diameter of 8 mm or more, in the suspected tumor drainage basin (Fig. 1.1). The role of positron emission tomography (PET) remains to be delineated and is plagued by false positives, but this may ultimately also prove useful in ruling out such gross disease. It should be kept in mind that the sentinel node technology represents an excellent technique for detection of micrometastases in patients felt to have a reasonably low risk of metastases, but is not as accurate at detecting grossly involved nodes.

Imaging studies, including CT with iodine contrast, MRI with gadolinium contrast, and ultrasonography, should be used to better identify grossly involved, nonpalpable nodes. CT with contrast is standard in North America, though ultrasound, if done in a detailed fashion, is a reasonable alternative. MRI with gadolinium contrast is a good option in iodine allergic patients. Central necrosis of the lymph nodes, although highly predictive, is a late finding. The uptake of 2-deoxy-2-[18F]fluoro-D-glucose as measured by PET has been reported as significantly more sensitive and only slightly less specific than MRI. However, foci of cancer smaller than 1 cm are below the resolution of PET as with CT and MRI.

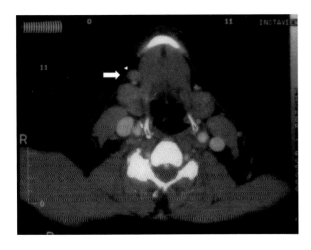

FIGURE 1.1 CT image reveals *prominent level* 1B LN in the region of the facial artery, in a patient with a cancer of the buccal mucosa (*arrow*). The occurrence of a prominent node or nodes in the expected pattern of drainage of the primary cancer would lead to interpretation as a positive node, despite borderline size, and would make the candidate a poor candidate for sentinel node biopsy.

SURGICAL TECHNIQUE

Step 1: Injection of the Primary Tumor

The injection is performed prior to the surgical procedure, generally on the morning of surgery, in the radiology suite. Injection is also sometimes performed late the day before, although the effect of this on the success rate of sentinel node identification remains to be delineated. While awake injection and imaging in radiology are the most commonly used techniques, as we extend this procedure to endoscopically accessible oropharyngeal, supraglottic, and hypopharyngeal lesions, it is likely that cooperative efforts with the nuclear radiologist and the use of portable cameras will allow for intraoperative endoscopic injection, with or without radiologic imaging, and gamma probe–guided sentinel node biopsy without the need for uncomfortable injections in an awake patient. Theoretical advantages of injecting under general anesthesia include better exposure of the primary and avoidance of motion of the patient related to discomfort. This may eventually further increase the reliability of this method. Taking into account that the radiolocalization of the detected hot spots does not represent the drainage of the primary, but the drainage of the tracer deposits, which are supposed to mimic the lymphatic drainage of the primary, the impact of a thorough and representative tracer injection becomes evident. Due to density and direction of the head and neck lymphatics, the primary may drain into several alternative lymphatic pathways, all representing first draining "sentinel" LNs.

Nevertheless, due to regulatory issues related to the injection of radioactive substances and the lack of widely available portable nuclear imaging, awake injection remains the most commonly used technique at present. It is important to ensure that the patient is comfortable so that an adequate preoperative injection is obtained. I use topical anesthetic, mild oral sedation, and lingual, inferior alveolar, and/or sphenopalatine nerve blocks to ensure patient comfort during manipulation and injection of the primary tumor. Direct injection of the tumor with local anesthetic should not be performed as it may affect uptake of the radionuclide and reportedly may even cause it to precipitate in the tissues. The injection technique involves narrow injection with a fine 25-gauge needle circumferentially encompassing the leading edge of the lesion and an additional injection in the center of the lesion (Figs. 1.2 and 1.3). Five tuberculin syringes with 1-mL aliquots of technetium-99 sulfur colloid, with a total radioactivity of 400 millicuries, would represent a standard dose for the morning of surgery. A slightly higher dose would be used the night before. These dosages are extrapolated from the practice for melanoma and have worked well for cancer of the oral cavity, but formal comparative evaluation of dosages and volumes for use in the oral cavity have yet to be performed.

I have used this technique for visible oral lesions. For submucosal lesions, it is well documented that a scar from a previous excisional biopsy can be injected to allow accurate sentinel node biopsy. Whether a previously excised oral lesion could undergo sentinel node excision by injection of an intraoral scar has yet to be determined. It is important to inject narrowly and not to inject the deep tissues. The radionuclide will extravasate more widely in the oral cavity around the site of injection than occurs in the skin and will usually go to the neck more quickly. There is no benefit to trying to inject a margin around the tumor, as this will lead to an unmanageable excess of radioactive nodes. I prefer to use unfiltered technetium-99 sulfur colloid. The presence of larger particles allows for retention of radioactivity in the proximal lymphatics. Retained particles at the site of primary injection are not a major issue as we recommend removal of the primary tumor first. However, it is also possible to obtain good results using filtered technetium sulfur colloid, and if there is a strong preference for addressing the lymphatics first, then this may be preferable as there is a better clearance of background radioactivity from the primary site. The more rapid migration of the filtered agent may also make it advantageous if injections of radionuclide are performed on the operating room table at the start of the procedure rather than prior to the surgical procedure.

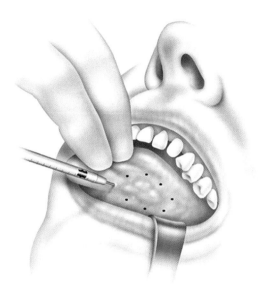

FIGURE 1.2
Schematic view of injection of a cancer of the tongue with radiotracer.

The use of blue dye concurrently with technetium sulfur colloid has become popular in sentinel node biopsy for melanoma. This is a reasonable technique for skin and certainly can help during the learning phase of the procedure, as the subtle blue-dyed lymphatic vessels can be traced toward the sentinel node. Furthermore, reinjection of the blue dye is performed in the operating room under anesthesia and can provide a measure of security against inadequacy of preoperative injection due to patient discomfort. My own preference, however, is to use the radionuclide alone. Numerous publications indicate that it is extremely unlikely to have blue sentinel nodes that are not also radioactive. Anaphylactic allergic reactions to isosulfan blue dye, though rare, can occur. For oral lesions in particular, I prefer to remove the primary first to eliminate radioactive background at the primary site. When the technique is performed in this sequence, the blue dye has usually run through to the distal lymphatics by the time the oral resection is completed and margins are sent, making the dye less useful. Finally, oral cavity resections have functional implications that force the surgeon to obtain adequate but relatively close margins compared to those often obtained for cutaneous melanoma. Blue staining of the oral tissues can lead to loss of the visual cues the surgeon uses to guide decisions regarding whether there is tumor involvement at a margin. Thus, for all of these reasons, I prefer not to use adjunctive blue dye, particularly for cancer of the oral cavity. However, other surgeons prefer to use adjunctive blue dye and obtain excellent results. The removal of sentinel nodes based solely on the blue dye technique is less accurate and should not be performed without also injecting radionuclide.

Step 2: Radiologic Lymphatic Mapping

After injection, nuclear imaging of the lymphatics is obtained (Fig. 1.4). SPECT technology, though not absolutely necessary, may eventually provide even better three-dimensional localization of the sentinel node (Figs. 1.5 and 1.6). The availability of both AP and lateral imaging will generally be adequate, however, to guide the surgeon. A dynamic phase should be acquired with serial images for 1 hour following injection. These images should be acquired for 1 minute each. Transmission images should be acquired for 1 to 2 minutes in each new movement of the camera. (Transmission images are obtained using a flat source place on the detector

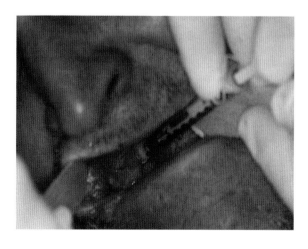

FIGURE 1.3
Transoral injection of a cancer of the buccal mucosa.

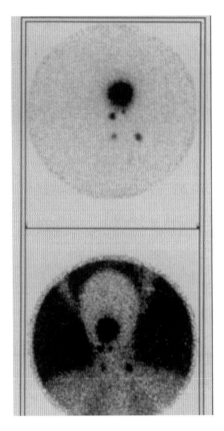

FIGURE 1.4 Standard nuclear imaging showing bilateral neck sentinel nodes after injection of a cancer of the tongue.

opposite the working detector. This is done to achieve better localization of any LNs that take up the radio-pharmaceutical, by superimposing them on a body image.) While it is possible to perform sentinel node biopsy with the intraoperative gamma probe alone, the radiologic image can be useful in providing a rough guide to the location of the sentinel node. It may provide for a more complete informed consent process by predicting unexpected drainage to the contralateral neck or other areas that were not expected to be involved.

Step 3: Removal of the Primary Tumor

I prefer to resect the primary tumor transorally first. If the injection field was sufficiently narrow, this usually eliminates or greatly reduces background radioactivity at the primary site that can confound the sentinel node identification. The usual, appropriate surgical margins, with frozen section control, should be obtained. The sentinel node technique can also be performed in conjunction with a mandibulotomy or other technique of exposure, as long as the primary tumor stage is T2 or less, and as procedure is extended to the oropharynx, this may become more common. In some situations, it may be necessary to perform the nodal biopsy prior to primary resection. However, for most appropriate oral cancers, the lesion will be accessible for resection prior to addressing the lymphatics. Removal of the primary tumor first is less important when the lymphatic basin is distant from the primary cancer and is often less of an issue for skin lesions (i.e., auricular scalp or nasal lesions). However, this can be important for lesions of the neck or preauricular skin where the lymphatics are immediately deep to the primary cancer. It is especially important in cancer of the floor of mouth due to the immediate proximity of the submandibular lymphatics.

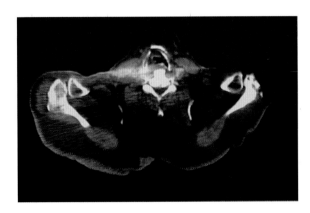

FIGURE 1.5 SPECT–CT fusion lymphoscintigram showing a sentinel node in the axial plane.

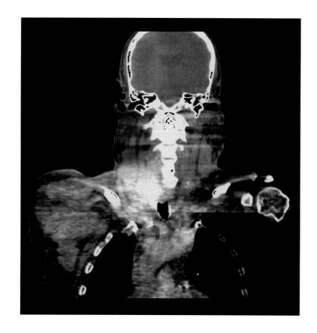

FIGURE 1.6
SPECT–CT fusion lymphoscintigram showing sentinel node in coronal plane.

Step 4: Gamma Probe–Guided Sentinel Node Biopsy

The handheld gamma probe is now used to confirm the location of the SLN(s), which previously were determined by lymphoscintigraphy (LS) (Fig. 1.7A). The skin is marked with the location of the nodes. Background readings should be taken of the precordium as a lower-limit background measurement (Fig. 1.7B), as well as

FIGURE 1.7
A: The gamma probe is passed with a slow smooth motion in radial fashion and angulation to map the location and depth of the radioactive LN. Rapid movements lead to falsely high auditory feedback. The probe should be angled away from the primary injection site. The site of the hot node(s) is marked.
B: Background reading is taken at the precordium. **C:** The gamma probe is drawn slowly over the neck seeking additional hot areas. This process is repeated after the hottest node(s) are removed. **D:** Blunt dissection toward the "hot spot" is followed by reinsertion of the gamma probe into the path of dissection and angulation in various directions seeking the hot LN.

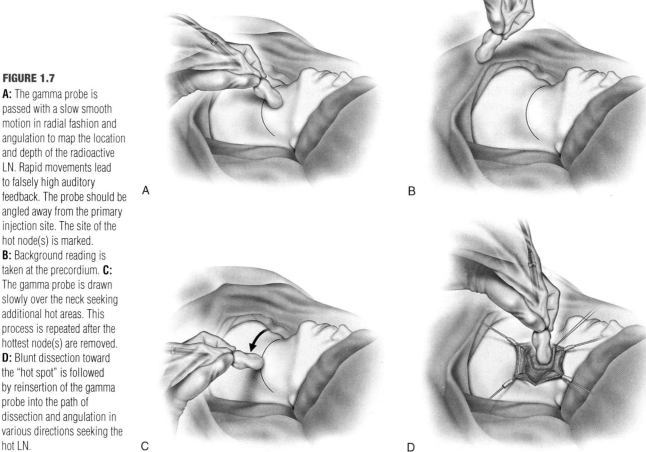

A

B

C

D

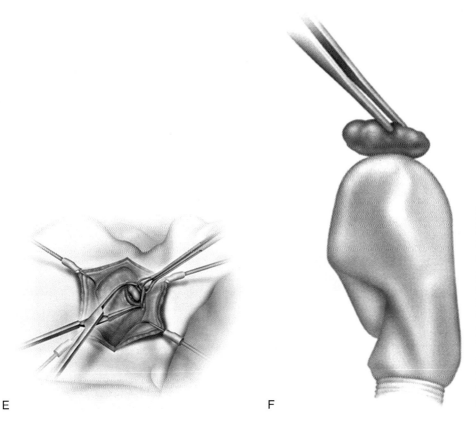

E   F

FIGURE 1.7 *(continued)*
E: The sentinel node is excised using a combination of blunt dissection and division of tissue using bipolar cautery. Unipolar cautery should be avoided when the proximity of neurovascular structures is not known. **F:** Ex vivo readings pointing away from the patient should confirm whether this is the radioactive node.

at the resected primary site as an upper limit of background. The latter is important in avoiding errors due to "shine through" from the primary injection site.

If the patient is to undergo sentinel node biopsy alone, with neck dissection planned only for positive findings intraoperatively or on permanent histopathology, the incision can be drawn narrowly over the node. However, the incision must be consistent with the possibility of subsequent neck dissection, and the planned incision for the formal lymphadenectomy should be considered. Alternatively, the incision can be drawn in the line of that to be used for neck dissection, although shorter in length, and flaps can be elevated. This latter approach is that used when immediate gamma probe–guided neck dissection is the plan, as on the ACOSOG validation trial. After the incision is made, subplatysmal flaps are elevated sufficiently to provide access to the hot area. The neck should first be carefully palpated, in order to identify palpable gross lymphatic disease that may not be physiologically functional and hence may not take up radioactivity. The finding of gross cancer involvement would, of course, contraindicate sentinel node biopsy and mandate formal neck dissection.

If no gross disease is identified, the surgeon will now localize the sentinel node(s). Use of the probe to locate the nodes is not intuitive, and it is best learned through instruction by a surgeon with experience in the technique. Initial readings are taken of the precordium and back table in order to assess the level of hematogenous radioactivity. Readings are also obtained from the resected tumor specimen and the bed of resection, in order to assess the level of anticipated background activity. The probe is slowly passed over the neck at a steady rate assessing the auditory input for radioactivity generated by the gamma probe (Fig. 1.7C). Care is taken to aim away from the primary resection bed. Since the probe measures radioactivity over time, rapid or unsteady movement will lead to higher readings and louder auditory input and should be avoided. Using the steady constant motion, the probe is moved radially across each hot spot allowing the surgeon to determine the direction in which to proceed, in three dimensions, in order to locate the sentinel node. The ability to use the probe to assess the three-dimensional location of the node is not intuitive and requires some instruction and practice. Using a fine hemostat or McCabe nerve dissector, the surgeon bluntly dissects toward the sentinel node. Bipolar cautery can be used to divide the tissues to provide wider exposure. I recommend avoidance of paralysis and caution in using unipolar electrocautery as the neurovascular structures in the neck are not specifically identified, although the spinal accessory and marginal nerves may often be visualized in the course of the procedure.

As a dissection cavity is opened, the gamma probe is introduced into this space along the plane of dissection and angled in various directions in order to guide the surgeon to the sentinel node (Fig. 1.7D). The sentinel node is excised by blunt dissection (Fig. 1.7E). Probe readings (counts per minute) are recorded for initial readings taken while the node is in the patient, as well as for "ex vivo" readings of the extracted node, away from the patient (Fig. 1.7F). Repeat readings in the resection bed are taken to ensure that there are no adjacent hot nodes that also need to be removed. Any LN exhibiting 10% or more of the radioactivity of the most radioactive node in the same anatomic area will be considered an additional SLN and will be harvested separately. If there are a large number of very radioactive nodes (i.e., more than 6), this essentially represents a failure of the technique and piecemeal removal of a large number of nodes is illogical in my opinion. The surgeon should proceed to selective neck dissection if indicated. In the case where there is a very hot sentinel node in a specific area, there may be a relatively hot node in a completely separate anatomic region (i.e., submental region versus level II jugular region) that does not reach 10% of the radioactivity of the hottest node. If this second node is truly in a separate area and is significantly greater than background (2 or more times background readings), it should still be harvested as a sentinel node, as it may represent a separate drainage pattern from a different portion of the tumor. Review of the lymphoscintigraphic imaging and knowledge of basic anatomic principles will allow the surgeon to judge whether such additional areas of borderline radioactivity need to be excised. When the SLN dissections are performed prior to resection of the OCSCCA or if significant radioactivity persists in the bed of resection, the use of intraoral lead shields can be helpful. The presence of a collimator on the gamma probe is recommended to reduce background signal from the primary tumor, and most modern probes have fine tips with collimators. With cancer of the posterior tongue, background activity can be avoided by using a transoral suture on the tongue to pull the primary bed away from the lymphatics.

The issue of dealing with background activity at the primary site is most marked for the level 1 nodes with cancer of the floor of the mouth. In this situation, the surgeon may need to perform some initial dissection, below the level of the marginal mandibular nerve, transecting the tissues down to the level of the mylohyoid muscle. In this manner, the LNs are mobilized away from the oral cavity, allowing for more accurate identification of the SLN(s) by placing the gamma probe into the tunnel thus created and directing the probe inferiorly away from the background radioactivity at the floor of mouth injection site. Each SLN is labeled, measured, described, and recorded separately as to location and total ex vivo counts per second.

Skin lesions of the periauricular region and scalp represent a unique technical challenge as they commonly drain to the parotid LNs. The proximity of the facial nerve branches and the dense nature of parotid tissue contraindicate blunt dissection searching for LNs within the substance of the parotid gland. In our experience, in many cases, nodes can be identified on the capsule of the parotid gland, which can be safely excised with a capsular dissection. These may be located on the tail of the parotid, anterior edge of the parotid, or region around the temporal vessels (for scalp lesions). Electromyographic intraoperative facial nerve monitoring is useful in such cases. If the gamma probe directs the surgeon to nodes deep within the parotid, then in many cases it is best to identify a distal branch of the facial nerve, or occasionally even the main trunk, and perform a localized excision of the hot portion of the gland, with identification of the facial nerve. Such a procedure might be termed a "gamma probe guided partial parotidectomy" and still simplifies the procedure relative to a formal lateral lobe parotidectomy with concurrent neck dissection. In this situation, it is particularly important to tag the tissue adjacent to facial nerve branches with permanent suture in order to provide for easy re-exploration if the sentinel node is positive. Similar marking of the location of the spinal accessory nerve would be advantageous if it is identified in the course of an upper jugular sentinel node biopsy.

Step 5: Rigorous Histopathologic Assessment of the Sentinel Node

For cutaneous lesions, particularly for melanoma, where formal lymphadenectomy is not standard, sentinel node biopsy is gaining wide acceptance. As mentioned previously, minimally invasive T1 oral lesions represent an emerging group for which the option of sentinel node biopsy might be considered if the surgeon's practice has been "watchful waiting" for such a lesion. However, in any situation where sentinel node biopsy alone is performed, exhaustive histopathologic evaluation of the sentinel node with fine sectioning and concurrent immunohistochemistry should be performed to rule out microscopic foci of cancer (Fig. 1.8) and allow for therapeutic neck dissection or radiation. If such an evaluation remains negative, close follow-up and consideration of serial radiologic imaging (CT, MRI, or serial ultrasound) should be considered.

FIGURE 1.8

Micrometastasis seen on hematoxylin and eosin stain **(A)**, juxtaposed with identical section stained with immunohistochemical cytokeratin stain **(B)**.

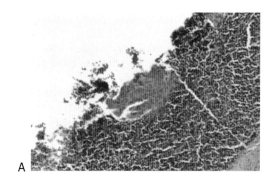
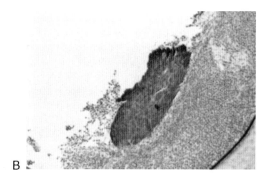

POSTOPERATIVE MANAGEMENT

The early postoperative management will generally be dictated by the resection of the primary site. Most patients who are candidates for sentinel node biopsy will have a limited resection of the cancer, which can be managed by inpatient observation, either in the intensive care unit or on a regular patient floor, depending on the level of concern regarding edema of the airway. Simple oral rinses and gentle oral cavity cleaning are all that is necessary. Perioperative corticosteroids are used to reduce edema.

For more extensive resections or for patients who are difficult to intubate, temporary tracheostomy may be the safest approach. If a tracheostomy is required, then the usual care by skilled nurses, with frequent saline irrigation, suctioning, and cleaning of the inner cannula, will be needed. The need for a tracheostomy should be infrequent, however, if appropriate lesions are being selected.

The neck wound from the sentinel node biopsy will be significantly smaller than a neck dissection wound and will have less drainage and edema. Depending on the number of LNs removed and the extent of dissection, a suction drain may or may not be advisable. If a suction drain is used, it will usually be removed within 3 days. The typical patient having this procedure, with a small primary cancer, would spend one night in the hospital and require little postoperative care.

The biggest postoperative issue is the need to rush the final histopathologic analysis, so that patients with micrometastases can be taken to surgery for neck dissection prior to the development of significant inflammation in the neck. Active investigation is ongoing in order to develop better techniques to evaluate the status of the sentinel node in "real time" during the initial procedure. Techniques such as rapid reverse transcriptase-polymerase chain reaction (RT-PCR) and step sectioning during frozen section have been studied, but effective, standardized "real time" assessment of the sentinel node is still not available. Thus, at this point, we must request rushed immunohistochemical evaluation of step sections and quickly return for completion neck dissection in the small percentage of patients that require this. Communication regarding this issue during the postoperative period is essential.

COMPLICATIONS

Complications are rare with this technique, and in fact, the minimally invasive nature of the procedure relative to the moderate morbidity of neck dissection is the impetus for the development of this technique. Nonetheless, as in any procedure, complications can occur. One concern with SLNB in the head and neck region is the theoretical risk of injury to the facial nerve and spinal accessory nerve during blunt dissection through narrow exposure. It is also possible that surgeons employing this technique might compromise on the completeness of the procedure in the parotid gland, which allows the avoidance of facial nerve dissection, but can imply an oncologic risk. The relatively few publications addressing this issue to date have reported incidences of even minor complications that are <1%. Theoretically in the hands of an inexperienced operator, the risk of injury to the facial or spinal accessory nerves may be greater with SLNB than with formal parotidectomy and selective neck dissection. Since the presence of sentinel node micrometastases may be recognized postoperatively, the potential risk of nerve injury related to reexploration of an inflamed, recently operated wound also needs to be considered.

RESULTS

Selective neck dissection remains the standard approach for the majority of cancers of the oral cavity, particularly for larger and significantly invasive T2, T3, and T4 lesions. The floor of the mouth is a problem site with current technology, due to interference from shine through, as the lymphatic basin is too close to the primary site, and the level I nodes cannot be safely addressed by SLNB for this anatomic subsite. Significant data already exist, however, to advocate SLNB as a reasonable alternative to selective neck dissection for smaller, thinner cancers of the oral cavity, other than floor of mouth, that fall in a category where watchful waiting might reasonably be chosen as an alternative, but where they are not so minimally invasive that the risk of metastases is negligible.

The sentinel node concept is discarded by some based on the misconception that selective neck dissection has no significant morbidity. Coming from a tradition of more radical neck procedures, the selective neck dissection is generally viewed as an intervention with negligible morbidity by many head and neck surgeons. In fact, although the morbidity of selective neck dissection is significantly less than that of modified radical and radical dissections, there is measurable morbidity in a variable percentage of patients, including issues with shoulder function secondary to temporary trapezius weakness followed by adhesive capsulitis of the shoulder, pain syndromes, contour changes, and lower lip mobility. This has been demonstrated in numerous quality of life studies and at least two objective functional assessments. Stoeckli et al. have also performed a formal quality of life assessment of sentinel node biopsy versus selective neck dissection showing significant benefit. The moderate morbidity of selective neck dissection has led some to suggest watchful waiting as an alternative for patients of lower risk. SLNB has developed as an intermediate option in response to this controversy. All of these complications are observed much less frequently with SLNB, although formal quality of life assessments have not yet been performed.

Another issue is our inability to achieve immediate diagnosis of positive sentinel nodes. Frozen section, even with multiple sections, is not sufficiently accurate, and tissue is better preserved for permanent sections. Thus, for the minority of patients with micrometastases identified in the sentinel nodes, we are sometimes dealing with issues of re-exploration and dissection of functionally important nerves in a recently operated wound. Ultimately rapid RT-PCR assessment of nodes may ultimately provide immediate information regarding the status of the sentinel node. As future studies are designed to safely evaluate the sentinel node biopsy technique, the opportunity should be taken to plan correlative studies to validate the role of these new technologies in tumor assessment.

SLNB will likely play an increasing role in the management of cancer of the oral cavity, given that there are lesions and situations where the "wait and see" approach continues to be advocated. It may provide an intermediate approach for small but moderately invasive T1 or smaller T2 lesions in whom watchful waiting is currently the major alternative to neck dissection. Although not discussed in this chapter, this technology also makes sense for lip cancers, periauricular skin cancers, adnexal cancers, nasal vestibular cancers, and other histologies and sites where the risk of metastases falls in a range of 5% to 15%—high enough to make watchful waiting risky but low enough to make selective neck dissection seem excessive. It appears unlikely that SLNB will ever replace selective neck dissection for very invasive, larger T2 and T3N0 lesions of the oral cavity.

Equally important is the evaluation for the significant unpredictability of lymphatic pathways observed for both cutaneous and oral lesions. In fact for lesions not involving the midline but within a few centimeters of it, LS and gamma probe–guided surgery may ultimately provide the solution in these patients, in whom we often struggle with the decision regarding contralateral neck management. Increased accuracy in the identification of micrometastases will ultimately lead to more accurate staging.

The sentinel node technique is likely to have an increasing role in the management of head and neck cancer in the future. Surgeons can gain experience in the use of this technique for cutaneous malignancies, early-stage oral cancers with intermediate invasiveness (i.e., approximately between 2 and 6 mm depth). The technique can also be practiced in the context of a gamma probe–guided neck dissection for more invasive cancers, preferably in the context of a clinical trial, allowing the patient to benefit from improved mapping of drainage patterns and more accurate staging through better identification of micrometastases. Pilot data on the use of this technique in the pharynx and larynx will continue to emerge. It is hoped that this chapter will provide a guide to the surgeons as they evaluate the neck, and allow for proper evaluation of the N0 neck with imaging, an understanding of the potential role of biologic markers in assessing risk, and the developing role of LS and sentinel node biopsy in detecting microscopic lymphatic metastases.

PEARLS

- Select early lesions without extremely deep invasion.
- Use preoperative CT or MRI with contrast to detect grossly involved LNs.
- Accurate radiotracer injection requires a comfortable patient; use sedation or lingual nerve block as indicated.
- Inject closely into normal tissue around the lesion.
- Manage background activity from the primary site.
- Tag identified nerves.
- Exhaustive step sectioning and immunohistochemistry
- Close follow-up and neck imaging if indicated

PITFALLS

- Counsel patients regarding potential reexploration for delayed positive findings in the sentinel nodes.
- Avoid large lesions as an excessive number of nodes will result.
- Use of the gamma probe is not intuitive, and training in its use is important.
- Do not inject local anesthetic directly into the primary tumor.
- Avoid blue dye for mucosal lesions (tissue/margin staining).
- Floor of mouth primary cancers may complicate identification of SLNs.
- Patiently remove additional nodes with radioactivity 10% or more of the most radioactive SLN.

INSTRUMENTS TO HAVE AVAILABLE

- Standard head and neck set
- Neoprobe or other handheld gamma counter

- Collimator tip attachment to reduce scatter and shine through false-positive readings
- Methylene blue dye and tuberculin 1-mL syringe if dual labeling method is to be used to identify "hot" and "blue" SLN
- Nerve stimulator

SUGGESTED READING

Chepeha DB, Taylor RJ, Chepeha JC, et al. Functional assessment using Constant's Shoulder Scale after modified radical and selective neck dissection. *Head Neck* 2002;24:432–436.

Civantos FJ, Moffat FL, Goodwin WJ. Lymphatic mapping and sentinel lymphadenectomy for 106 head and neck lesions: contrasts between oral cavity and cutaneous malignancy. *Laryngoscope* 2006;112(suppl 109):1–15.

Civantos FJ, Zitsch RP, Schuller DE, et al. Sentinel lymph node biopsy accurately stages the regional lymph nodes for T1-2 oral squamous cell carcinomas (OSCC): results of a prospective multi-institutional trial. *J Clin Oncol* 2010;28: 1396–1400.

Ferris RL, Xi L, Seethala RR, et al. Intraoperative qRT-PCR for detection of lymph node metastasis in head and neck cancer. *Clin Cancer Res* 2011;17(7):1858–1866.

Murer K, Huber GF, Haile SR, et al. Comparison of morbidity between sentinel node biopsy and elective neck dissection for treatment of the N0 neck in patients with oral squamous cell carcinoma. *Head Neck* 2011;33(9):1260–1264.

2 SELECTIVE NECK DISSECTION

Robert L. Ferris

INTRODUCTION

Neck dissection has evolved to be more targeted and less invasive over the past 100 years since Crile described the classical radical neck dissection (RND). Another conceptual advance held that modified RND was technically feasible and oncologically sound, removing only lymphatic structures and retaining the sternocleidomastoid muscle (SCM), accessory nerve, and/or internal jugular vein (IJV). The potential then arose for removing less than all five levels of the ipsilateral neck for mucosal or cutaneous squamous cell carcinoma, with potential application of this "selective neck dissection (SND)" to thyroid or salivary carcinomas as well. Over the past 20 years, the SND has become more widely accepted, first as a staging procedure and more recently as a therapeutic approach to early (N1) lymph node metastasis.

The advent of this development toward SND was supported by the seminal contribution of JP Shah (1990) reporting on the specific levels in the neck where metastatic lymph nodes were observed, originating from certain subsites within the oral cavity, oral pharynx, larynx, or hypopharynx. Reporting on the patterns of metastasis in over 1,000 RNDs (all five levels dissected), it became clear that targeted SND could be adopted removing only three or four of the five cervical levels in selected patients based on the site of the primary cancer (Fig. 2.1A and B). As a staging procedure, the SND was found retrospectively to have removed microscopic N1 metastasis in more than 30% of cN0 patients. Thus, one or two metastatic lymph nodes, <3 cm in size and without extracapsular spread (ECS), can be adequately treated by SND, removing appropriate cervical levels according to the patterns of spread from the original primary site of the cancer.

Besides its oncologic value, SND has been demonstrated to reduce the morbidity and cosmetic deformity associated with more extensive modified radical neck dissection (MRND) or RND, due to avoidance of manipulation, mobilization, or transection of the spinal accessory nerve, which is the major morbidity of neck dissection. Thus, currently SND is the minimum procedure that most appropriate in most patients with head and neck squamous cell carcinoma. For the N0-N1 neck, the SND provides crucial staging information, documenting the presence and extent of metastatic disease in the neck. Furthermore, it provides information regarding the presence of ECS a very poor prognostic factor warranting adjuvant therapy with chemoradiation. After SND, patients without high-risk features such as multiple lymph nodes positive (>3) or ECS can then undergo observation or (reduced) dose postoperative radiotherapy.

HISTORY

It is crucial to identify the site and extent of the primary cancer (mucosal, cutaneous, salivary, or thyroid) to guide appropriateness for SND. It is also important to inquire about associated features including dysphagia, mass in the neck, hoarseness, or other symptoms associated with the cancer in the upper aerodigestive tract. Any prior oncologic treatment or history of neck surgery should be elicited. For a squamous cell carcinoma with an unknown primary mucosal site, it is crucial to establish whether a prior tonsillectomy has

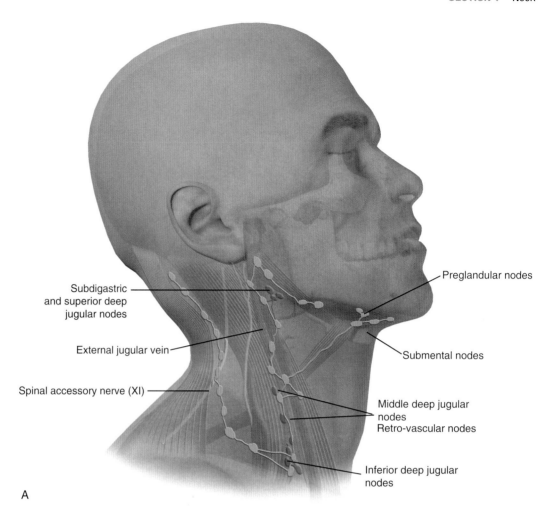

Subdigastric
and superior deep
jugular nodes

External jugular vein

Spinal accessory nerve (XI)

Preglandular nodes

Submental nodes

Middle deep jugular
nodes
Retro-vascular nodes

Inferior deep jugular
nodes

A

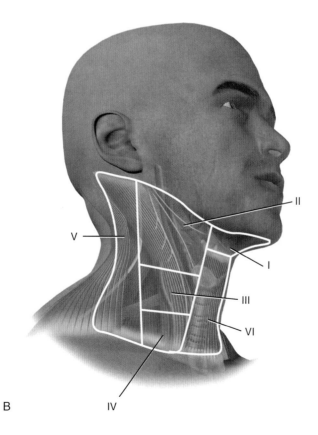

II

V

I

III

VI

IV

B

FIGURE 2.1
A: Lymphatic drainage of the
head and neck. **B:** Levels of
the cervical lymph nodes.

been performed. A history of cutaneous malignancy should not be overlooked, since aggressive squamous cell carcinoma of the skin, particularly in elderly or immunosuppressed individuals, may metastasize to the cervical lymph nodes.

PHYSICAL EXAMINATION

A thorough examination of the head and neck should be performed in the office, palpating the neck for the presence of enlarged nodes, fixed lymphadenopathy, fixation of the overlying skin to the lymph nodes, or other signs of gross metastasis. Preoperative documentation is crucial and should be combined with radiographic imaging. I prefer a contrast-enhanced computed tomography (CT) scan of the neck from the skull base to the clavicles, since this will include retropharyngeal nodes. The rate of level IIB metastasis is very rare (1%) in the clinically and radiographically negative neck; however, the rate increases (10% to 15%) for metastasis to level IIB, when clinically positive lymph nodes are observed preoperatively. The SND would then include level IIB in the dissection. Indications for SND are preoperative clinical N0-N1 as a diagnostic and staging procedure. Postoperative identification of pathologic N1 status may be adequately treated with SND alone, in the absence of ECS. When a SND identifies N2b metastasis, multiple positives nodes >2, are a standard indication for adjuvant radiotherapy. More extensive lymph node metastasis should be discovered preoperatively since SND is not sufficient therapy in situations of clinical stage N2-N3.

INDICATIONS

An SND is indicated in the absence of palpable cervical metastases (i.e., in the elective surgical treatment of the N0 neck). Early metastatic cancer (cN1) is also an indication for SND.

CONTRAINDICATIONS

The SND is not indicated in the following situations:

- Patients with multiple clinically obvious cervical lymph node metastases, particularly when they are found to involve or to be closely related to the spinal accessory nerve
- Patients with a bulky metastatic tumor mass or with multiple matted nodes in the superior aspect of the neck

PREOPERATIVE PLANNING

Imaging

Various radiographic techniques may be used prior to SND. I believe that the CT scan using IV iodinated contrast is the most helpful preoperative test prior to SND. The size, number, and three-dimensional relationship of any suspicious lymph nodes can be identified and documented. It is fast, is relatively inexpensive, and emits a low dose of radiation. Ultrasonography (US) of the neck is appropriate particularly if the surgeon has access to this instrument in the clinic. US can identify suspicious lymph nodes, as well as size, number, and potential for ECS. It is also inexpensive and does not deliver radiation, therefore providing several advantages. A disadvantage is the lack of the transferable three-dimensional planar axial imaging for review by multiple individuals over time, since it is operator dependent. Magnetic resonance imaging has similar advantages to CT during, but is used less often, due to greater expense and time to perform, reducing patient compliance and surgeon comfort with the images. Positron emission tomography–computed tomography (PET–CT) has become increasingly used for pretreatment staging of cancer of the head and neck and is often more accurate than contrast-enhanced CT alone. However, PET–CT is more useful for identifying occult distant metastasis, whereas false positives and false negatives reduce its utility in accurately staging the clinically negative (cN0) neck. In this situation, SND is the most accurate test for determining the pathologic status of the neck (pN status) and is superior to PET–CT in sensitivity and specificity.

Fine Needle Aspiration Biopsy

Fine needle aspiration biopsy (FNAB) is integral to the preoperative planning for SND and should be used (and repeated if necessary) to document cytologically the presence of cancer in a suspicious lymph node(s). Necrotic or cystic lymph nodes may emanate from the oropharynx (tonsil/base of tongue) or primary thyroid cancers, and repeat FNAB may be necessary with image guidance. Open biopsy should be strongly discouraged, unless frozen section is planned, with conversion to immediate SND if positive.

SURGICAL TECHNIQUE

The SND is performed similarly to the comprehensive, type III MRND, with the exception that all cervical levels (I–V) are not removed in the SND. In all cases of SND, no nonlymphatic structures are routinely removed, thus preserving the SCM, IJV, and spinal accessory nerve. An example is shown in Figure 2.2 for SND appropriate for cN0/cN1 oropharyngeal, laryngeal/hypopharyngeal primary cancers. The SCM should not be divided, but rather is retracted posteriorly to permit access to the cervical levels to be dissected. In some situations, early-stage metastasis to the neck (N1) with ECS may be attached to the SCM or jugular vein, and in these rare instances, these structures may need to be partially removed. However, this is quite rare, and in these situations, conversion to a comprehensive MRND would seem prudent.

For cosmetic reasons and for wide access to the neck structures, I prefer a hockey stick incision beginning at the mastoid tip with the posterior–inferior corner squared off. The incision course is inferiorly in a vertical direction behind the SCM, to permit the incision to be hidden postoperatively. At the lower extent, a right angle is created, carrying the incision horizontally in a prominent skin crease in the supraclavicular interiorly toward the midline. This incision may be longer than other surgeons advocate; however, I find that it provides ideal access to all cervical levels, including level IA, and is cosmetically pleasing, since a shirt collar would hide this incision better than ones placed in a higher, mid-neck location. The posterior–inferior corner of the incision can be marked with a 21-gauge needle dipped in methylene blue on either side of the incision to permit accurate reapproximation; however, I find that a sharp, 90-degree corner is simple to reapproximate, avoiding a dog-ear at either edge of the incision.

I prefer performing SND with the hemostatic (Shaw) scalpel (no. 15 blade), set at 110°C for the skin incision. Others may use a no. 15 blade on a scalpel or a monopolar cautery set on cutting. The Shaw hemostatic scalpel is set on 220°C, for the dermal layer, and then I increase the temperature of the blade to 300°C, for the remainder of the procedure. After either technique of skin incision, the dissection is carried down into a subplatysmal plane to permit the incised flap to be elevated with an adequate blood supply (within the platysma). During flap incision and elevation over the SCM, care is taken to avoid damage to the greater auricular nerve

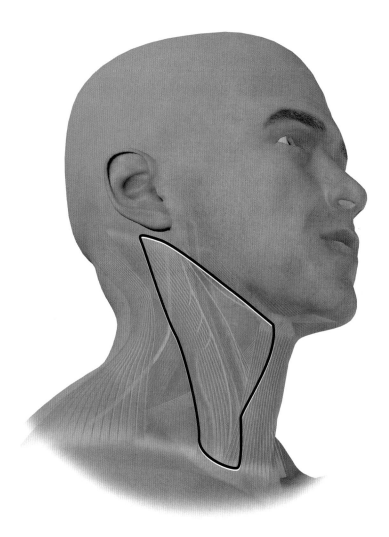

FIGURE 2.2

SND for laryngeal/ hypopharyngeal primary cancers (levels II, III, IV).

and external jugular vein, which course over the SCM muscle but deep to the platysma. While injury to the greater auricular nerve may have limited consequences, damage to the external jugular vein will cause significant bleeding, which can reduce the tissue planes visible to the surgeon, and eliminates a potential source of microvascular anastomosis for venous drainage, if this is planned as part of the procedure. Elevation of the subplatysmal skin flap is performed in one sweeping motion in a superior and anterior direction, since the incision is placed at the posterior and inferior extent of dissection. Again this streamlines this portion of the procedure, reducing the manipulation with skin hooks and expediting this necessary, although noncritical portion of the surgical procedure. Care is taken in the most anterior and superior flap elevation to avoid injury to the marginal mandibular branch of the facial nerve (Fig. 2.3). For cancers of the oropharynx, larynx, and hypopharynx (Fig. 2.2), level I is not usually dissected and therefore the inferior border of the submandibular gland is the upper extent of the dissection, avoiding injury to the marginal mandibular nerve. The skin flaps should be retracted with hooks or a suture secured to the drapes with a hemostatic clamp to assist in retraction and visualization, freeing up the surgical team and assistants to help with more important aspects of the SND.

The SND proceeds with an incision over the anterior border of the SCM, along its entire length. The surgeon and first assistant grasp this fascia with traction and countertraction in opposing directions (anterior or posterior), elevating it to demonstrate the fascial plane of dissection. Thus, the superficial layer of the deep cervical fascia is incised and the SCM is "unwrapped" and is progressively retracted with an Army - Navy retractor. The SCM is skeletonized anteriorly until the cervical plexus is encountered at the posterior border of the SCM. Approximately one-third of the way inferior to the insertion of the SCM, the spinal accessory nerve (cranial nerve XI) is identified from anterior to the SCM, where it courses deep through the muscle. In some patients, a branch of the accessory nerve penetrates the SCM or runs parallel to it from the cervical rootlets (C2-C4). If possible, this should be preserved along with the spinal accessory nerve, since retraction trauma to the spinal accessory nerve is the major cause of morbidity of the SND. If the nerve is traumatized, stretched, or inadvertently cut, the SCM and/or trapezius muscles will atrophy to a firm and fibrotic structure. Great care must be observed when the second assistant is retracting the upper portion of the SCM during SND, since pressure or stretch injury will induce potentially permanent neuropraxia, weakness, and loss of range of motion of the ipsilateral shoulder, constituting the shoulder syndrome. This includes adhesive capsulitis and deltoid atrophy, preventing abduction and generating a great deal of morbidity postoperatively.

Incision of the cervical sensory rootlets or the deep neck fascia in the posterior floor of the neck over the scalene and splenius muscles should be avoided, since this is not necessary in the SND procedure. Hemostasis should be achieved sequentially with the Shaw scalpel at 300°C, taking care not to rush through this portion of the procedure, since additional time for hemostasis is necessary if bleeding is encountered from small vessels,

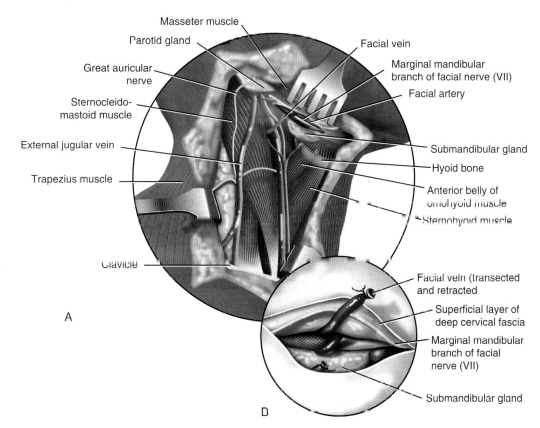

FIGURE 2.3 A,B: Preservation of the marginal mandibular branch of the facial nerve in level I.

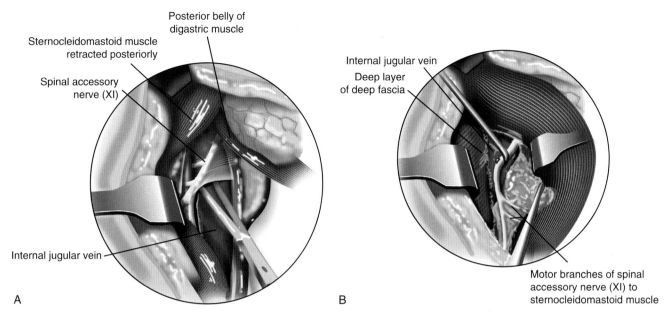

FIGURE 2.4 A: Mobilization of the spinal accessory nerve (CN XI) in level II. **B:** Transposing nodal packet from Level IIB underneath CN XI.

using the Shaw, monopolar, or bipolar cautery. No branches of the jugular vein run posteriorly, except inferiorly where the transverse cervical artery and vein are encountered in the supraclavicular fossa, although these should be deep to the standard SND.

Once the submandibular gland is mobilized at its superior and posterior/deep extent, the posterior belly of the digastric muscle is encountered and is a convenient landmark, which is followed back to the jugular vein in level II, where the spinal accessory nerve crosses superficially 70% of the time. The digastric muscle is retracted superiorly, to directly visualize the spinal accessory nerve and the IJV and enable the fibroadipose level II tissues to be connected with the level I and submandibular gland portion of the neck dissection (Fig. 2.4). This enables the superior extent to be mobilized off the surface while the jugular vein and spinal accessory nerve are under direct vision and can be carefully dissected in the inferior and anterior direction; likewise, the omohyoid is generally preserved in the SND and often serves as the inferior extent of dissection. If level IV is being dissected, this fibroadipose tissue is mobilized, taking care to avoid injury to the IJV, the transverse cervical plexus of vessels, or the thoracic duct on the left side. The level IV tissue is transposed around the omohyoid muscle taking care to avoid injury to the jugular vein, which runs immediately deep to the omohyoid. At this point, the fibroadipose SND specimen is transected at the anterior extent at the strap muscles prior to their attachment to the larynx. I prefer to mark level II for the pathologist with a suture since this is the superior extent of the specimen.

During an SND, paralytic agents should not be given by the anesthesiologist, and thus, cautery dissection or hemostasis near the spinal accessory nerve will lead to muscle and shoulder spasms. In this region, it is ideal to use the Shaw blade with a wet, cold sponge draped over the nerve with the nondominant hand of the surgeon to keep it cool and safe from the hot Shaw blade. If level IIB is dissected, the spinal accessory nerve should be mobilized carefully with a tenotomy scissor (Fig. 2.4) enabling the submuscular recess (level IIB) fibroadipose tissue to be incised and mobilized from the splenius capitus muscle with fascia still covering it. The level IIB packet of lymph nodes is grasped with an Allis clamp and transposed underneath the mobilized spinal accessory nerve. Alternatively level IIB can be dissected separately from the superior and posterior direction of the accessory nerve landmarks and sent separately, to avoid mobilization of the accessory nerve and its surrounding vasa nervorum. The jugular chain lymph nodes are then retracted with 6-prong blunt rakes anteriorly and superficially over the surface of the IJV, while the Shaw scalpel is used to incise and transpose successively this fibroadipose package over the surface of the jugular vein (Fig. 2.5). There are no posterior venous branches, but as the fibroadipose tissue is retracted and the dissection ensues over the surface of the IJV, the facial vein confluence is encountered superiorly and should remain deep to the dissection. The facial vein confluence may have been divided previously if a level IA and IB dissection with submandibular gland excision were performed (levels I–IV SND). However, in the setting of oropharynx, larynx, and hypopharynx cancers, where levels II–IV dissection are performed, the facial confluence should be preserved to improve venous drainage of the head and neck and avoid a large vein ligation, since a postoperative Valsalva or other high-pressure event can lead to the formation of a hematoma.

The incorporation of a level I dissection into the SND for carcinoma of the oral cavity is performed as follows. The inferior border of the submandibular gland is incised and a plane of this fascia is kept intact as the gland is depressed with the nondominant hand of the surgeon. Often the marginal mandibular branch of the facial nerve can be visualized but should not be specifically dissected since this can lead to irreversible

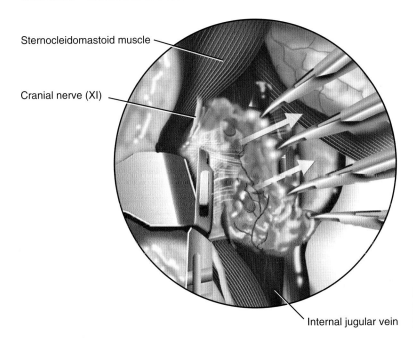

Sternocleidomastoid muscle

Cranial nerve (XI)

FIGURE 2.5

Dissection of the fibrofatty tissue along the jugular chain.

Internal jugular vein

neurapraxia. The submandibular fascia containing the marginal mandibular branch of the facial nerve is successively elevated off of the submandibular gland, taking care to include the facial lymph nodes which may drain primary cancers of the floor of mouth and tongue. The submandibular fascia is elevated to the level of the mandible and the level IB dissection ensues. Often the facial artery must be divided twice as the gland in the fibrofatty level I tissue is retracted inferiorly and the posterior direction leads to encountering the artery a second time. During the superior and interior extension of the submandibular gland excision, the mylohyoid is retracted anteriorly to expose the submandibular ganglion and submandibular duct, which are ligated successively to avoid injury to the lingual and hypoglossal nerves.

Note that if level I is included, this is obvious to the pathologist due to the presence of the submandibular gland. While some authors advocate preservation of the submandibular gland, I prefer to excise it so that the optimal oncologic procedure is performed, removing all level I pre- and postvascular nodes. In addition, the gland is often devascularized and without adequate nerve supply and thus may not be functional. Previously some surgeons advocated obtaining a frozen section of any suspicious lymph nodes so that SND would be converted to MRND in this case. I prefer to make the best assessment of clinical node positivity using clinical and radiographic examination preoperatively, so that the surgical plan is clear to the team and to the patient without intraoperative decision making based on altering the extent of surgery in such a setting.

At the end of the procedure, copious irrigation, with or without antibiotic solution, is performed and hemostasis obtained with the Shaw hemostatic scalpel or the bipolar cautery. I use a no. 10 flat Jackson-Pratt (JP) suction drain, placed through a separate stab incision in the posterior or inferior skin flap in the conspicuous location. A pressure dressing or a gauze wrap should be avoided so is not to obscure a hematoma. The drain can sometimes be removed on postoperative day (POD) 1 but most commonly on POD 2. In patients who have undergone previous irradiation, planning may be necessary to discharge the patient with the drain on POD 1 or 2, since inpatient hospitalization is generally not necessary after recovery from anesthesia (24 to 36 hours). Postoperatively assessment of the function of the marginal mandibular branch of the facial nerve, tongue weakness and sensation, and spinal accessory nerve/shoulder function should be noted and documented. All patients who undergo SND should have a consultation with a physical therapist (PT/OT), experienced in shoulder strength and range-of-motion exercises. On the Head and Neck Service at the University of Pittsburgh, we have designed a detailed, printed handout of exercises for each patient to perform at home, after instruction and consultation with the PT/OT team. A Valsalva maneuver is applied to identify a chyle leak and to establish whether hemostasis is sufficient. A flat 10-mm JP drain is usually sufficient. The platysma layer is reapproximated with Vicryl sutures, and the skin is closed with monofilament suture or staples.

POSTOPERATIVE MANAGEMENT

Drains are maintained on low suction and are usually kept in place for 1 to 2 days to prevent a seroma or hematomas and to monitor for a chyle leak. A common sequela of SND is related to mobilization or manipulation of the spinal accessory nerve. The resulting denervation of the trapezius muscle, one of the most important shoulder abductors, causes destabilization of the scapula with progressive flaring of it at the vertebral border, as well as drooping, and lateral and anterior rotation of the shoulder. The loss of the trapezius function decreases the patient's ability to abduct the shoulder above 90 degrees at the shoulder. Paralysis of the trapezius muscle causes a clinical syndrome characterized by weakness and deformity of the shoulder girdle, usually accompanied by pain. Consequently, patients who have undergone a SND with spinal accessory nerve injury must be evaluated by a physical therapist early in the postoperative period. Aggressive and prompt physical and occupational therapy are recommended since they are useful in improving range of motion and avoiding adhesive capsulitis.

COMPLICATIONS

The carotid sheath should, at all times, be deep to the plane of the dissection. Injury to the phrenic and accessory nerves or other deep cervical structures can be avoided by positive identification. Occasionally a nonlymphatic structure must be resected if clinical evidence of ECS leads to a metastatic node adherent to it. A small injury to the IJV should not warrant its ligation, since a 7-0 Prolene suture can repair small, inadvertent injury and retain postoperative venous drainage and avoid edema. In SND, left-sided IV dissection puts the thoracic duct at risk and may occur even in a right-sided dissection in the minority of cases. During a left-sided SND encompassing level IV lymphadenectomy, double clamping and ligating with silk sutures low in the neck will avoid inadvertent shearing or leak of chyle from the main or accessory thoracic duct(s). Bipolar cautery may be used as can the Shaw scalpel, to seal smaller lymphatic vessels coursing in the region of the duct; however, silk ligation is more effective as a prevention maneuver. Valsalva with the assistance of the anesthesiologist is useful to confirm the integrity of the thoracic duct, so that in the presence of a leak, figure of 8 sutures using 3-0 Vicryl material should be placed. In rare instances, tissue sealant can be instilled, since immediate control of thoracic duct injury is most effective in order to avoid a later return to the operating room.

Thus, complications after SND, such as hematoma, chyle leak, and damage to cranial nerves X to XII and the marginal mandibular branch of CN7, may occur. Avoidance of injury, as with the rest of head and neck surgery, requires a detailed surgical knowledge of the anatomy and preoperative assessment of the topographic location of any suspicious lymph nodes, since oncologic excision is the fundamental goal of the SND, while maintaining complications at a minimum. The oncologic results of SND, in appropriately selected patients with cN0-cN1 disease, are as good as comprehensive neck dissection (MRND or RND). Indeed in pN1 necks after SND, the rate of recurrence in the absence of ECS or multiple positive lymph nodes is as low as other more extensive and comprehensive neck dissections. Performed correctly by an experienced head and neck surgeon, SND is a highly useful and oncologically effective procedure, with minimal morbidity.

RESULTS

SND is oncologically efficacious for all cN0 and selected cN1 cervical lymph node metastasis. Recurrence rates are approximately 5% inside or outside the dissected field, and the goal is therapy for early metastatic cancer and accurate staging to guide the use of adjuvant radiotherapy/chemoradiotherapy, as indicated. Mobilization or cautery near the spinal accessory nerve may result in temporary or permanent neuropraxia ("shoulder syndrome"), warranting delicate dissection around this structure. However, compared with MRND and RND, this procedure is cosmetically superior and, in appropriate cases, oncologically equivalent.

PEARLS

- Individuals performing SND should be comfortable with more comprehensive MRND and RND in the event that more extensive metastasis is discovered intraoperatively and conversion is necessary.
- Effective assistance during neck dissection results from experienced individuals providing countertraction of the important lymphatic and nonlymphatic structures so that the cervical fascia is unwrapped from these nonlymphatic structures, which are retained in the patient.
- Maintaining appropriate cervical fascial planes yields an avascular dissection and assists in a more effective and pleasant oncologic procedure.
- Careful identification and meticulous preservation of the spinal accessory nerve are crucial to the oncologic and functional result after SND.
- Avoiding the use of a sharp hemostat during dissection of the IJV will prevent many inadvertent traumatic injuries, including shearing of small or medium side venous branches of the IJV.

PITFALLS

- Unless level I is to be dissected, dissecting into the cervical fascia over the submandibular gland can lead to injury to the marginal mandibular branch of the facial nerve. Despite the best oncologic surgery, injury to this small nerve branch leads to embarrassing cosmetic defects postoperatively, which are quite visible to the patient and family.

- Overly aggressive retraction of the nerve often leads to permanent neuropraxia and (shoulder syndrome) adhesive capsulitis, with the attendant decrease in range of motion and shoulder strength.
- Routine inclusion of level IIB in the SND, with its attendant mobilization of the spinal accessory nerve, will cause unnecessary morbidity (shoulder syndrome) without providing sufficient oncologic benefit.

INSTRUMENTS TO HAVE AVAILABLE

- Shaw hemostatic scalpel (no. 15 blade)
- Monopolar and bipolar cautery
- Fine-tip, elongated Crile clamps
- 6-prong blunt rakes

SUGGESTED READING

Medina JE, Byers RM. Supraomohyoid neck dissection: rationale, indications, and surgical technique. *Head Neck* 1989;11(2):111–122.
Pillsbury HC III, Clark M. A rationale for therapy of the N0 neck. *Laryngoscope* 1997;107(10):1294–1315.
Simental AA Jr, Duvvuri U, Johnson JT, et al. Selective neck dissection in patients with upper aerodigestive tract cancer with clinically positive nodal disease. *Ann Otol Rhinol Laryngol* 2006;115(11):846–849.

3 SUPERSELECTIVE NECK DISSECTION FOR UPPER AERODIGESTIVE TRACT CARCINOMA

K. Thomas Robbins

INTRODUCTION

The superselective neck dissection (SSND) is a lymphadenectomy procedure in which there is compartmental *removal* of the lymph node–bearing tissue from two or less levels of the neck. It is viewed as a subcategory of the selective neck dissection (SND), which itself is defined as a lymphadenectomy that *preserves* the nonlymphatic structures of one or more levels of the neck.

Variations in neck dissections are common and have been practiced throughout the history of the procedure. Even Crile, who is credited the most for describing the radical neck dissection, in his landmark article included variations comparable to the contemporary SND. However, it was not until the 1970s that such operations were reported as a separate entity and referred to as a modified neck dissection, which ultimately encouraged a new philosophy in the management of metastases to the neck resulting in the SND procedure becoming the procedure of choice for the majority of neck dissections being performed today.

The SND is based on the patterns of lymphatic spread by metastatic cancer. In most situations, it involves the removal of lymph nodes from at least three neck levels because the risk is usually high for this number of levels. However, under more specific conditions, the number of levels of the neck at high risk may be less than three. In this situation, a more targeted neck dissection that encompasses less than three levels may be feasible. Thus, the SSND would be a surgical option.

HISTORY

It is important to rule out any symptoms indicating that the patient is not a surgical candidate. This would include complaints suggestive of extensive cancer at the primary site such as intractable pain, referred otalgia, severe dysphagia, and marked weight loss. One should look for clinical evidence of distant metastases such as complaints related to the chest.

PHYSICAL EXAMINATION

Whereas unresectable cancer in the primary site, extension of neck metastasis to involve the deep muscles of the neck or encasing the carotid artery, and evidence of distant metastases are all important exclusions to make on physical examination, definitive evidence is usually provided by imaging studies.

INDICATIONS

When used as a component of the primary treatment, the most common application of the SSND is in the treatment of supraglottic carcinoma. Tumors arising from this site have a high propensity to metastasize to the regional lymph nodes in levels IIA and III. Studies have shown that patients with supraglottic cancer, regardless of the T classification, rarely have evidence of metastases outside of these two levels provided that there is no clinical evidence of neck metastases at the time of diagnosis. Ambrosh et al. performed neck dissections limited to levels II and III in the majority of patients with cancer of the supraglottic larynx and a clinically negative neck undergoing transoral laser resection although it was only later that this targeted procedure became referred to as an SSND. When SSND is used as part of the primary treatment, it is important to point out that the presence of positive lymph node metastasis found within the neck dissection specimen is an indication for postoperative adjuvant radiation therapy.

In addition to the SSND being applicable as a component of the primary treatment for head and neck cancer, it also has a role in patients whose primary treatment approach is nonsurgical, namely, radiation therapy combined with chemotherapy. The use of chemoradiation has expanded over the past decade to become a common treatment approach for patients with advanced cancer of the head and neck. However, there remains an ongoing uncertainty related to the optimal management of metastases to the neck associated with cancer of the head and neck. Initially, the common philosophy was to perform a neck dissection on all patients who presented with bulky lymph node metastasis regardless of the response to the initial chemoradiation, the so-called planned neck dissection. However, after reports emerged indicating a high rate of control of metastasis to the neck when neck dissection was not performed among patients who had a clinical complete response to chemoradiation, the use of the planned neck dissection came into question. Thus, there is an emerging trend to perform neck dissection only for patients who do not achieve a clinical complete response in the neck. Under such circumstances, the procedure is referred to as a salvage neck dissection.

While the traditional philosophy was to remove lymph node groups in all five neck levels, more recent reports have demonstrated efficacy of the SND. Proponents of SND rely on the concept that the pattern of lymph node metastases in the cervical region is predictable and that neck levels that were not involved prior to treatment are very unlikely to harbor residual metastasis following chemoradiation. With this growing acceptance of the postchemoradiation SND, the rationale for its use presents the opportunity to include the option of performing a more targeted SND, namely, the SSND, one that removes the lymph nodes only at the levels in the neck, which are at the greatest risk for harboring clinically positive disease. For example, in patients for whom the residual lymph node metastasis is limited clinically to a single neck level following chemoradiation, there is evidence to indicate that removing only the lymph nodes in that level is feasible and safe.

CONTRAINDICATIONS

In addition to the general contraindications for undergoing surgery based on the medical status of the patient, the SSND should not be performed based on factors specific to the disease process. In its application for use as part of the primary treatment for patients with N0 disease, there is no evidence to support its efficacy for cancers arising in upper aerodigestive tract sites other than the supraglottic larynx. However, it is possible that its use may be expanded to other primary sites should additional data indicate lymph node metastasis confined to two or less levels of the neck. For patients with N+ disease, the SSND is contraindicated when used as part of the primary therapy.

In the context of using SSND following chemoradiation, the data do not support its use if there is residual nodal disease in multiple neck levels. Additionally, the procedure should be used with caution among patients whose initial lymph node metastasis involved more than two levels prior to therapy even though the residual adenopathy following chemoradiation may be confined to only one level in the neck.

PREOPERATIVE PLANNING

Routine laboratory investigation is important to rule out any systemic disease that may require special consideration. Imaging studies are also critical: computed tomography (CT) scans with contrast; magnetic resonance imaging studies may be indicated to substitute or complement CT scans; and FDG–PET studies. Typically, the FDG–PET is fused with CT scans in which case contrast can also be given to improve the imaging studies on CT alone. Specific analysis is necessary to define the cancer at the primary site as well as metastasis in the neck and to rule out any distant metastatic deposits. For patients who are being considered for SSND as part of the primary treatment concurrent with surgical removal of the primary lesion, the imaging studies should demonstrate the absence of metastatic cancer in the neck. However, for patients who are being considered for SSND following chemoradiation, the evidence of residual disease in the neck by imaging studies must be either absent or confined to a single level of the neck.

SURGICAL TECHNIQUE

As with most neck dissections, the patient is placed in the supine position with a shoulder role and draped in a manner to expose the important landmarks such as the suprasternal notch, clavicle, inferior auricle, mastoid

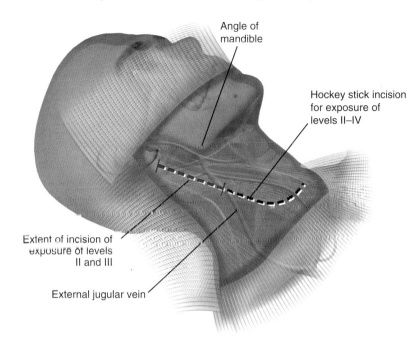

Angle of
mandible

Hockey stick incision
for exposure of
levels II–IV

Extent of incision of
exposure of levels
II and III

External jugular vein

FIGURE 3.1

Lateral view of the neck to
demonstrate the important
landmarks of the surface
anatomy to remain visible
in the surgical field and the
placement of the incision to
adequately expose levels II
and III.

process, and mentum. If the dissection involves both heminecks, each side is draped in a fashion to expose the landmarks on each side. The incision itself does not have to be as long as the ones used for the more traditional neck dissections, including SND. However, it should be placed in a manner by which it could be extended if the need arises during the procedure to convert the SSND into a more extensive procedure. Since the majority of SSNDs are performed for metastases associated with carcinoma arising in the pharynx and larynx, the neck levels most frequently targeted are II and III. Therefore, the following description is specific for this procedure.

The incision is made in the lateral neck extending vertically from the mastoid tip to the level of the cricoid cartilage or slightly inferior. In essence, this corresponds to the upper two-thirds of the classical hockey stick incision typically used for an SND in which levels II–IV are removed (Fig. 3.1). The cervical flap is then raised initially in the subplatysmal plane medially and laterally in a similar plane that lies superficial to the external jugular vein and the branches of the greater auricular nerve. The flap should be raised in order to identify the lateral border of the sternothyroid muscle medially, the angle of the mandible and the infraparotid region superiorly, and the level of the omohyoid muscle inferiorly. Next, the fascia is incised along the anterior border of the sternocleidomastoid muscle (SCM) to mobilize its medial aspect and allow retraction laterally in order to expose the internal jugular vein (IJV) and the fibroadipose tissue surrounding it. In this approach described, it is not necessary to sacrifice the greater auricular nerve and the external jugular vein.

At this point, the exposure should be sufficient to identify the anatomical boundaries of levels II and III. Next, it is important to identify the upper third of the spinal accessory nerve (SAN) and skeletonize it between its entry point into the sternocleidomastoid inferiorly and its superior location as it lies close to the IJV near the skull base. In following the SAN superiorly, it is important to identify the posterior belly of the digastric muscle and skeletonize its inferior border. By retracting this muscle, one can better visualize the superior aspect of the SAN and the adjacent IJV. Next to be performed is the removal of the contents of each neck level, which is essentially the fibroadipose tissue encompassing the lymph nodes of the upper and middle jugular chain and the superior third of the SAN. The goal is to remove the contents in continuity as a compartmental packet of fibroadipose tissue. The dissection can be started at any boundary but is typically begun superolaterally in the submuscular recess (sublevel IIB). Therefore, it is necessary to skeletonize the SAN along its distance of exposure. By gently retracting the SAN medially and the SCM laterally, the contents of sublevel IIB can be removed. After the fibroadipose tissue of sublevel IIB is mobilized and freed from the underlying muscular floor (supraspinous muscle), its contents are passed deep to the SAN. The dissection is then carried medially and inferiorly along the same muscular plane (levator medius and lateralis) until the lateral aspect of the IJV is exposed. Care is taken not to dissect laterally toward the posterior triangle in order to preserve the motor and sensory branches of the cervical plexus. The same dissection plane along the floor of the sublevels IIA and IIB is then extended inferiorly to the level of the superior belly of the omohyoid muscle. The contents of levels II and III are then swept medially over the IJV and the medial to it. Superiorly, the dissection is carried along the fascia overlying the carotid sheath which allows protection of the superior aspect of the IJV and carotid artery, vagus nerve, and hypoglossal nerve. Inferiorly the dissection stops at the junction of the omohyoid muscle crossing the IJV. However, because the juguloomohyoid nodes often lie slightly deep to this muscle, it is important to mobilize the superior border of the muscle and

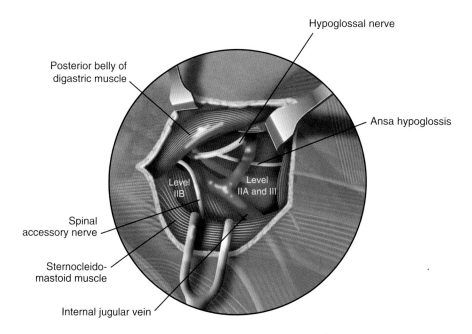

FIGURE 3.2

Exposure of the surgical bed following removal of levels II and III.

remove any nodes that lie deep to it. Medially, the dissection is extended to the lateral border of the sterno-hyoid muscle below and above by the vertical plane defined by the posterior aspect of the submandibular gland. Usually, the anterior jugular vein, the facial vein, and any communicating venous branches can be preserved (Fig. 3.2).

For bilateral procedures, a contralateral incision is made in a similar fashion, essentially representing a mirror image of the existing ipsilateral incision (Fig. 3.3). It is not necessary to connect the incisions, which is usually done for cases in which the bilateral neck dissections are more extensive. In fact, there is a distinct advantage to preserving the tissue planes in the midline of the neck and thereby optimizing blood supply and lymphatic drainage.

Closure of the surgical bed includes placing a suction drain through a separate stab incision laterally and inferiorly and approximating the wound edges using at least two layers of sutures. Since the amount of dead space is limited, the drain can usually be removed within 24 hours. Most patients are kept in the hospital over-night, although selected patients may be discharged the same day.

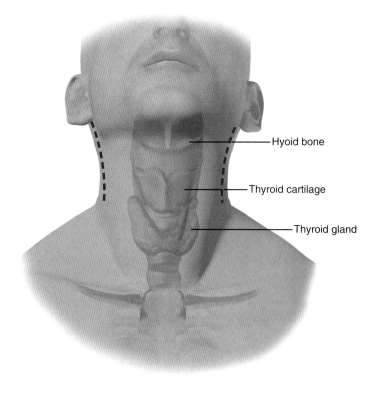

FIGURE 3.3

Placement of the incisions for bilateral SSND. It is not necessary to connect the incisions on each side of the neck if the cancer at the primary site is removed transorally.

POSTOPERATIVE MANAGEMENT

If the decision is made to use a neck drain, it can usually be removed the following day. For patients who have an SSND as an isolated procedure following chemoradiation, it is often feasible to discharge the patient from hospital the same day without a neck drain. Most patients require analgesia only for low to moderate pain. Range-of-motion shoulder and neck exercises are useful since the SAN is exposed and skeletonized.

COMPLICATIONS

Similar to the more traditional neck dissection procedures, complications may occur that include injury to nerves (SAN, hypoglossal, marginal mandibular, vagus), blood vessels (IJV, carotid artery), as well as infection and bleeding. However, the procedure of SSND itself has the advantage over more extensive neck dissections, including SND, of less morbidity because the surgical field is limited to only two levels and the incision can be short, usually approximately 8 cm. For patients who require bilateral neck dissections, two separate neck incisions can be made and it is not necessary to connect the two surgical fields. The end result following SSND is that there is a limited surgical field, which reduces the likelihood of developing extensive fibrosis of the soft tissues of the neck. The recovery from the surgery is rapid, and there is less risk to surrounding vital structures. All of these advantages become even more important in considering the long course of treatment with chemotherapy and radiation over many weeks that most patients are required to undergo.

RESULTS

When SSND is applied in the treatment of lymph node metastasis as part of the initial therapy, the published results support its use primarily for cancers arising in the supraglottic larynx. Ambrosch et al. reported the results of 711 dissections performed for carcinoma of the upper aerodigestive tract for patients undergoing transoral laser resection (Ambrosch, 1995). This included a subset of patients with cancers arising from the oropharynx, larynx, and hypopharynx. The majority of patients within this subset who had clinical N0 disease had a neck dissection that only included levels II and III. This more limited intervention, which is now referred to as an SSND, was based on observations by the authors that there was a low incidence of metastases in level IV for tumors specific to these sites. With regard to the status of the surgical pathology of the neck dissections, there were, respectively, 296 and 148 dissections of levels II–III performed on patients who were node negative and node positive. For the entire group of patients reported in the series, adjuvant radiation therapy was given in 36/249 (14.5%) patients with histopathologically uninvolved lymph nodes, and 158/254 (62.2%) patients with histologically proven lymph node metastases. The percentages of patients irradiated based on pN categories were as follows: pN1, 45.5%; pN2a, 72.7%; pN2b, 67.7%; and pN2c, 88.0%. The 3-year recurrence rate following combined therapy versus surgery only was a respective 0.0% and 5.5% for patients with N0 disease, 3.0% and 6.3% for patients with an N1 neck, and 7.0% and 24.0% for patients with an N2 neck. Clearly, the use of adjuvant radiation therapy diminished the risk of recurrence in the neck among patients with all three categories of N classification. While the authors used SSND as an intervention for selected patients with hypopharyngeal and oropharyngeal tumors, its use is best documented for supraglottic carcinoma based on studies documenting a very low incidence of levels IV and V metastases among patients with an N0 neck (Ferlito).

In a comparison study of clinical versus pathologic analysis of neck level–specific metastases to determine the feasibility of SSND following cathode ray tube, the findings in 177 patients (239 heminecks) with N+ disease treated with RADPLAT were compared (Robbins et al., 2007). The protocol included 4 weekly intraarterial infusions of cisplatin (150 mg/M2) and concurrent radiation therapy (2 Gy/day × 35 fractions over 7 weeks). Comparisons were made between the clinical presence of neck level–specific metastasis at postchemoradiation restaging and subsequent evidence of pathologic disease following neck dissection. Tumor sites included oropharynx (81), hypopharynx (39), larynx (27), oral cavity (19), and others (11). Pretreatment nodal classification included N1 (39), N2a (15), N2b (44), N2c (48), and N3 (31). Response of lymph node metastasis based on clinical evaluation (physical examination, radiologic studies) was as follows: CR, 89 (50%); PR, 81 (46%); PD, 4 (2%); and unevaluable, 3 (2%). Among the necks that were restaged as a partial response, 73 had clinical evidence of residual adenopathy, which involved only one level in the neck. Fifty-seven patients subsequently had a salvage neck dissection, for whom the pathologic findings were correlated with the postchemoradiation staging for neck level–specific metastases. Only 2 of the 57 evaluable patients had evidence of pathologic lymph node metastasis extending beyond the single neck level, one of whom had disease in the contiguous neck level. The correlations supported the hypothesis that SSND is feasible among patients whose residual lymph node metastasis is confined to a single level. In addition to the anatomical pathologic study, shown in another analysis of clinical outcomes following neck dissection after chemoradiation, namely, RADPLAT, was the absence of regional recurrence noted among a small subset (seven patients) in which an SSND was performed (Robbins et al., 2005). Most recently, the treatment outcomes were reported of a larger series of 35 SSNDs, among which 23 were performed in patients who had a complete response in the neck and 12 were performed in patients who did not have a complete response following chemoradiation, and thus categorized as salvage neck dissection procedures (Robbins et al., 2012). In this latter group, all patients achieved a CR at the primary site. There were 8 neck specimens in which there was residual metastatic cancer found on pathologic examination. This involved one specimen in the complete response group (4%) and seven specimens in the partial response group (67%). Only one of the pathologic positive nodal metastases exhibited extracapsular spread (ECS). Over a median follow-up of 33 (range: 8 to 72) months, there were 8 recurrences, all of which occurred either at the primary site or at distant sites. There were no isolated recurrences in the neck, however, there was one patient who was diagnosed with a recurrence in the primary site and neck simultaneously. The projected 5-year disease-specific survival rate for the group was 60%.

The data show that SSND is an effective treatment strategy applicable to a specific subset of patients following chemoradiation for advanced cancer of the head and neck. With this latter application, it may be viewed as an adjuvant therapy rather than part of the primary treatment. It is based on the principle that neck levels with clinically absent metastases prior to treatment, which then receive a therapeutic dose of radiation along with concurrent chemotherapy, should have a very low risk for having occult residual metastases following treatment. This should obviate the need to surgically remove the nodes from these levels, even though other neck levels had clinically positive metastasis.

PEARLS

- Preservation of sensation by the greater auricular nerve can usually be achieved by raising the skin flaps in the subplatysmal plane medially and then extending the neck incision laterally to extend the corresponding surgical plane over the greater auricular nerves and external jugular vein. Lateral retraction on the SCM may result in a neuropraxia of these nerve branches, but recovery of sensory function is expected.
- Injury to the mandibular branch of the facial nerve is best prevented by raising the neck flaps in the subplatysmal plane. The use of paralytic agents for anesthesia should be withheld until the nerve has been identified and isolated. The mandibular nerve is at risk to be injured in its lateral course during dissection of level IIA. Careful retraction on the upper neck flap is important to avoid compression of this nerve.
- The SAN is identified as the SCM is retracted laterally. Careful placement of retractors on the SCM should be done in order to avoid pressure on the SAN.
- In patients who have extensive fibrosis surrounding the metastasis overlying the IJV, careful dissection using a fine hemostat to separate the lymph node away from the vein is usually possible. However, the inability to identify a surgical plane between the IJV and the lymph node requires removal of the IJV. The necessity to perform this removal does not necessarily indicate the need to perform a more extensive removal of the lymph nodes in other levels.
- Patients who have evidence of shoulder dysfunction following neck surgery should begin range-of-motion exercises and other physiotherapy techniques immediately. The majority of patients will recover as long as the spinal accessory is intact.

PITFALLS

- Place the shorter neck incision in a line that corresponds with the direction of its extension in case the additional neck levels need to be incorporated.
- Direct pressure on the SAN when retracting on the SCM may result in frozen shoulder syndrome.
- When performing a postchemoradiation SSND, be certain that the cancer at the primary site has completely resolved.

INSTRUMENTS TO HAVE AVAILABLE

- Standard head and neck tray.
- Fine tip hemostats and dissecting scissors.
- Bipolar cautery.

SUGGESTED READING

Shah JP. Patterns of cervical lymph node metastasis from squamous carcinomas of the upper aerodigestive tract. *Am J Surg* 1990;160(4):405–409.

Robbins KT, Medina JE, Wolfe GT, et al. Standardizing neck dissection terminology. Official report of the Academy's Committee for Head and Neck Surgery and Oncology. *Arch Otolaryngol Head Neck Surg* 1991;117(6):601–605.

Ambrosch P, Kron M, Pradier O, et al. Efficacy of selective neck dissection: a review of 503 cases of elective and therapeutic treatment of the neck in squamous cell carcinoma of the upper aerodigestie tract. *Arch Otolaryngol Head Neck Surg* 2001;124:180–187.

Robbins KT, Doweck I, Samant S, et al. Effectiveness of superselective and selective neck dissection for advanced nodal metastases after chemoradiation. *Arch Otolaryngol Head Neck Surg* 2005;131(11):965–969.

Robbins KT, Shannon K, Vieira F. Superselective neck dissection after chemoradiation: feasibility based on clinical and pathologic comparisons. *Arch Otolaryngol Head Neck Surg* 2007;133(5):486–489.

Robbins KT, Dhiwakar M, Vieira F, et al. Efficacy of super-selective neck dissection following chemoradiation for advanced head and neck cancer. *Oral Oncol* 2012;48:1185–1189.

4 MODIFIED RADICAL NECK DISSECTION

James Y. Suen

INTRODUCTION

In 1906, George Crile described the classical radical neck dissection (RND). It was the primary operation for surgical management of metastatic cervical lymph nodes for many decades. Starting in the late 1960s and later, Bocca and Pignataro, O. Suarez, Ballantyne, Jesse, and Suen began to describe modifications of the RND and demonstrated that the control and cure rates were equal to the RND.

The technique of the modified radical neck dissection (MRND) includes removal of all cervical node levels (I, II, III, IV, and V) (Fig. 4.1) with preservation of one or more of the following: the spinal accessory nerve, the sternocleidomastoid muscle (SCM), and the internal jugular vein (IJV).

Cancer in the neck may represent either a primary cancer or metastasis from a cancer usually primary in the upper aerodigestive tract or the skin of the face or neck. Primary cancers in the neck arise from the tail of the parotid gland, the thyroid, the submandibular gland. Lymphoma is frequently encountered in the neck.

Other sites to consider that can metastasize to the neck include lungs, breast, cervix, prostate, and other intra-abdominal organs.

HISTORY

It is important to ask if the patient has a history of having had a skin cancer of the head and neck removed in the past or has a persistent sore area in the upper aerodigestive tract. Also it is important to inquire about hoarseness, dysphagia, and weight loss.

Question whether the patient has had other cancers, such as lung, breast, intra-abdominal, or prostate. These cancers can spread via lymphatics, and usually metastasize to the left supraclavicular lymph nodes.

PHYSICAL EXAMINATION

A complete examination of the head and neck must be performed. The location of the enlarged nodes can guide you to the primary site. It is important to check the thyroid gland for nodules.

The size, number, and mobility of the lymph nodes are important to note. Fixation to the skin or underlying structures may be a contraindication to this procedure.

INDICATIONS

1. N2a, N2b, N3a, and N3b cervical lymph node metastasis. N1 if surgery is the only treatment planned.

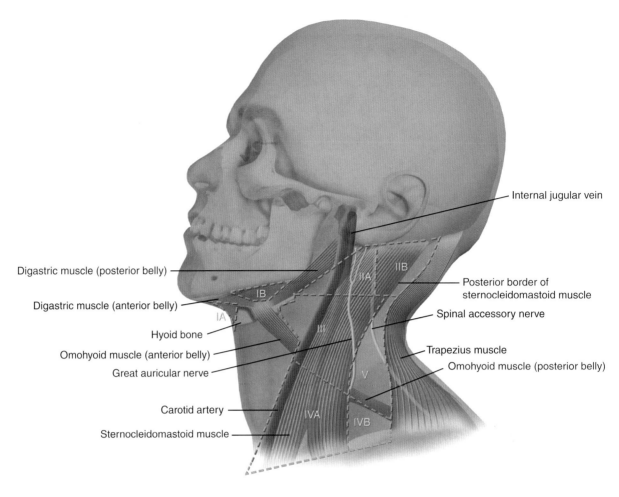

Internal jugular vein

Digastric muscle (posterior belly)

Posterior border of sternocleidomastoid muscle

Digastric muscle (anterior belly)

Spinal accessory nerve

Hyoid bone

Trapezius muscle

Omohyoid muscle (anterior belly)

Omohyoid muscle (posterior belly)

Great auricular nerve

Carotid artery

Sternocleidomastoid muscle

FIGURE 4.1 Cervical lymph node nomenclature and lymph node levels.

CONTRAINDICATIONS

1. Life expectancy of <3 months
2. Uncontrollable cancer at the primary site
3. Lymph nodes fixed deeply and unchanged by irradiation and/or chemotherapy
4. Surgeon who is inexperienced with the MRND

PREOPERATIVE PLANNING

Imaging Studies

a. Ultrasound (US), if the surgeon is experienced using it. US can identify the size and number of cervical lymph nodes and is inexpensive.
b. Computed tomography (CT) scan can be very helpful. It can identify size and numbers of cervical lymph nodes and their internal architecture. It can be performed quickly and is less expensive than a magnetic resonance imaging (MRI) scan.
c. MRI can also provide the same information regarding cervical lymph nodes. It is more expensive and takes a longer time to perform.
d. Positron emission tomography–computed tomography (PET-CT) can identify unknown primaries and will usually identify metastatic cervical lymph nodes. It is also capable of identifying distant metastases or second primary cancers, particularly thyroid. This scan is very expensive and takes several hours to complete.

Biopsy

A fine needle aspiration biopsy (FNAB) should identify the histology, if there is an experienced pathologist reading it. Some metastatic lymph nodes may be necrotic, and if the FNAB samples only the necrotic fluid, the diagnosis may be missed.

With FNAB being available, it is unusual to need an open biopsy. Lymphoma may be difficult to diagnose by this technique and might require removal of a lymph node.

SURGICAL TECHNIQUE

The MRND should remove essentially the same lymph nodes as an RND (Fig. 4.2). The SCM is in the middle of the dissection and makes the surgery more difficult. The SCM can be divided at the inferior attachment to the clavicle to make the surgery easier, or it could be resected with the lymph nodes. The SCM muscle should be removed if tumor is adherent to it or invading into it.

An incision should be planned so that all the lymph nodes can be accessed. My preference is a "hockey-stick" incision. This incision begins at the mastoid tip and should be carried almost straight down to just above the clavicle; the incision should be curved medially to the midline. Before I start the incision, I place scratch marks, with a knife, on each side of the incision mark and place these at several spots. With a long incision, it is easier to match these points up for accurate closure of the skin.

The incision is usually made with a monopolar needle-tip cautery through the skin and dermis, then I switch to the blade-tip Bovie. The blade tip is useful for dissecting while in the off position. During the flap incision and elevation, I watch for the external jugular vein that can bleed significantly. This vein can be preserved or ligated.

After completing the incision, I elevate the skin flap both posteriorly and anteriorly. Posteriorly, I elevate back until the trapezius muscle is encountered. Anteriorly, I elevate the flap just beneath the platysma muscle and carry it to the midline. If the primary cancer is in the oropharynx, hypopharynx, larynx, or thyroid, it is unlikely for the lymph nodes to involve the submandibular triangle, so I do not resect that level.

After the flaps are elevated, I retract them with a suture or with hooks on a rubber band (Lone Star hooks) to keep them out of the way (Fig. 4.3).

I make an incision into the superficial fascia over the SCM muscle along its entire length and grasp the fascia with hemostats to retract it away from the muscle (Figs. 4.4 and 4.5). This process is referred to as "unwrapping" the SCM muscle; I then dissect deep to it until the nerves of the cervical plexus are encountered at the posterior border of the muscle (Fig. 4.6). During this dissection, the SCM muscle must be retracted laterally. The spinal accessory nerve can be identified where it is deep to the muscle in the upper one-third (Fig. 4.6). There is a branch of the spinal accessory nerve that innervates the SCM muscle, and I prefer to save it. If the nerve to the muscle is cut inadvertently, the SCM muscle will atrophy and with time will become very firm and fibrotic.

While dissecting the fascia off of the muscle, the muscle must be retracted. The blade-tip cautery or the Shaw knife or a regular no. 10 Bard Parker knife blade can be used. Hemostasis must be controlled with the monopolar or bipolar cautery as vessels are encountered. I prefer the bipolar cautery because it does not cause the muscle to contract when touched.

Once the dissection reaches the nerves of the cervical plexus, the decision must be made whether to dissect around the nerves or remove them. If the cervical plexus nerves are cut at the posterior edge of the SCM muscle,

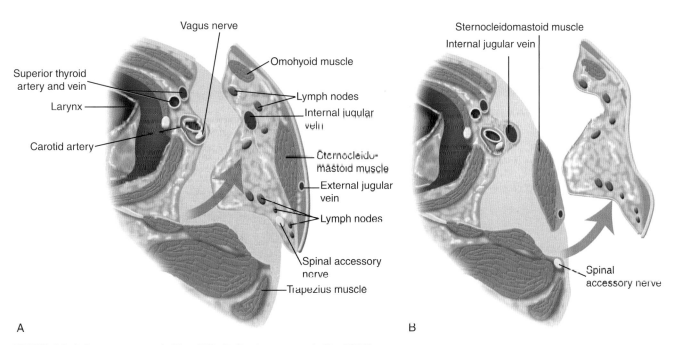

A

B

FIGURE 4.2 A: Structures removed with an RND. **B:** Structures removed with a MRND.

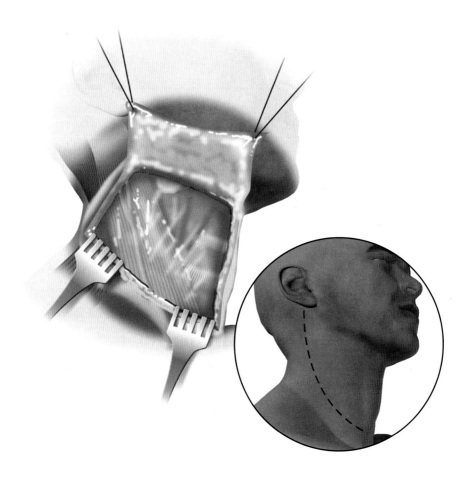

FIGURE 4.3
Technique of MRND. Flap
elevated and contents of the
neck exposed.

they must be cut again as the dissection comes forward toward the carotid sheath. The spinal accessory nerve is in a vulnerable position in the posterior triangle and should be protected and saved.

Dissecting the posterior triangle is not easy from this anterior approach. If there are clinically positive nodes in that area, it would be better to go posterior to the SCM muscle and dissect the fascia and contents off of the posterior edge of the SCM and off of the trapezius muscle. In the inferior aspect of the posterior triangle,

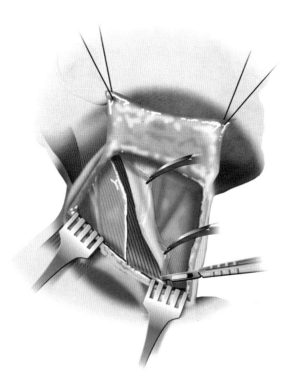

FIGURE 4.4
Technique of MRND. Incision
and elevation of the superficial
fascia off of the SCM.

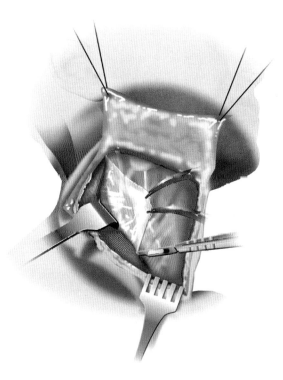

FIGURE 4.5 Fascia dissected from the medial aspect of the SCM.

there are many veins and these should be ligated or clipped with hemoclips. At the superior aspect of the posterior triangle, above the spinal accessory nerve, the tissue should be dissected and removed, especially if there were clinically positive nodes in the upper jugular chain (Fig. 4.6). This tissue can be removed separately and submitted as superior, posterior triangle tissue, "level IIB."

After the posterior cervical contents and the tissues deep to the SCM muscle are dissected off of the deep cervical muscles (splenius capitis and levator scapulae), the carotid sheath is encountered. At this point, the IJV is being retracted medially over the carotid artery, and the artery may be encountered first. Around the carotid artery, jugular vein, and vagus nerve, I would recommend dissecting with a hemostat right on the vessels and a knife (Fig. 4.7). The cautery can injure these vessels and cause significant bleeding.

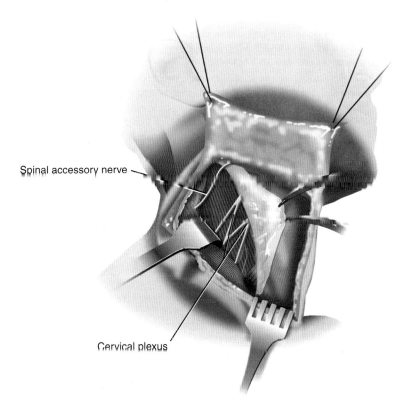

Spinal accessory nerve

Cervical plexus

FIGURE 4.6

Nerves of the cervical plexus at the posterior edge of the SCM. Tissue around the spinal accessory nerve is dissected out.

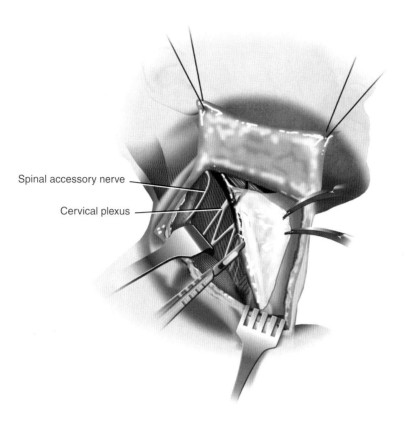

Spinal accessory nerve

Cervical plexus

FIGURE 4.7
Dissecting tissue off of the internal jugular vein.

At this point, clinically positive lymph nodes will probably be found, and care must be taken to dissect the lymph nodes off of the vessels and without crushing them. Traction on the lymph nodes and the normal structures is important to facilitate the dissection.

Once the tissue is dissected off of the carotid sheath, it should be dissected to the strap muscles and can then be removed (Fig. 4.8). At the superior aspect of the dissection just above the bifurcation of the carotid artery, the hypoglossal nerve should be identified and preserved. If the jugular vein is accidentally cut, I prefer to repair it rather than take the vein. If the nodes are adherent to the jugular vein, it is better to remove the vein.

Dissection of the supraclavicular nodes on the left side of the neck can potentially cause injury to the thoracic duct. Care must be taken to avoid it and to be liberal with bipolar cautery to seal the smaller lymphatic vessels going into the thoracic duct.

I like to orient the tissue removed by placing it on a paper diagram of a neck, so the pathologist can tell if the nodes are from the upper, mid, or lower neck when processed. I staple the tissue to the diagram so it cannot move.

After completing the MRND, I irrigate the neck and look for any bleeding that needs to be controlled. A medium or large Hemovac drain is placed into the neck and secured with a suture at the exit point and the incision closed.

POSTOPERATIVE MANAGEMENT

The drain is connected to a Hemovac suction. I usually do not use a pressure dressing after neck dissection. The drain remains for at least 3 or 4 days, or if the patient has had previous irradiation, I may leave it for about 7 days.

I also check for weakness of the tongue (CN12), hoarseness (CN10), and function of the trapezius muscle (CN11) in case they were injured during surgery.

Most patients who undergo an MRND only should be able to be discharged from the hospital on the first or second postoperative day.

COMPLICATIONS

Potential complications include hematoma, or chyle leak, and permanent nerve damage to cranial nerves 10, 11, and 12 and the mandibular branch of the facial nerve. Knowing the anatomy and being meticulous will minimize complications.

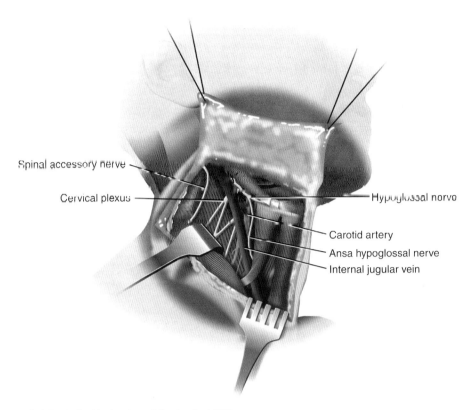

Spinal accessory nerve

Cervical plexus

Hypoglossal nerve

Carotid artery

Ansa hypoglossal nerve

Internal jugular vein

FIGURE 4.8 Residual anatomy following the MRND.

RESULTS

Results are difficult to assess because many variables are involved, such as surgeon's experience, whether surgery is the only treatment being used, postoperative radiation or chemo/radiation, and whether the MRND is done for salvage after radiation or for neck recurrence after previous selective neck dissection.

In my experience of performing over 1,000 MRNDs in 37 years, I feel that the control rate for metastatic cancer to the cervical lymph nodes is as good as an RND.

PEARLS

- If you are inexperienced in MRND surgery, remove the SCM muscle and the cervical plexus nerves with the dissection to get better exposure and to avoid missing metastatic lymph nodes.
- Proper traction and countertraction during surgery is important to facilitate the dissection.
- Stay in the proper tissue planes when elevating the flaps.
- When the dissection is on the carotid sheath, use a hemostat to find the tissue planes to remove all nodal disease off of the carotid artery and the IJV.
- Find and preserve the spinal accessory nerve throughout its entire length. Be careful with traction on the nerve, because it can be injured permanently if too much traction is applied.
- Prevent a vasovagal response by avoiding pressure on the carotid sinus.
- If tumor is adherent to the IJV, resect the vein with the dissection.
- Keep a large suction drain in the neck for at least 3 days.

PITFALLS

- Operating around the SCM muscle may result in missing metastatic lymph nodes.
- Saving the cervical plexus nerves makes it more difficult to do an en bloc resection of the nodes.
- Operating to remove the lymph nodes around the spinal accessory nerve can be frustrating, and inadvertently one may cut the IJV or permanently injure the nerve.
- Dissecting the lymph nodes off of the IJV, the vein may be lacerated resulting in significant bleeding.
- Avoid the use of monopolar cautery on the major blood vessels for the same reason.
- To avoid a seroma or hematoma, do not remove the suction drain too early.

INSTRUMENTS TO HAVE AVAILABLE

- Needle point cautery tip for the skin incision
- Protected, Teflon-coated cautery blade tip for the rest of the dissection
- A Shaw scalpel can make the dissection easier, but this knife is easy to have tissue adhere to the edge making it dull and it has to be wiped clean frequently.
- Have a good bipolar cautery for bleeders on the muscles and around the carotid sheath.
- Have some parotid dissecting hemostats available while removing the nodes and tissues off the vessels of the carotid sheath.

SUGGESTED READING

Lindberg RD. Distribution of cervical lymph node metastasis from squamous cell carcinoma of the upper respiratory and digestive tracts. *Cancer* 1972;29:1446.

Bocca E. Critical analysis of the techniques and value of neck dissection. *Nuovo Arch Ital Otol* 1976;4:151.

Bocca E, Pignataro O, Sasaki CT. Functional neck dissection. *Arch Otolaryngol* 1980;106:524.

Suen JY, Wetmore SJ. Cancer of the neck. In: Suen JY, Myers EN, eds. *Cancer of the Head and Neck*. New York: Churchill Livingstone, 1981:185.

Suen JY, Goepfert H. Standardization of neck dissection nomenclature [Editorial]. *Head Neck Surg* 1987;10:75.

5 ROBOTIC MODIFIED RADICAL NECK DISSECTION FOR THYROID CANCER; SURGICAL TECHNIQUE USING GASLESS, TRANSAXILLARY APPROACH

Sang-Wook Kang

INTRODUCTION

The higher socioeconomic status enjoyed today has resulted in quality of life being viewed as a major issue. This trend has greatly influenced medical disciplines, and many medical and surgical therapies have been modified based on quality of life considerations. Accordingly, minimally invasive surgery in various surgical fields has rapidly developed and spread due to increased concerns about issues, such as incision scars, degree of pain, and time required to return to work after surgery.

In the head and neck area, well-differentiated thyroid carcinoma (WDTC) is the most common malignancy and, unlike other cancers of the head and neck, usually has a favorable prognosis. Furthermore, the incidence of early-stage cancer of the thyroid has markedly increased due to the institution of various health-screening programs, and the proportion of thyroid cancer in young women, who are particularly sensitive to cosmesis, is increasing. Accordingly, trials on endoscopic or minimally invasive techniques in thyroid surgery have been continuously conducted with a main aim of avoiding visible scars on the neck, and many early satisfactory results have already been reported for these techniques.

Papillary carcinoma of the thyroid (PTC)—the most common type of WDTC—usually has a mild biologic course, but nevertheless, it frequently metastasizes to the cervical lymph nodes (LNs). In cases of metastasis to the lateral neck nodes (LNM) from PTC, bilateral total thyroidectomy with modified radical neck dissection (MRND) for metastatic lateral cervical nodes is the treatment of choice. However, although conventional open MRND is the safest and most efficient type of surgical treatment, a desperately long incision scar on the neck is inevitable. In view of the favorable nature and high prevalence of PTC in women, the avoidance of unsightly scarring in the neck area necessitates minimally invasive and remote approaches to lateral neck dissection. Accordingly, I have applied endoscopic techniques to thyroidectomy and MRND procedures for PTC with LNM. Furthermore, the incorporation of dexterous robotic technology in surgery of the neck enables more precise and meticulous endoscopic movement during the complex procedure required for MRND. Recently, a robotic MRND technique for cancer of the thyroid with LNM was introduced and produces excellent cosmetic results. In addition, the technical feasibility and safety of robotic MRND have been reported, and the technique has been found to be capable of complete compartment-oriented dissection.

In the early 20th century, George Washington Crile first described a systematic surgical approach to en bloc neck dissection for cancers of the head and neck, and subsequently, Martin and his colleagues refined Crile's original methods and substantially expanded the concept of radical neck dissection to its current format. Later many surgeons, including Suárez, Bocca, and Gavilán, attempted to modify, standardize, or establish the surgical extent of neck dissection. During the 1960s, surgeons at the MD Anderson Hospital (Jesse, Ballantyne, and Byers) began to selectively remove, based on location of the primary lesion, only the neck LN groups at highest risk of metastasis.

Recently, profound comprehension of the pathophysiology of cancers of the head and neck and intensive treatment experience resulted in alternative surgical options for cervical LN metastasis, such as selective or superselective neck dissection in accordance with primary tumor biology to reduce surgical morbidity while preserving oncologic safety.

In carcinoma of the thyroid, MRND type III (actually, selective neck dissection [levels II–VI]) is the current treatment of choice for the management of WDTC with LNM. In this chapter, I will describe in detail robotic MRND methods for the management of WDTC with LMN.

HISTORY

The patient should be questioned about a history of dysphagia, weight loss, or skin cancer removed in the past, or a persistent sore area in the upper aerodigestive tract. Also it is important to inquire about hoarseness, dysphagia, or weight loss. Question whether the patient has had other cancers, such as lung, breast, intra-abdominal, or prostate in addition to thyroid cancer. These cancers can spread via lymphatics and usually go to the left supraclavicular LNs.

PHYSICAL EXAMINATION

A complete examination of the head and neck should be performed. The location of the enlarged nodes can often guide you to the primary cancer. It is important to check the thyroid gland for nodules.

The size, number, and mobility of the LNs are important. It is also critical to note fixation to the skin, or underlying structures which may be a contraindication to this procedure.

INDICATIONS

The eligibility criteria for robotic MRND are as follows: (1) WDTC with clinical LNM (cases with a minimum of 1 or 2 metastatic LNs in the lateral neck), (2) a primary tumor size of ≤4 cm, and (3) minimal invasion of the anterior thyroid capsule and strap muscles by the primary cancer.

The role of the robotic procedure for the management of cancer of the thyroid with LMN remains controversial. For experienced surgeons, this approach may be well suited for cases with limited LNM from WDTC, but its role in cases of more locally advanced cancer is uncertain, and thus, robotic MRND is clearly contraindicated in such cases.

The exclusion criteria that should be applied are (1) definite tumor invasion to an adjacent organ (recurrent laryngeal nerve, esophagus, major vessels, or trachea), (2) multiple LN metastases in multiple levels of the lateral neck, or (3) perinodal infiltration at a metastatic LN.

CONTRAINDICATIONS

1. Life expectancy of <3 months
2. Uncontrollable cancer at the primary site
3. Fixed LNs unchanged by irradiation and/or chemotherapy
4. Surgeon who is inexperienced with robotic surgery and open MRND

PREOPERATIVE PLANNING

WDTC should be diagnosed in all patients by preoperative fine-needle aspiration biopsy (FNAB). High-resolution staging ultrasonography (US) and computed tomography of the neck can be performed for preoperative staging of the disease. All patients with clinically palpable lateral neck nodes or a lateral LN with a suspicious ultrasound appearance by preoperative staging US should undergo US-guided FNAB.

The presence of metastasis to a lateral neck node can be determined by US-guided FNAB histology or by measuring thyroglobulin (Tg) levels in FNAB washout fluid (FNA-Tg > 10 ng/mL, >mean + 2 SD of FNA-Tg measured in node-negative patients, or >serum-Tg) from lateral neck LNs.

Extent of Dissection for Modified Radical Neck Dissection

The optimal management of PTC remains the subject of considerable debate. Nevertheless, the most important initial consideration is the complete surgical resection of the cancer of the thyroid and metastatic LNs. Radioactive iodine treatment can be administered later for ablation of any remaining thyroid tissue, and TSH suppression

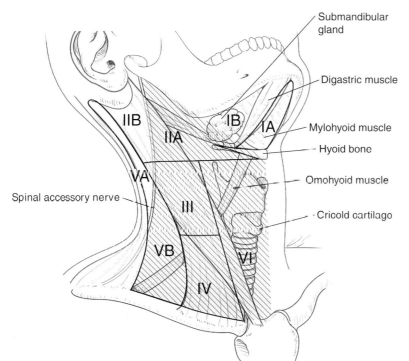

FIGURE 5.1

The anatomic landmarks used to divide the lateral and central LN compartments into levels I–VI; the area with a deviant crease line is where LN dissection is made during MRND.

therapy can be added according to risk. The surgical extent of PTC can be classified using the two LN–bearing compartments to which PTC usually metastasizes, that is, the central and lateral compartments. Routine prophylactic lateral neck dissection in PTC patients is controversial, because lateral neck areas may be treatable by second surgery. However, therapeutic lateral neck dissection in PTC patients with clinically determined LMN is always necessary.

The surgical approaches used most commonly in cases with LNM from PTC are bilateral total thyroidectomy with central compartment neck dissection and concurrent MRND (type III, sparing sternocleidomastoid muscle [SCM], spinal accessory nerve, and the internal jugular vein [IJV]). The submental, submandibular, parotid, and retroauricular nodes are virtually never dissected, and level IIB and VA lymph nodes are not routinely dissected either in cancer of the thyroid with LNM, because its rarely metastasizes to levels I or IIB, or VA.

However, if an enlarged or suspicious cervical LN is encountered by palpation or by preoperative US in these areas, these compartments are also included in en bloc dissection. Thus, the usual extent of surgical dissection for MRND in WDTC with LNM are levels IIA, III, IV, VB, and VI, which applies to robotic and open MRND procedures (Fig. 5.1).

SURGICAL TECHNIQUE

Patient Preparation

With a patient in a supine position under general anesthesia, the neck is slightly extended by inserting a soft pillow under the shoulder and turning the face away from the lesion. The lesion-side arm is stretched out laterally and abducted about 80 degrees from the body (Optimally expose the axillary and lateral neck areas). The landmarks for dissection are the sternal notch and the midline of the anterior neck medially, the anterior border of trapezius muscle laterally, and the submandibular gland superiorly (Fig. 5.2).

Development of Working Space

A 7- to 8-cm vertical skin incision is placed in the axilla along the anterior axillary fold and the lateral border of the pectoralis major. A subcutaneous skin flap is made over the anterior surface of the pectoralis muscle from axilla to the clavicle and the sternal notch. After crossing the clavicle, a subplatysmal skin flap is made. The flap is dissected medially over the SCM muscle toward the midline of the anterior neck. Laterally, the trapezius muscle is identified and dissected upward along its anterior border. The spinal accessory nerve is identified and traced carefully along its course until it passes on the undersurface of the SCM muscle. The subplatysmal skin flap is elevated upward to Erbs point, and after exposure of this landmark, the dissection proceeds deep to the

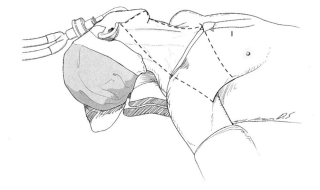

FIGURE 5.2

Patient position and superficial landmarks for flap dissection.

posterior surface of the SCM muscle to the submandibular gland superiorly. After subplatysmal flap dissection, the posterior branch (clavicular head) of the SCM is transected at the level of clavicle-attachment point (to completely expose the junction area between the IJV and subclavian vein). The dissection of the SCM muscle fascia begins at the posterior edge of the muscle and proceeds in a medial direction beneath the two heads of the muscle. The external jugular vein is ligated where it crosses the SCM muscle and the dissection proceeds upward until the submandibular gland and the posterior belly of the digastric muscle are exposed. The superior belly of the omohyoid muscle is divided at the level of the thyroid cartilage, and the thyroid gland is then detached from the strap muscles.

After flap dissection, the patient's face is turned to face forward. A long and wide retractor blade (Chung retractor) designed for MRND is inserted through the axillary incision and placed between the thyroid and the strap muscle (Fig. 5.3). The entire thyroid gland and levels IIA, III, IV, VB, and VI area are fully exposed by elevating the two heads of the SCM muscle and the strap muscles. A second skin incision for the fourth robotic arm is made on the anterior chest wall, 6 to 8 cm medially and 2 to 4 cm superiorly from the nipple (Video 5.1).

Docking and Instrumentation

The patient cart is placed on the lateral side of the patient (opposite to the main lesion). The operating table should be positioned slightly oblique with respect to the direction of the robotic column to allow direct alignment between the axis of the robotic camera arm and the surgical approach route (from axilla to anterior neck, usually the direction of retractor blade insertion).

Four robotic arms are used for the operation. Three arms are inserted through the axillary incision: The 30-degree dual channel endoscope is placed on the central camera arm through a 12-mm trocar; the Harmonic curved shears is are placed on the right arm of the scope through a 5-mm trocar, and the 5-mm Maryland dissector (Intuitive Inc.) is placed on the left side arm of the scope. The ProGrasp forceps (Intuitive Inc.) is placed on the fourth arm and inserted through the 8-mm anterior chest trocar. To prevent collisions between the robotic arms, the introduction angle is important. In particular, the camera arm should be placed in the center of the

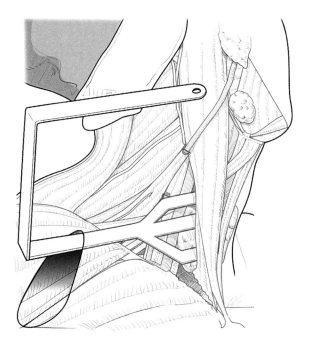

FIGURE 5.3

Insertion of the external retractor. Initial position of retractor for thyroidectomy and neck dissection of levels III, IV, VB.

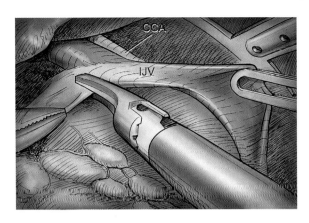

FIGURE 5.4 Level III/IV dissection. The IJV is drawn medially using the ProGrasp forceps, soft tissues and LNs are pulled in a lateral direction by Maryland dissector and detached from the anterior surface of the IJV to the posterior aspect of IJV until the common carotid artery and vagus nerve are identified. CCA, common carotid artery; IJV, internal jugular vein.

axillary skin incision. The camera is inserted in the upward direction (the external third joint should be placed in the lowest part [floor] of the incision entrance, and the camera tip should be directed upward). The Harmonic curved shear and 5-mm Maryland dissector arms should be inserted through in the opposite manner (in the downward direction). Finally the external three joints of the robotic arms should form an inverted triangle.

Robotic Total Thyroidectomy with Central Compartment Neck Dissection

Robotic total thyroidectomy with central compartment node dissection has been well described in the previous chapter, and thus, no detailed description of the procedure is provided here. The procedure is conducted in the same manner as double-incision robotic thyroidectomy.

Robotic MRND

After total thyroidectomy with central compartment neck dissection, lateral neck dissection is started at the level III/IV area around the IJV. The IJV is drawn medially using the ProGrasp forceps, soft tissues and LNs are pulled in the lateral direction using the Maryland dissector and detached from the anterior surface of the IJV to the posterior aspect of IJV until the common carotid artery, and vagus nerve are identified. Smooth, sweeping lateral movements of the Harmonic curved shears can establish a proper plane and delineate vascular structures from specimen tissues (Fig. 5.4). Skeletonization of the IJV progresses superiorly from the level IV to the upper level III area. During this procedure, the superior belly of the omohyoid muscle is cut at the level of the thyroid cartilage. Packets of LNs are then drawn superiorly using the ProGrasp forceps, and LNs are meticulously detached from the junction of the IJV and subclavian vein. Careful dissection is performed to avoid injury to the thoracic duct. Difficulty may be experienced reaching the straight Harmonic curved shears to the deepest point of level IV due to obstruction by the clavicle. In these cases, increasing the height of the external third joint of the robotic arm with the Harmonic curved shears and increasing the introduction angle of the shears usually resolves this problem. In general, the transverse cervical artery (a branch of the thyrocervical trunk) courses laterally across the anterior scalene muscle, anterior to the phrenic nerve. Using this anatomic landmark, the phrenic nerve and transverse cervical artery can be preserved without injury or ligation (Fig. 5.5). Further dissection is followed along the subclavian vein in a lateral direction. After clearing level IV area, the inferior belly of omohyoid muscle is cut at the point where it meets trapezius muscle. The distal external jugular vein (which can join the IJV or subclavian vein) is ligated with Hem-o-Lok clips® at the inlet to the subclavian vein. Dissection then proceeds upward along the anterior border of trapezius muscle while preserving the spinal accessory nerve (Fig. 5.6). After finishing levels III, IV, and VB node dissections, redocking is needed to improve the

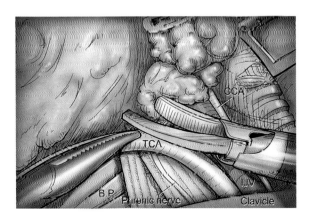

FIGURE 5.5 Level IV, V dissection. Transverse cervical artery (a branch of the thyrocervical trunk) is skeletonized by detaching level IV, V lymph nodes identifying anterior scalene muscle, phrenic nerve, and brachial plexus. CCA, common carotid artery; IJV, internal jugular vein; TCA, transverse cervical artery; BP, brachial plexus.

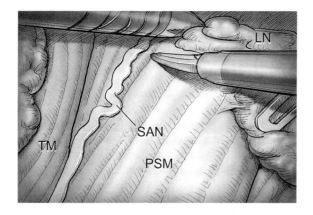

FIGURE 5.6
Level V dissection. After clearing level IV area, the dissection proceeds upward along the anterior border of trapezius muscle while preserving the spinal accessory nerve. PSM, posterior scalene muscle; SAN, spinal accessory nerve; TM, trapezius muscle; LN, lymph nodes.

operation view for the dissection of the level II LN. The external retractor is removed and reinserted through the axillary incision toward the submandibular gland (Fig. 5.7). The second docking procedure is performed in the same manner as the first docking, and thus, the operative table should be repositioned more obliquely with respect to the direction of the robotic column to allow alignment between the axis of the robotic camera arm and the direction of retractor blade insertion. Drawing the specimen tissue inferolaterally, the soft tissues and LNs are detached from the lateral border of the sternohyoid muscle, submandibular gland, anterior surfaces of carotid arteries, and the IJV. Level IIA dissection proceeds to the posterior belly of digastric muscle and the submandibular gland superiorly (Fig. 5.8; Video 5.2). After the specimen has been delivered, a 3-mm closed suction drain is inserted, as described for robotic thyroidectomy above. The wound is closed cosmetically (Fig. 5.9).

POSTOPERATIVE MANAGEMENT

Postoperative pain can be controlled by the usual medication regimen for pain control.

The routine period of drain placement after the operation differs from surgeon to surgeon according to their each one's own experience and preference. However, if the drainage amount is <50 mL/day, the drain can be safely removed without any risk of postoperative seroma.

Discharge and outpatient hospital follow-up plan are based on the surgeon's experience and preference.

COMPLICATIONS

In the head and neck region, neck dissection is one of the most complex and precision-requiring procedures. A long cervical scar and postoperative neck discomfort are inevitable consequences of the procedure. Previously, nobody dared to apply a minimally invasive surgical technique to neck dissection, mainly because of its complexity and the risks of complications. Although, several reports have been issued on endoscopic

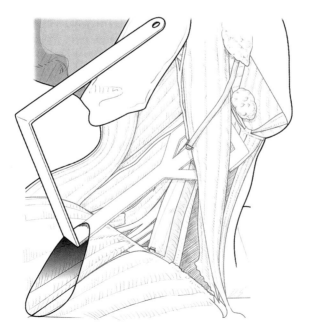

FIGURE 5.7
Repositioned external retractor for level II dissection.

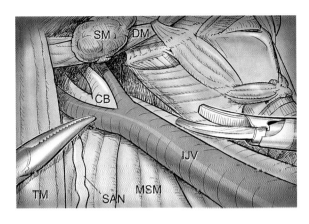

FIGURE 5.8 Level II dissection. The level IIA dissection proceeds to the posterior belly of digastric muscle and the submandibular gland superiorly. SM, submandibular gland; DM, digastric muscle (posterior belly); CB, bifurcation of common carotid artery; IJV, internal jugular vein; MSM, middle scalene muscle; SAN, spinal accessory nerve; TM, trapezius muscle.

approaches to functional neck dissection or MRND, these approaches had many technical and instrumental limitations. However, the technical dexterity of surgical robots has markedly reduced operational difficulties and perioperative morbidities during robotic MRND.

The complications after robotic MRND are similar to those after conventional open or endoscopic MRND (Table 5.1). Hypoparathyroidism (transient/permanent), recurrent (inferior) laryngeal nerve injury, and superior laryngeal nerve injury can occur after central compartment neck dissection, and chyle leakage, nerve injuries (spinal accessory, ramus mandibularis, sympathetic [Horner syndrome], phrenic, brachial plexus), hemorrhage/seroma, and wound infection can occur after lateral neck dissection.

Through the 3D camera in magnified view, critical nerves and thoracic ducts are more vividly identified and preserved during robotic MRND than during open or endoscopic methods. Furthermore, multiarticulated instruments and a stable robotic platform reduce the risks of major vessel or thoracic duct injury.

If the surgeon is experienced with the manipulation of robotic instruments and of the open MRND procedure, robotic MRND has no technique-specific complication.

RESULTS

The dexterities of cutting-edge robotics have markedly advanced endoscopic and minimally invasive surgery. Using this technology, the most exacting procedures in the head and neck area can be managed using an endoscopic approach with excellent cosmesis (Fig. 5.10A and B). Already, satisfactory early surgical outcomes and excellent technical feasibilities have been reported for the management of WDTC with LNM by robotic MRND. Furthermore, robotic MRND using the transaxillary approach can allow complete compartment-oriented LN dissection without injury to any major vessel or nerve and without compromising surgical oncologic principles.

With advances in instrumentation and more experience, robotic MRND is sure to become as accepted alternative means of surgery in low-risk WDTC patients with LNM.

PEARLS

* Prior to starting the robotic procedure for thyroid gland or neck dissection, the surgeon should be experienced at the open procedures of thyroid gland surgery and neck dissection.
* The surgeons should also be educated and trained enough, for example, in an animal or cadaveric laboratory, to manipulate robotic instruments before performing actual operations.

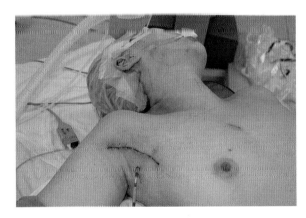

FIGURE 5.9 Axillary wound in the immediate postoperative period. The wound is closed cosmetically through continuous subcuticular suture using absorbable suture material.

TABLE 5.1	**Perioperative Complications Following Robotic MRND for Thyroid Cancer**

Chyle leakage (thoracic duct injury)
Hemorrhage/seroma
Hypoparathyroidism (transient/permanent)
Nerve injuries (during lateral neck dissection)
Recurrent (inferior) laryngeal nerve injury
Spinal accessory, ramus mandibularis, sympathetic (Horner syndrome), phrenic, brachial plexus
Superior laryngeal nerve injury
Wound infection

- One of the most important requirements for successful robotic thyroid surgery or neck dissection is the development of adequate working space.
- During initial experiences in robotic surgery, stepwise extensions of the surgical procedure favor successful surgery.
- Before starting robotic MRND, surgeons should have sufficient experience of robotic thyroidectomy and be familiar with operative anatomies.

PITFALLS

- During robotic procedures using the transaxillary approach, if a patient has an especially prominent clavicle, the Harmonic curved shear (nonarticulated instrument) may not reach the deepest point of the level IV LN area (just beneath the area where the IJV joins the subclavian vein) due to obstruction by the clavicle.
- Patients with a long neck and narrow shoulders are difficult candidates for level IIB area dissection using the robotic procedure due to frequent collisions between robotic instruments. In such cases, the remote centers of each robotic instrument do not have enough working space.
- To resolve the above two problems, a small retroauricular skin incision instead of the second incision in the anterior chest wall could be a suitable alternative for robotic neck dissection of the level IIB and deepest level IV area.

INSTRUMENTS TO HAVE AVAILABLE

- Patient position
  - Arm board
  - Soft pillow
- Development of working space
  - Electrocautery with regular and extended-sized tip
  - Vascular Debakey or Russian forceps (extended length)
  - Army Navy retractor × 2
  - Right-angled retractors × 2
  - Breast-lighted retractor × 2
  - Endoscopic clip appliers
- Maintenance of working space
  - Chung retractor (special set of retractors for MRND, Fig. 5.11A)
  - Table mount and suspension device (BioRobotics Seoul, Korea, or Marina Medical, Sunrise, FL) (Fig. 5.11B)

FIGURE 5.10

A: Postoperative incision scar after robotic MRND (3 weeks after the operation). **B:** The axillary scar is completely hidden in a natural arm position.

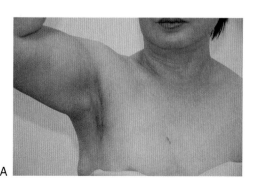
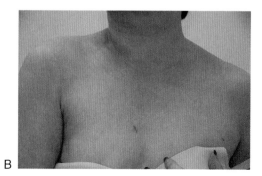

A   B

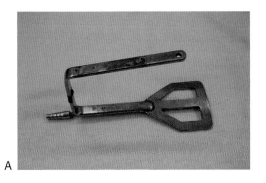

A

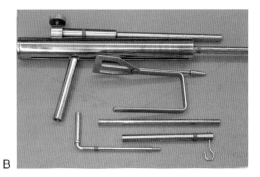

B

FIGURE 5.11
Special set of Chung retractors for MRND; (**A**) wide and long blade of external retractor, (**D**) table mount and suspension devices.

* Robotic procedure
  * 5-mm Maryland dissector
  * 8-mm ProGrasp forceps
  * 5-mm Harmonic curved shears
  * Dual channel 30-degree endoscope (used in the rotated down position)
  * Endoscopic graspers and forceps
  * Endoscopic suction irrigator

Disclaimer

The authors declare that they have no proprietary, commercial, or financial interests that could be construed to have inappropriately influenced this study.

SUGGESTED READING

Kang SW, Jeong JJ, Nam KH, et al. Robot-assisted endoscopic thyroidectomy for thyroid malignancies using a gasless transaxillary approach. *J Am Coll Surg* 2009;209(2):e1–e7.
Holsinger FC, Sweeney AD, Jantharapattana K, et al. The emergence of endoscopic head and neck surgery. *Curr Oncol Rep* 2010;12(3);216–222.
Kang SW, Lee SH, Ryu HR, et al. Initial experience with robot-assisted modified radical neck dissection for the management of thyroid carcinoma with lateral neck node metastasis. *Surgery* 2010;148(6):1214–1221.
Ryu HR, Kang SW, Lee SH, et al. Feasibility and safety of a new robotic thyroidectomy through a gasless, transaxillary single-incision approach. *J Am Coll Surg* 2010;211(3);e13–e19.
Lee S, Ryu HR, Park JH, et al. Excellence in robotic thyroid surgery: a comparative study of robot-assisted versus conventional endoscopic thyroidectomy in papillary thyroid microcarcinoma patients. *Ann Surg* 2011:253(6);60–66.

6 RADICAL NECK DISSECTION

Jesus Medina

INTRODUCTION

The radical neck dissection is a comprehensive cancer operation that removes the lymph node–bearing tissues of one side of the neck, from the inferior border of the mandible to the clavicle and from the midline to the anterior border of the trapezius muscle. Included in the resected specimen are lymph node groups I through V, the spinal accessory nerve, the internal jugular vein, and the sternocleidomastoid muscle (Fig. 6.1).

The first description of this operation was published by Crile in 1906. It was Martin et al. in the 1950s who championed the concept that a cervical lymphadenectomy for cancer was inadequate unless all the lymph node–bearing tissues of one side of the neck were removed and that this was not possible without resecting the sternocleidomastoid muscle, internal jugular vein, and spinal accessory nerve because of the close association of the lymphatics with these structures.

As a result of Martin's influence, the radical neck dissection was for many years the only dissection of the lymph nodes performed in patients with cancer of the head and neck.

HISTORY

The clinician should record:

- The frequency and duration of symptoms related to the primary tumor, such as pain, otalgia, odynophagia, hoarseness, dysphagia, cough, and hemoptysis
- The occurrence and extent of weight loss and all other comorbidities
- History of risk factors such as the quantity of tobacco and alcohol consumed each day
- History of previous treatment to the head and neck with radiation (total dose and portals) or surgery

PHYSICAL EXAMINATION

Physical examination should include:

- Examination of all the areas of the oral cavity, pharynx, indirect laryngoscopy, or fiberoptic examination of the larynx if necessary
- Palpation of the neck bilaterally, recording the location (levels I-VI), size, mobility, and relationship of the node(s) to adjacent structures. This should include bimanual palpation of the submandibular area.
- Documentation of the presence or absence of trismus and of actual or potential airway compromise, which may have bearing on the management of the airway during induction of anesthesia

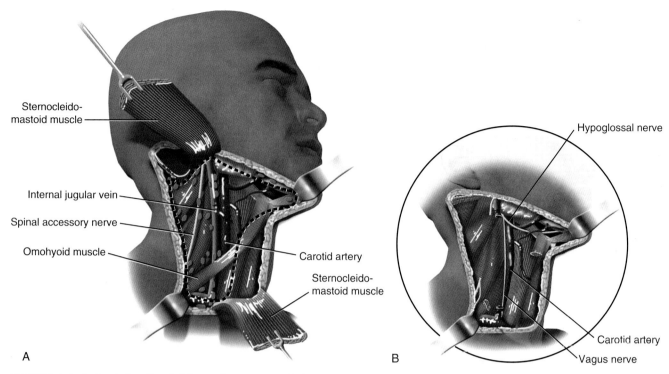

Sternocleido-
mastoid muscle

Internal jugular vein

Spinal accessory nerve

Omohyoid muscle

Carotid artery

Sternocleido-
mastoid muscle

Hypoglossal nerve

Carotid artery

Vagus nerve

A

B

FIGURE 6.1 Radical neck dissection. **A:** Intraoperative appearance. **B:** Postoperative appearance.

INDICATIONS

The radical neck dissection is indicated in the following situations:

- Patients with multiple clinically obvious cervical lymph node metastases, particularly when they involve the lymph nodes of the posterior triangle of the neck and are found to involve or to be closely related to the spinal accessory nerve
- Patients with a bulky metastatic tumor mass or with multiple matted nodes in the superior aspect of the neck
- When a neck dissection is performed to remove residual disease in the neck following an ill-advised incisional biopsy of a cervical lymph node containing metastatic cancer. In such cases, extensive undermining during the biopsy procedure, postoperative inflammation, and ecchymosis often obscure the relationship of the tumor to the sternocleidomastoid muscle, spinal accessory nerve, or internal jugular vein, making their preservation problematic.

CONTRAINDICATIONS

A radical neck dissection is not indicated in the following circumstances:

- In the absence of palpable cervical lymph node metastases (i.e., in the elective surgical treatment of the N0 neck)
- When the diagnostic evaluation of the patient reveals (a) frank involvement of the wall of the carotid artery in patients whose preoperative evaluation indicates intolerance to carotid ligation and the location and extent of the cancer in the neck, that is, near the skull base, precludes reconstruction of the carotid and (b) involvement of the base of the skull, paraspinal muscles, transverse processes of the cervical vertebrae, and the brachial plexus

PREOPERATIVE PLANNING

In patients with advanced metastases to the neck requiring a radical neck dissection, the preoperative evaluation must include comprehensive imaging studies that address:

- Resectability. In this regard, CT and MRI imaging are used to define the relationship of the metastatic cancer to critical structures such as the common and the internal carotid artery, the cervical spine, the vertebral artery, and the brachial plexus. If the common or the internal carotid artery is suspected of involvement by cancer, a systematic preoperative evaluation should include four-vessel cerebral angiography to determine the status of the contralateral carotid artery and to assess intracerebral collateral circulation. In addition, an attempt should be made during the angiography to measure carotid back pressure and to assess dynamically the collateral circulation by using balloon occlusion techniques while monitoring the patient for evidence of neurologic deficits under normotensive and hypotensive conditions.

● The presence of metastases in lymph nodes that are not routinely removed with a radical neck dissection such as the retropharyngeal, paratracheal, and upper mediastinal nodes

● The possibility of distant metastases. A positron emission tomography–computed tomography (PET-CT) scan is a useful study in this regard and in staging the disease.

SURGICAL TECHNIQUE

The patient is positioned on the operating table with the neck extended, if necessary, with a rolled up towel or blanket under the shoulders and the head turned toward the opposite side and stabilized with a foam doughnut.

The incisions most commonly used to perform a radical neck dissection are outlined in Figure 6.2. Skin flaps are elevated in a subplatysmal plane. However, depending upon the size and extent of the tumor in the neck, the platysma may be left over the area involved by tumor as the skin flaps are elevated in a supraplatysmal plane. Skin that is infiltrated with cancer or the scar of a previous open biopsy should be left on the specimen.

Dissection of the Submandibular Triangle

● As the superior cervical flap is elevated, it is important to keep the plane of dissection superficial to the fascia that covers the submandibular gland; this facilitates identification of the ramus mandibularis of the facial nerve. This nerve lies deep to the fascia but superficial to the facial vessels, which are exposed and divided. The submandibular prevascular and retrovascular lymph nodes, which are usually immediately below or medial to the nerve, are likewise exposed (Fig. 6.3). When these nodes are involved by tumor, it is preferable to leave the platysma attached to them. In such cases, it may not possible, nor desirable, to expose and preserve the ramus mandibularis.

● The next step is to incise the fascia and adipose tissue along and medial to the inferior border of the mandible. As this is done, it is usually necessary to divide the submental artery at the angle between the anterior belly of the digastric and the inferior border of the mandible and the nerve to the mylohyoid.

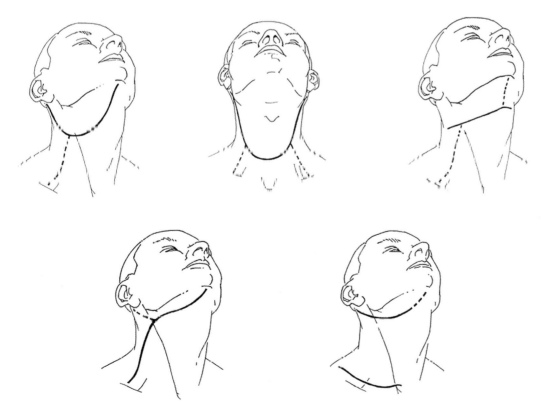

FIGURE 6.2
Various incisions to perform radical neck dissection.

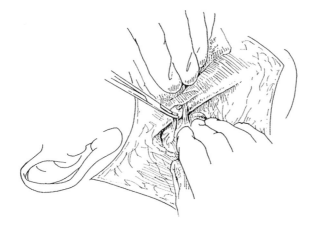

FIGURE 6.3
Facial vessels being divided below marginal branch of VII nerve.

- The fascia of the anterior belly of the digastric muscle is incised and the fibroadipose tissue lateral to the mylohyoid muscle is dissected. A "clean" dissection of this area is important because it contains the preglandular lymph node(s), which can be the first echelon of lymphatic drainage for cancer of the floor of the mouth and oral tongue. When the dissection reaches the posterior border of the mylohyoid, this muscle is retracted forward with a Richardson retractor. This exposes three structures that are somewhat parallel but in different planes; from lateral to medial and from superior to inferior, they are the lingual nerve, Whartons duct, and the hypoglossal nerve. The submandibular ganglion located inferior to the lingual nerve and Whartons duct is divided.
- With the submandibular gland mobilized, the contents of the submandibular triangle are dissected in a posterior direction. The facial artery is exposed as it crosses anteriorly, under the posterior belly of the digastric (Fig. 6.4). The artery is divided and ligated completing the dissection of the submandibular triangle.

Superior Lateral Dissection

- The tail of the parotid gland may be dissected and retracted superiorly or transected if necessary to provide an adequate tissue margin above a large or a high level II lymph node (jugulodigastric) involved with tumor; the posterior facial vein and the greater auricular nerve are divided. The sternocleidomastoid muscle is incised close to its insertion on the mastoid process. Incising the fibroadipose tissue medial to the muscle exposes the splenius capitis muscle posteriorly and the levator scapulae muscle anteriorly.
- Depending upon the location and the extent of the cancer in the neck, it may be necessary to include the posterior belly of the digastric muscle in the dissected specimen. If the digastric muscle is not removed, it is retracted superiorly with an Army Navy or a similar retractor. Blunt and sharp dissection immediately deep to it exposes the superior most portion of the internal jugular vein, the spinal accessory nerve, and the hypoglossal nerve. At this point in the dissection, if the location and extent of the tumor permit it, the internal jugular vein and the spinal accessory nerve are divided (Fig. 6.5).

Posterior Dissection

- The dissection continues posteriorly and inferiorly along the anterior border of the trapezius muscle. The fibroadipose tissue of the posterior triangle of the neck is then dissected anteriorly and inferiorly in a plane immediately lateral to the fascia of the splenius capitis and the levator scapulae muscles (Fig. 6.6).

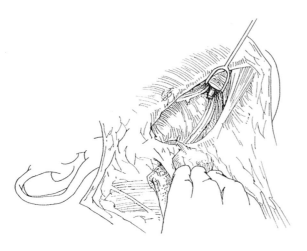

FIGURE 6.4
Submandibular triangle with facial artery across posterior belly of the digastric muscle.

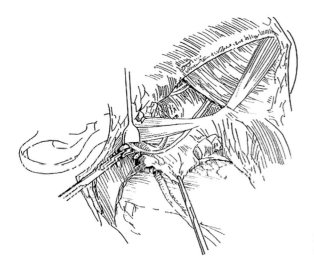

FIGURE 6.5 Superior dissection. Internal jugular vein is divided and ligated.

- The spinal accessory nerve and the transverse cervical vessels are divided as they cross the anterior border of the trapezius muscle. During this portion of the operation, it is important to preserve the branches of the cervical plexus that innervate the levator scapulae muscle, unless the extent of the disease in the neck precludes it.

Inferior Dissection

- The sternocleidomastoid muscle and the superficial layer of the deep cervical fascia are incised just superior to the superior border of the clavicle, in a layer-by-layer fashion. The external jugular vein and the omohyoid muscle are divided (Fig. 6.7).
- After several "fascial" layers are incised, the fibroadipose tissue in this region can be gently pushed superiorly exposing and preserving the brachial plexus, the scalenus anticus muscle, and the phrenic nerve.

Medial Dissection

- The dissection continues anteriorly as the specimen is dissected off of the scalenus medius muscle, the brachial plexus, and the scalenus anticus muscle. Care must be taken not to injure the phrenic nerve. In this area of the neck, the thoracic duct on the left side or an accessory duct on the right often needs to be divided and ligated. The duct is anterior or superficial to the anterior scalene muscle and the phrenic nerve and posterior to the carotid artery and the vagus nerve. To avoid a chyle leak through contributing lymphatic channels, the adipose tissue in this region is clipped using Ligaclips and then transected.
- As the dissection continues in a cephalad direction, the cutaneous branches of the cervical plexus are divided. After this is done, only a relatively thin layer of tissue remains to be incised before the vagus nerve, the common carotid artery, and the internal jugular vein are exposed (Fig. 6.8).
- Depending upon the location of the cancer in the neck, the internal jugular vein can be divided first near its superior or its inferior end. If the tumor mass is located in level II or level III, the vein is divided first superiorly, immediately below to the posterior belly of the digastric muscle. The specimen is then dissected in an inferior direction, separating it from the vagus nerve, the carotid artery, and the superior thyroid vessels

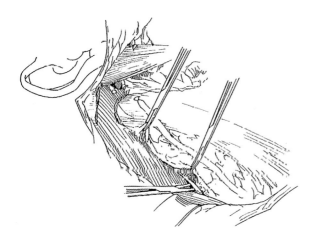

FIGURE 6.6 Posterior dissection.

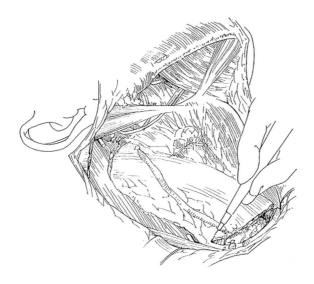

FIGURE 6.7
Inferior dissection.

The medial limit of the dissection is marked by the strap muscles. The final step of the dissection is the ligation and division of the inferior end of the internal jugular vein. However, if the metastatic lymph nodes are located high in the jugulodigastric region, especially if the cancer is extensive and may require removal of the external carotid artery or the hypoglossal nerve, the internal jugular vein is first divided inferiorly, and the dissection is carried in a superior direction along the common carotid artery. "Freeing up" the surgical specimen from the inferior aspect of the neck allows easier and safer dissection of the tumor in the superior lateral portion of the neck off of the internal and external carotid artery and the hypoglossal nerve.

Closure of the Wound

- After copious irrigation and meticulous hemostasis, the wound is usually closed in two layers; the first one approximates the platysma anteriorly and the subcutaneous tissue laterally, and the second one approximates the skin. In general, it is best to avoid continuous suturing in the wound closure, since a seroma, a chyle collection, an abscess, or a pharyngocutaneous fistula may require the wound to be partially opened, for drainage.
- One or two suction drains are left in place; they should not rest immediately on the carotid artery or in the area of the thoracic duct. Bulky pressure dressings are not necessary.

POSTOPERATIVE MANAGEMENT

- Drains are maintained on low suction and are usually kept in place for 7 to 10 days to prevent seromas, particularly in the area of the posterior triangle of the neck.
- Patients undergoing bilateral radical neck dissection can develop inappropriate secretion of antidiuretic hormone (ADH). Monitoring urine and serum osmolarity will help to guide postoperative fluid replacement.
- A common sequela of the radical neck dissection is related to the removal of the spinal accessory nerve. The resulting denervation of the trapezius muscle, one of the most important shoulder abductors, causes

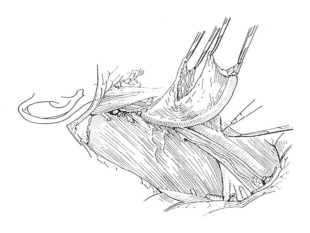

FIGURE 6.8
Medial dissection.

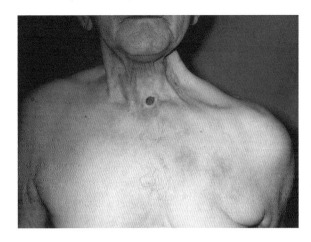

FIGURE 6.9 Shoulder drooping following radical neck dissection.

destabilization of the scapula with progressive flaring of it at the vertebral border, as well as drooping, and lateral and anterior rotation of the shoulder. The loss of the trapezius function decreases the patient's ability to abduct the shoulder above 90 degrees at the shoulder. Paralysis of the trapezius muscle causes a clinical syndrome characterized by weakness and deformity of the shoulder girdle, usually accompanied by pain (Fig. 6.9). Consequently, patients who have undergone a radical neck dissection must be evaluated by a physical therapist early in the postoperative period. Aggressive and prompt physical and occupational therapy are recommended since they are useful to improve range of motion and to strengthen alternative muscles to compensate for the loss function of the trapezius muscle.

COMPLICATIONS

- *Hematoma.* It usually occurs immediately after surgery. If detected early, milking the drains may result in evacuation of the accumulated blood and resolve the problem. If this is not accomplished immediately or if blood reaccumulates quickly, the patient should be returned to the operating room and the wound explored under sterile conditions, the hematoma evacuated, hemostasis obtained, and the drains replace.
- *Chyle Leak.* Management depends on the time of onset of the leak, the amount of chyle drainage in a 24-hour period, and on the presence or absence of accumulation of chyle under the skin flaps. When the daily output of chyle is high (400 to 600 mL. in a day or 200 to 300 mL/day for 3 days), especially when the chyle fistula becomes apparent immediately after surgery, it is preferable to explore the wound early. Surgical exploration is also warranted when chyle accumulates under the skin flaps either because of inadequate drain size or because of the volume or consistency of the chyle causes partial or complete obstruction of the drains. On the other hand, chylous fistulae that become apparent later in the postoperative period, after enteral feedings are resumed, or those that drain <400 mL of chyle per day, are initially managed conservatively with closed wound drainage and diet modifications aimed at decreasing chyle drainage while maintaining nutritional support.

In cases where surgery fails to stop a chyle leak, administration of octreotide (100 µg given subcutaneously three times a day) and percutaneous lymphangiography–guided cannulation and embolization of the thoracic duct may be effective.

- *Facial and Cerebral Edema After Bilateral Radical Neck Dissection.* Synchronous bilateral radical neck dissections, in which both internal jugular veins are ligated, can result in the development of facial edema, cerebral edema, or both. The facial edema can be dramatically severe (Fig. 6.10). These problems result from the combination of a mechanical factor of venous drainage as well as inappropriate secretion of ADH. These complications can be prevented by preserving at least one external jugular vein and by curtailing the volume of fluids administered intraoperatively.
- *Carotid Artery Rupture.* The most feared and most commonly lethal complication after neck dissection is exposure and rupture of the carotid artery. Therefore, every effort must be made to prevent it. If the skin incisions have been designed properly, the carotid seldom becomes exposed in the absence of a salivary fistula. Fistula formation and flap breakdown are more likely to occur in the presence of malnutrition, diabetes, and prior radiation therapy, which impair healing capacity and compromise vascular supply. Faced with any of these risk factors, the surgeon must use flawless surgical technique in closing oral and pharyngeal defects. In addition, perioperative antibiotics and, more importantly, use of free or pedicled vascularized flaps that provide skin for closure of mucosal defects and variably bulky muscle are important in preventing this complication.

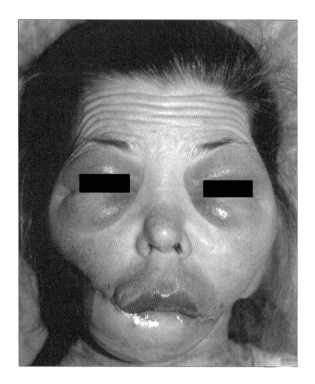

FIGURE 6.10
Severe facial and palpebral edema following bilateral radical neck dissections.

RESULTS

The rate of recurrence in the ipsilateral side of the neck after therapeutic radical neck dissection is often related to control of the primary cancer. The number of lymph nodes involved by cancer has been found to correlate with the incidence of cancer recurrence in the neck and survival. Patients with four or more involved nodes had significantly worse prognosis than patients with only one node involved. The location and number of lymph node levels involved is also a factor involved in recurrence after radical neck dissection. Strong, in a landmark paper from Memorial Sloan-Kettering, reported a series of 204 patients treated by radical neck dissection alone. The recurrence rate in the neck was 36.5% in patients with histologically positive nodes at one level of the neck and 71% in patients with positive nodes at multiple levels. The presence of tumor spread beyond the capsule of a lymph node is a major determinant for prognosis and need for postoperative chemoradiation. Several investigators have shown that the recurrence rate in the neck after radical neck dissection is significantly higher when extracapsular spread of tumor is demonstrated. The efficacy of a therapeutic radical neck dissection must be considered in relationship with the adjuvant use of radiation therapy. Studies from various institutions have shown that the combined use of radical neck dissection and postoperative radiation therapy can decrease recurrence in the ipsilateral neck and prevent recurrence in the contralateral side in patients with cervical lymph node metastases who have one or more of the factors associated with increased risk of recurrence (i.e., multiple histologically positive nodes and extracapsular spread of tumor).

PEARLS

- Identification of the marginal mandibular nerve decreases the potential for damaging this structure.
- Preserve the nerves to the levator scapula whenever feasible.
- Always orient the surgical specimen for the pathologist.

PITFALLS

- Avoid trifurcate incisions.
- Chyle leak may ensue, particularly on the left side in level IV while dissecting the fibroadipose tissue adjacent to the inferior end of the internal jugular vein. To avoid this, use clips liberally before dividing the fibroadipose tissue that may contain lymphatics.
- Avoid continuous suturing in the wound closure, since a portion of the wound may need to be opened to drain blood or chyle.

INSTRUMENTS TO HAVE AVAILABLE

- Scalpel
- Mosquito clamps
- Hemostats
- Skin hooks
- Richardson retractors
- Army Navy retractors
- Monopolar and bipolar cautery
- Vascular clamps and clips

SUGGESTED READING

Crile G. Excision of cancer of the head and neck. *JAMA* 1906;47:1780–1786.

Martin H, DelValle B, Erhlich H, et al. Neck dissection. *Cancer* 1951;4:441–449.

O'Brien CJ, Smith JW, Soong SJ, et al. Neck dissection with and without radiotherapy—prognostic factors, patterns of recurrence and survival. *Am J Surg* 1986;152:456–463.

Snow GB, Balm AJM, Arendse JW. Prognostic factors in neck node metastasis. In: Larsen D, Ballantyne AJ, Guillamondegui OM, eds. *Cancer in the Neck: Evaluation and Treatment*. New York, NY: Macmillan Publishing Company, 1986:53–63.

Strong EW. Preoperative radiation and radical neck dissection. *Surg Clin North Am* 1986;49(2):271–276.

7 ROBOT-ASSISTED NECK DISSECTION VIA MODIFIED FACE-LIFT OR RETROAURICULAR APPROACH

Yoon Woo Koh

INTRODUCTION

Cervical lymph node metastasis is frequently encountered in the management of cancer of the head and neck, and its inappropriate treatment is often associated with treatment failure. Since the establishment of the basis for radical neck dissection by George Washington Crile in the early 20th century, the cultivation of neck dissection techniques has been directed toward the preservation of vital structures and the minimization of neck levels covered by neck dissection (e.g., modified radical neck dissection, functional neck dissection, selective neck dissection, superselective neck dissection, and sentinel lymph node biopsy). Elective neck dissection in the clinically N0 neck is performed not only to remove occult metastatic deposits in the regional lymph nodes at the time of initial treatment but also to provide pathologically proven nodal stage, which helps in determining whether adjuvant therapy is required. With all the efforts to optimize the surgical extent based on the distribution of lymph node metastasis and thereby reduce the surgical morbidity, the scar on the neck after neck dissection has been accepted as unavoidable. However, since disfiguring scars may be a great burden for both surgeons and patients, I sought to develop a surgical technique to hide the scar of neck dissection and recently reported our technique of robot-assisted neck dissection carried out through a modified face-lift or retroauricular approach.

HISTORY

In a situation of a known primary cancer, history taking for identifying nodal metastasis may not be of great importance because imaging studies (e.g., ultrasonography, CT, or MRI) can detect the nodal metastasis more precisely. However, the presence of pain/tenderness and the growth rate of a mass in the neck should be asked to add useful information for determining the necessity of fine needle aspiration biopsy (FNAB), which can confirm the preoperative diagnosis of cancer in the lymph node. History of previous neck surgery or parotid surgery should be sought.

PHYSICAL EXAMINATION

After the evaluation of the primary cancer, palpation of the neck is mandatory especially in the area of primary lymphatic drainage. The location of the mass and its size, fixation to the surrounding structures, consistency, and pulsation should be described. Function of the facial, lingual, vagus, spinal accessory, hypoglossal, and phrenic nerves should be evaluated preoperatively. Any findings indicative of previous neck or parotid surgery should be assessed. The length and circumference of the neck are major determinants of good exposure. Though the patient who has a long slim neck provides the best exposure, I have accomplished the robot-assisted neck dissection successfully in less favorable situations. Therefore, the somatometry does not provide the absolute contraindication.

Somatometry means: classification of persons according to body form and relation of types to physiological and psychological characteristics.

INDICATIONS

Indications for robot-assisted neck dissection are: (1) patients who have biopsy-proven cancer of the head and neck, for example, early cancer of the oral cavity that requires an elective neck dissection including levels I, II, and III or early cancers of the oropharynx or hypopharynx that need elective selective neck dissection including levels II and III; (2) patients who have not previously been treated for cancer of the head and neck; (3) patients who have a resectable primary cancer (T1 or T2); and (4) patients who lacked clinically suspicious metastatic neck nodes (cN0). Recently, I extended the indication up to cN1 without suspected extracapsular spread in accordance with the accumulation of experience.

CONTRAINDICATIONS

Contraindications for robot-assisted neck dissection are as follows: (1) patients expressing refusal after the explanation for the advantages and disadvantages of the procedure, (2) patients undergoing chemoradiation for primary treatment due to refusal of surgery, (3) patients in whom the primary cancer had recurred, (4) patients with distant metastasis at the time of initial presentation, (5) patients who were suspected of having extracapsular spread in the cervical lymph nodes, (6) patients who have advanced nodal stage more than N2, (7) patients who have had a cervical skin incision for the removal of primary cancers, or (8) patients who needed free flap reconstruction for a primary surgical defect. Recently, I have begun to gather data in patients in whom robot-assisted neck dissection and free flap reconstruction via modified face-lift or retroauricular approach were performed simultaneously. Therefore, the necessity for free flap reconstruction is a relative contraindication.

PREOPERATIVE PLANNING

Imaging Studies

CT and MRI are the most useful imaging studies and can reveal the size, number, location, and extent of cervical lymph node metastasis. It is especially important to define the extracapsular spread of cervical lymph node metastasis because the oncologic safety of the procedure can be violated due to the spillage of malignant cells during the manipulation of lymphoadipose tissues in robot-assisted neck dissection. PET–CT can also be useful for detecting occult metastasis in cN0 neck and for demonstrating distant metastasis.

Fine-Needle Aspiration Biopsy

To confirm the cervical lymph node metastasis, FNAB should be performed; the sensitivity and specificity of which are over 92% and 94%, respectively, according to the study of Frable. A successful FNAB is dependent on the skills of the radiologist and pathologist. The result of FNAB is one of the prime determinants in selecting the option for treatment of cervical lymph node metastasis.

SURGICAL TECHNIQUE

This technique is indicated for dissection of levels I, II, and III (supraomohyoid neck dissection), which is frequently performed as part of the treatment for cN0 cancer of the oral cavity. It could also be applied to levels II and III dissection for cN0 squamous cell carcinoma of the oropharynx and hypopharynx in the context of superselective neck dissection. The concept of this approach was originally presented by Terris et al. as a modified face-lift incision for parotidectomy in 1989, and the early cases were performed through the same incision. However, I found out that a retroauricular incision without preauricular extension provided enough space for the surgical exposure of levels I, II, and III and now the procedure is conducted entirely through a retroauricular approach. Recently I have accumulated experience with this approach for the endoscopic removal of benign masses in the upper neck including the submandibular gland. However, according to our experience, straight and rigid endoscopic instruments may have limitations in approaching the site of dissection in narrow and angled working space, and the endoscopic view may be hindered by the surrounding tissues or the instruments. In order to obtain sufficient surgical exposure and instrumentation to secure oncologic safety and prevent injury of vital neurovascular structures, I used the robotic surgical system for dissection in combination with conventional technique under direct vision.

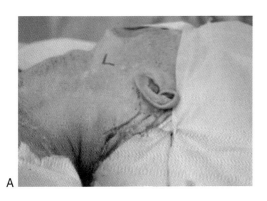
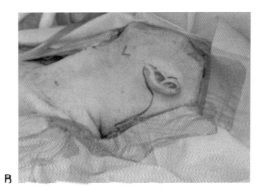

FIGURE 7.1
Skin incision. **A:** Retroauricular approach. **B:** Modified face-lift approach

Description of Technique

Skin Incision and Flap Elevation

The patient is placed in the supine position under general anesthesia with the neck slightly extended by inserting a soft pillow under the shoulder. The patient's head is turned to the opposite direction of the primary lesion. The retroauricular incision is made starting from the inferior aspect of the retroauricular sulcus, moved superiorly to the midpoint of the sulcus, and then smoothly angulated downward 0.5 cm inside the hairline (Fig. 7.1A). The modified face-lift incision is extended from the retroauricular incision to the natural preauricular fold and continued behind the tragus (Fig. 7.1B). There have been reports of using a linear hairline incision for retroauricular approach to perform endoscope-assisted submandibular gland resection. However, an incision prolonged to the retroauricular sulcus may relieve the tension of the skin flap compared to that of a linear incision along the hairline only. The skin of the retroauricular sulcus shows more elasticity compared to that of the scalp at the hairline, and extension of incision to this area provides sufficient height (>4 cm) for the entrance to the surgical field. Moreover, instrumentation may be conducted in closer proximity than a linear hairline incision.

The skin flap is elevated along the subplatysmal plane (Fig. 7.2) just above the sternocleidomastoid (SCM) muscle using a monopolar cautery under direct vision and is continued to the midline of the anterior neck and superiorly to the inferior margin of the mandible and inferiorly to the level of the omohyoid muscle. Two assistants put traction on the skin flap using the Army-Navy or right-angle retractors.

Neck Dissection Under Direct Vision via a Modified Face-Lift or Retroauricular Approach

Before docking the robotic arms, dissection of fibroadipose tissues accessible under direct vision is performed by the conventional technique. The marginal branch of the facial nerve is first identified using the distal facial artery and vein as landmarks and is preserved by carefully dissecting it from the surrounding fibroadipose tissues and thereby thoroughly dissecting the perifacial lymph nodes (Fig. 7.3A). Distal facial artery (Fig. 7.3B) and vein are identified along the inferior border of mandible and ligated using the Harmonic curved shears (Harmonic Ace 23E; Johnson & Johnson Medical, Cincinnati, OH). Fibroadipose tissues of level II and upper III lateral to the carotid sheath can be identified through direct vision and dissected with monopolar cautery and Harmonic curved shears for vascular ligation. After identifying the spinal accessory nerve (SAN) by using the transverse process of the atlas as a landmark, skeletonization of the SAN is performed (Fig. 7.3C). After dissection of level IIb (Fig. 7.3D) and part of levels IIa and III from the SCM muscle lateral to the carotid sheath, a self-retaining retractor (Chung retractor, originally made for transaxillary robotic thyroidectomy) is introduced, and the skin flap is elevated (Fig. 7.4A). Recently I developed a retractor modified from the Chung retractor by decreasing the length of axis and removing the projecting suction hole (Fig. 7.4B and C).

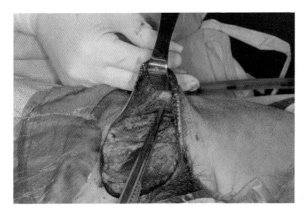

FIGURE 7.2 Subplatysmal elevation of the skin flap.

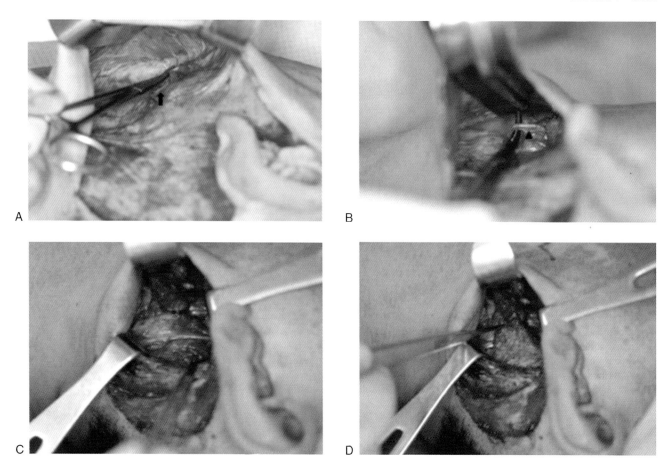

FIGURE 7.3 Intraoperative view under direct vision. **A:** Marginal branch of the facial nerve (*arrow*). **B:** Distal facial artery (*arrowhead*). **C:** Skeletonization of the SAN. **D:** Dissection of level IIb.

Instrumentation gets more convenient without unnecessary collisions, and the smoke during dissection may be cleared by the patient-side assistant.

 Robot-Assisted Neck Dissection Technique (Video 7.1)

Three robotic arms are inserted via the retroauricular approach: a 30-degree dual channel endoscope (Intuitive, Inc., Sunnyvale, CA) is placed on the central camera arm, a 5-mm spatula monopolar coagulator or a Harmonic

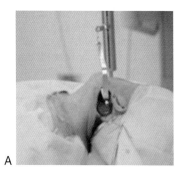
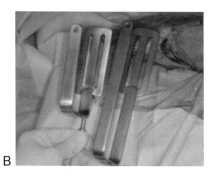

FIGURE 7.4

Self-retaining retractors. **A:** Chung retractor. **B:** Modified retractor with shorter length. **C:** Modified retractors with shorter length or no suction hole. The four on the left are for neck dissection or submandibular gland resection, and the two on the right are for thyroidectomy.

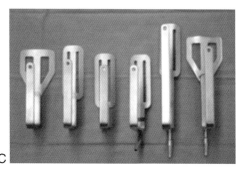

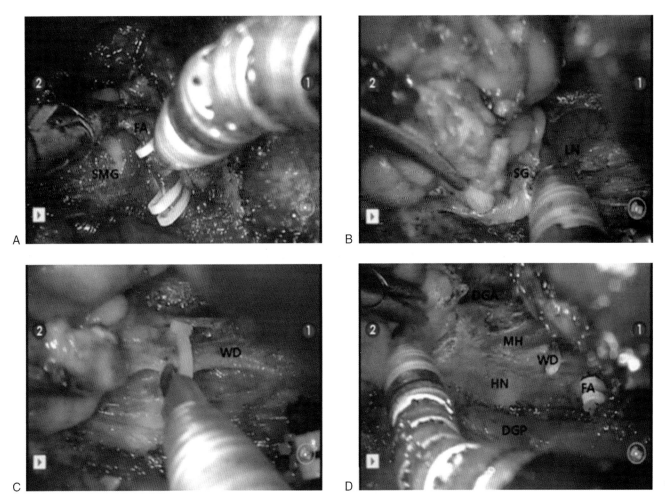

FIGURE 7.5 Level I. **A:** Ligation of proximal facial artery. **B:** Separation of the submandibular ganglion from the lingual nerve. **C:** Sealing of Wharton duct. **D:** Completion of level I dissection. SMG, submandibular gland; FA, facial artery; SG, submandibular ganglion; LN, lingual nerve; WD, Wharton duct; DGA, anterior belly of digastric muscle; MH, mylohyoid muscle; HN, hypoglossal nerve; DGP, posterior belly of digastric muscle.

curved shears (Intuitive, Inc.) is placed on the right arm, and a 5-mm Maryland dissector (Intuitive, Inc.) on the left arm of the scope. In some cases, an endoscopic alligator forceps may be manipulated by a patient-side assistant to expose the surgical view.

Recently, I have used mainly the monopolar coagulator for dissection. Dissection of level I is conducted in a lateral to medial fashion. The posterior belly of the digastric muscle is first identified, and then the proximal facial artery is sealed with a Harmonic curved shears or doubly ligated using a vascular clip performed by the assistant (Fig. 7.5A). The submandibular gland is dissected along the inferior border of the mandible taking great care to avoid thermal injury to the marginal mandibular branch of the facial nerve. After identification of the mylohyoid muscle, the submandibular ganglion (Fig. 7.5B) and Whartons duct (Fig 7.5C) are sealed with preservation of the hypoglossal and lingual nerve. The remaining lymphoadipose tissues attached to the mylohyoid muscle are dissected followed by dissection of level Ia. After the completion of level I dissection (Fig. 7.5D), posterior belly of the digastric muscle is pulled superiorly using the Army Navy retractor so that the superior portion of level IIa may be exposed. Fibroadipose tissues of levels IIa and III are drawn up with the Maryland forceps, and the monopolar cautery or the Harmonic curved shears dissect them from the fascial carpet and carotid sheath preserving the cervical plexus and phrenic nerve (Fig. 7.6A). During the level IIa dissection, the hypoglossal nerve is easily identified and preserved (Fig. 7.6B). The superior thyroid and lingual artery anterior to the carotid sheath are identified and preserved (Fig. 7.6C). The SCM muscle is retracted posteriorly by the assistant using an Army Navy retractor to expose the surgical field, and the specimen is pulled medially by a Yankauer suction or an endoscopic alligator forceps. After removing the fibroadipose tissue from level I to III (Figs 7.6D and 7.7A), the surgical field is irrigated, and close inspection under the endoscopic view for any site of hemorrhage should be done. Tiny bleeding points on the skin flap should not be neglected. A closed suction drain is inserted posterior to the hairline, and the skin is closed with simple interrupted suture technique. The levels of neck dissection may be extended to levels IV and V in selected cases of cN1 by adding a transaxillary incision and performing a two-channel approach. This technique called the "transaxillary and retroauricular approach" has been recently reported.

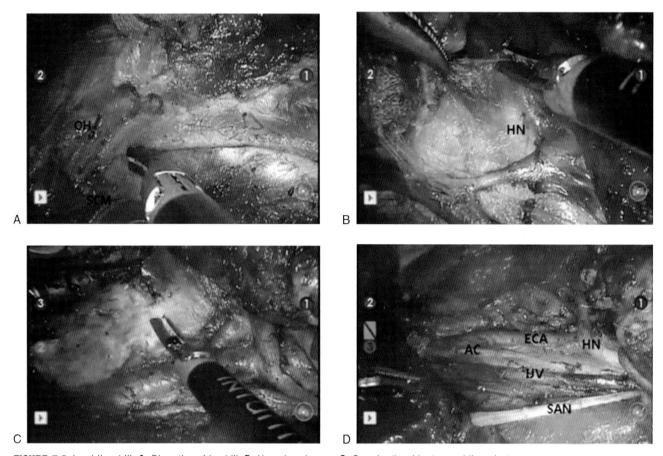

FIGURE 7.6 Level II and III. **A:** Dissection of level III. **B:** Hypoglossal nerve. **C:** Superior thyroid artery and lingual artery. **D:** Completion of level I to III dissection. OH, omohyoid muscle; SCM, sternocleidomastoid muscle; HN, hypoglossal nerve; ECA, external carotid artery; AC, ansa cervicalis; IJV, internal jugular vein; SAN, spinal accessory nerve.

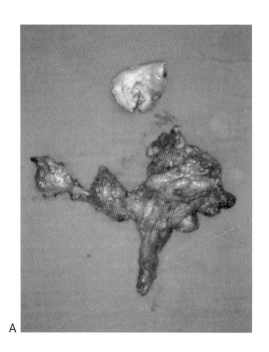

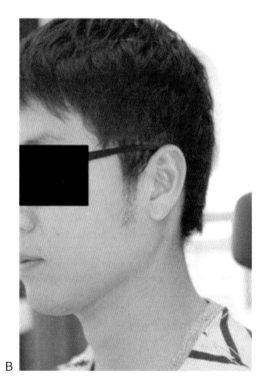

FIGURE 7.7
A: Surgical specimen. **B:** Postoperative scar.

TABLE 7.1   Possible Complications Associated with Robot-Assisted Neck Dissection via Modified Face-Lift or Retroauricular Approach
• Hair loss   • Hematoma   • Infection   • Keloid/scar formation   • Necrosis or discoloration of the skin flap   • Nerve injury marginal branch of facial, greater auricular, hypoglossal, lingual, spinal accessory, vagus nerves

POSTOPERATIVE CARE

The neck should be monitored for any signs of postoperative hemorrhage or infection, and the Hemovac should be checked to see whether it is functioning properly. The drain is removed when the drainage volume falls to 20 mL or less. Any change of skin color or signs of skin flap necrosis should be detected.

COMPLICATIONS

The complications of this surgical procedure are listed in Table 7.1, which are all well known in conventional neck dissection. To prevent injury of the marginal branch of the facial nerve, it should be thoroughly identified using the distal facial artery as a landmark, and special care should be given not to make any thermal injury during the dissection. Since an external retractor may be used by the assistant to expose the submandibular area, care should be given not to put traction on the nerve. In addition, the operator should take care not to traumatize the nerve during the frequent change of instruments during dissection under direct vision or robotic instrumentation.

As it is for any open surgery of the neck, complications may be prevented with comprehensive understanding of the anatomy of the neurovascular structures. However, since the surgical field is relatively narrow compared to that of an open conventional technique, thorough experience in conventional neck dissection should be a requisite. Necrosis of the retroauricular skin flap could be prevented by limiting the upper end of the flap to the level of the external auditory meatus and avoiding an acute angle.

RESULTS

Dissection of the lymphoadipose tissues of levels Ib, II, and III located lateral to the carotid sheath was quite feasible under direct vision using the modified face-lift or retroauricular approach. However, identification of the marginal branch of the facial nerve and the SAN and dissection of lymphoadipose tissues from these structures may take some time in the less experienced surgeon.

Compared to my personal experience with endoscopic resection of the submandibular gland via the retroauricular approach, robot-assisted dissection of level Ib was much more convenient using the multiarticulated EndoWrist of robotic arms. Surgical exposure and instrumentation for the upper and medial aspect of the submandibular gland could be conducted without any difficulty. My clinical data from our department showed that there were no significant differences between the robot-assisted neck dissection and the conventional open technique considering the postoperative complications, amount and duration of drainage, and hospital stay. However, the operation time was longer in the robot-assisted group although the time tended to decrease with accumulation of experience. Satisfaction score of the patients related to the cosmetic results was obviously higher in the robot-assisted group since the scar was hidden by the auricle and hair (Fig. 7.7B).

PEARLS

- The key point of this surgical technique is acquiring an adequate working space. In my experience, the height of the skin flap raised after introducing the self-retaining retractor should be at least 4 cm. If the height is not acquired, the retroauricular incision should be extended to a modified face-lift incision, or the hairline incision may be extended to caudal direction.
- Identify the greater auricular nerve and the external jugular vein to maintain the subplatysmal skin flap. Before proceeding with elevation of the skin flap to the mandible, identify the platysma muscle and make sure you are in the correct surgical plane.
- Digital palpation and identification of the distal facial artery just below the mandible provide an anatomical landmark to identify the marginal branch of the facial nerve.

- A patient-side assistant should be trained to provide a good surgical view during the robotic dissection, using the Army Navy retractor, Yankauer suction, and endoscopic alligator forceps. Sometimes, robotic arms only are not enough for adequate surgical view and instrumentation.
- A modified face-lift incision may be more convenient to acquire an adequate working space for a beginner in this procedure. In addition, identification of the marginal branch of the facial nerve seems to be easier with the extended incision.
- Since robot-assisted dissection of level I may be somewhat more complex including the risk of marginal branch injury and dissection or ligation of the facial artery, submandibular ganglion, and Wharton duct, a beginner may initially try an elective dissection of levels II and III for cN0 oropharyngeal or hypopharyngeal cancer treated with transoral approach or transoral robotic surgery.
- I recommend beginners to conduct endoscopic or robot-assisted submandibular gland excision via retroauricular approach in advance. The experience will be helpful in level I dissection.

PITFALLS

- Damage to the retroauricular hair follicles during skin incision and flap elevation will cause loss of hair and visible scar postoperatively.
- Thermal injury to the marginal branch of the facial nerve during skin flap elevation will lead to functional deficit in the movement of the lower lip.
- Elevation of the skin flap without identification of the platysma muscle may lead to thinning of the skin flap, which could result in postoperative skin depression or even penetration of the skin.

INSTRUMENTS TO HAVE AVAILABLE

- Harmonic scalpel (Harmonic Ace 23E; Johnson & Johnson Medical, Cincinnati, OH)
- Modified Chung retractor, usually applied in robotic thyroidectomy via the transaxillary approach but reduced in length for the purpose of this operation
- Army Navy retractor
- Right-angled retractor, which progressively lengthens to facilitate elevation of the skin flap
- Bovie tip (electrocautery tip): conventional size of spatula type and also additional tips, which progressively lengthen
- Hemoclip or Hem-o-lok for Harmonic scalpel for ligating uncontrollable vessels such as branches of internal jugular vein

ACKNOWLEDGMENT

Thanks to Eun Chang Choi for his assistance in the preparation of this manuscript.

SUGGESTED READING

Ferlito A, Silver CE, Rinaldo A. Elective management of the neck in oral cavity squamous carcinoma: current concepts supported by prospective studies. *Br J Oral Maxillofac Surg* 2009;47:5–9.

Kang SW, Lee SH, Ryu HR, et al. Initial experience with robot-assisted modified radical neck dissection for the management of thyroid carcinoma with lateral neck node metastasis. *Surgery* 2010;148:1214–1221.

Kim WS, Lee HS, Kang SM, et al. Feasibility of robot-assisted neck dissections via a transaxillary and retroauricular ("TARA") approach in head and neck cancer: preliminary results. *Ann Surg Oncol* 2012;19(3):1009–1017.

Koh YW, Chung WY, Hong HJ, et al. Robot assisted selective neck dissection via modified facelift approach for early oral tongue cancer: a video demonstration. *Ann Surg Oncol* 2012;19(4):1334–1335.

8 POSTEROLATERAL NECK DISSECTION

Jeffrey N. Myers

INTRODUCTION

The posterolateral neck dissection is an operation that is typically used in the management of cutaneous cancers of the posterior scalp, auricle, or upper neck either electively to stage the clinically node-negative neck or therapeutically to treat the node-positive neck. In contemporary practice, this operation is most often used to treat a clinically node-negative neck that has been found to have microscopically positive nodal disease in one or more of the regional nodal basins. While a description of this operation was first published in 1962, Drs. Goepfert, Jesse, and Ballantyne of the MD Anderson Cancer Center wrote a definitive description of this procedure and their results with it in 1980. Typically, this operation involves the removal of the lymph nodes in the postauricular, suboccipital, spinal accessory and the jugular lymph node basins (Fig. 8.1). In experienced hands, this operation provides excellent oncologic, functional, and cosmetic results.

HISTORY

As the majority of patients undergoing this procedure will have skin cancer as the primary indication for the procedure, a history of prior skin cancers, including their histologic type, location, and treatment, will be very useful for treatment planning. In addition, sun exposure and family history are relevant to tumor management and surveillance after treatment. An occupational history is also useful, as this operation even when performed without complication can lead to decreased shoulder function for up to 10 to 18 months following surgery. Typically this is manifested by decreased range of motion and strength on shoulder abduction, which can be improved greatly with early intervention by a trained physical therapist with anticipated return to baseline.

PHYSICAL EXAMINATION

Visual evaluation and palpation of the extent of the primary tumor and nodal metastasis are traditionally part of the initial assessment of the patient for whom posterolateral neck dissection is being considered. This includes inspection of the scalp, auricle, and neck and palpation of the entire neck with particular attention to the postauricular, suboccipital, spinal accessory and jugular nodal basins. The number and size of each involved node should be recorded and used as part of the clinical staging. Previous surgery in this area should be noted.

INDICATIONS

This operation is indicated in the management of cutaneous cancers of the posterior scalp, auricle, or the superior aspect of the neck either electively to stage the clinically node-negative neck or therapeutically to treat the node-positive neck. It is used most often to treat a clinically node-negative neck that has been found to have microscopically positive nodal disease in one or more of the regional nodal basins on sentinel lymph node biopsy.

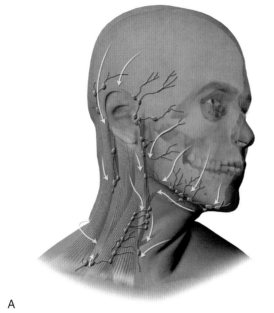
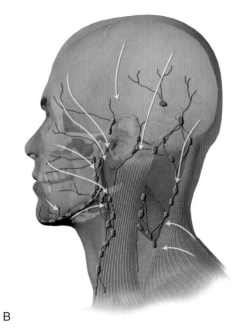

A   B

FIGURE 8.1
A,B: Nodal drainage pathways for cutaneous malignancies of the lateral face, scalp, and neck. **C:** posterolateral neck dissection specimen.
(A and B. Adapted from Balch CM, Houghton AN, Milton GW, et al., eds. *Cutaneous Melanoma*. 2nd ed. Philadelphia, PA: Lippincott; 1992, with permission.
C. Adapted from Eduardo M, Diaz MD Jr, John R, et al. The Posterolateral neck dissection technique and results. *Arch Otolaryngol Head Neck Surg* 1996;122:477–480, with permission.)

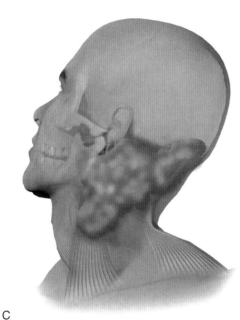

C

CONTRAINDICATIONS

This operation is contraindicated in patients for whom the procedure would neither prolong survival nor provide significant palliation. This may include patients with disseminated metastatic cancer. Additionally, those patients with extensive lymph node metastasis with involvement of the deep muscles of the neck, vertebrae, or carotid artery are advised to consider systemic therapy options that could help decrease the risk of distantly metastatic disease and potentially make the local–regional disease burden more manageable by resection. Patients deemed to be medically high risk for general anesthesia, who have microscopic nodal disease, can often be managed successfully with radiation therapy alone.

PREOPERATIVE PLANNING

Imaging Studies

Cross-sectional imaging of the head and neck region is typically obtained to define the location and extent of the primary cancer and the presence of regional nodal metastases. This is most often accomplished with an axial computed tomography (CT) scan with contrast. However, a magnetic resonance imaging (MRI) or positron emission tomography/computed tomography (PET/CT) may also be used. Systemic imaging may be indicated based on the histology and clinical stage of disease. For patients with melanoma or Merkel cell carcinoma with thick primary tumors or extensive lymph node metastasis, a PET/CT and brain MRI or brain MRI with CT scans of the head and neck, chest, and abdomen should be obtained.

Fine Needle Aspiration Biopsy

Patients found to have palpable lymph node metastasis may be recommended to have a fine needle aspiration biopsy (FNAB) of an involved node if the results will change the patient's management. Such a case would be if the presence of histologically confirmed lymph node metastasis is part of the inclusion criteria for a protocol of neoadjuvant systemic therapy. In cases where the finding of lymph node metastasis is indeterminate by cross-sectional imaging criteria, ultrasound-guided FNAB may be used to confirm or rule out the presence of regional lymph node metastasis to facilitate treatment planning.

SURGICAL TECHNIQUE

Anesthesia

Because of the extent of this procedure, I recommend that the operation be performed under a general inhalational anesthetic. The endotracheal tube is optimally placed and secured at the oral commissure contralateral to the neck that is being dissected. Typically, I perform the procedure with a paralytic agent used throughout the entire operation. This prevents excess stimulation of motor nerves by electric dissection. Even in the presence of paralyzing agents, these motor nerves are readily identified through reliable anatomic landmarks and the stimulation provided by electrical dissection.

Positioning

When bilateral posterolateral neck dissections are performed, consideration should be given to placing the patient in the prone position. As this occurred in only 3 of 55 patients reported in a large series, this is a rare positioning for this operation. Most patients are placed in the supine position with the ipsilateral upper extremity tucked at the patient's side and the operating table turned at a 90-degree angle such that the side of the dissection is facing out. A shoulder roll is placed under the patients shoulders to extend the neck, and the head is turned toward the anesthesiologist.

Draping

The neck, shoulder, upper chest, and, if needed based on the location of the primary, the ear or scalp are prepped. Towels are then used to square off the operative field including exposure of the posterior neck to the nuchal line, the clavicle, the anterior neck to the midline, and the superior aspect of the auricle. Inclusion of the auricle and/or scalp in the operative field should be considered, based on the location of the primary tumor.

Incision

The incision is designed to provide optimal visual access to facilitate the removal of all the lymph node groups to be dissected while preserving vital structures and cosmesis. The location of the primary tumor and incisions used for prior procedures such as a lymph node biopsy may in part dictate the design of the incision. When these are not considerations, I often employ an S-shaped incision in which a horizontal limb is oriented along the occiput from the midline to the postauricular region where it then descends vertically just anterior to the anterior border of the trapezius to an inferior cervical skin crease, which the incision should follow horizontally anterior to the anterior border of the sternocleidomastoid muscle (SCM) (Fig. 8.2).

Flap Elevation

After making the incision with a scalpel or cautery, the superior flap is elevated to the pinna anteriorly, the superior aspect of the auricle superiorly, and the midline medially. The posterior–inferior flap is elevated to the midline in the superior half of the neck and the anterior border of the trapezius muscle in the lower half of the neck all the way to the clavicle. The anterior flap is elevated to the anterior border of the omohyoid muscle. When elevating the superior and posterior flaps, care should be taken to elevate a very thin flap in a subcutaneous plane, which leaves the majority of the subcutaneous adipose tissue on the specimen, as the lymph nodes can be found within the subcutaneous adipose tissue in this portion of the neck. All of the flaps are secured with skin hooks.

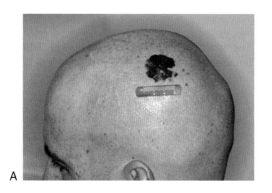

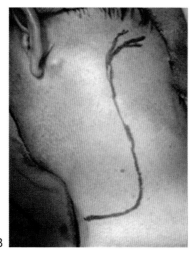

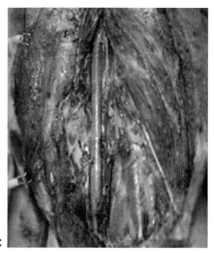

FIGURE 8.2
A: Patient with left parietal scalp melanoma. **B:** Design of incision for left posterolateral neck dissection. **C:** Left neck after left posterolateral neck dissection.

Nodal Dissection

The superficial layer of deep cervical fascia is incised from the mastoid tip to the clavicle along the anterior aspect of the SCM, and this fascia is elevated on both the medial and lateral aspects of the muscle. This fascia and the external jugular lymph nodes should be entirely removed as they are important components of the specimen in cutaneous malignancies of the scalp, ear, and/or face. While dissecting along the anterior aspect of the SCM, the spinal accessory nerve must be identified and skeletonized throughout its entire course from its exit deep to the posterior belly of the digastric muscle to its entry into the SCM. Dissection on the lateral aspect of the muscle from anterior to posterior brings one to the underside of the SCM where the spinal accessory nerve can be seen exiting the muscle. The nerve is followed to the trapezius muscle and skeletonized throughout its course in the operative field to ensure its preservation.

The fibroadipose lymph node–bearing tissue of the postauricular and suboccipital regions is then dissected off of the underlying bone and muscle in a posterior–inferior direction. The prior delineation of the SCM helps to prevent detachment of the SCM insertion from the mastoid/occipital skull during the dissection of these posterior–superior nodes. The suboccipital lymph nodes lie along the course of the occipital artery, and branches of this artery will need to be divided in order to remove this nodal group.

At this point I use two one-half inch Penrose drains that are wrapped around the superior and inferior aspects of the SCM, pulled anteriorly, and secured to the drapes to provide exposure of the posterior portion of the neck (Fig. 8.3A).

The internal jugular vein (IJV) is then identified just above the clavicle and the posterior aspect of the vein is delineated. The fibroadipose lymph tissue overlying the deep layer of deep cervical fascia is then divided very carefully from the IJV to the trapezius just above the clavicle. Using gauze sponges to gently spread this tissue, the specimen is elevated off of the deep layer of deep cervical fascia to expose the phrenic nerve and brachial plexus. Care is taken at this time to avoid injury to these nerves and to prevent avulsion of the transverse cervical vessels or injury to the thoracic duct. Fibroadipose node–bearing tissue is removed from the inferior–lateral portion of the neck where the trapezius and clavicle meet. Extreme caution must be exercised in this region to avoid injury to the inferior–lateral branches of the brachial plexus and the terminal aspect of the spinal accessory nerve. This tissue should be clamped and oversewn with 2-0 silk ties. The dissection then extends from lateral to medial, elevating the nodal tissue off of the trapezius to the midline in the upper half of the neck and the anterior border of the trapezius in the lower neck. Some surgeons advocate resection of the superior aspect of

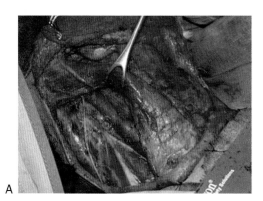
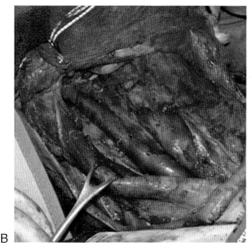

FIGURE 8.3 A: Posterior exposure of right neck for dissection is facilitated by anterior retraction of sternocleidomastoid. **B:** Anterior exposure of right neck for dissection facilitated by posterior retraction of the muscle. Retraction of the muscle is typically accomplished using two Penrose drains. One drain is placed around the superior aspect and the other around the inferior aspect of the muscle. The drains are secured to the drapes with large hemostats.

the trapezius from C1 to C4, in order to remove nodes deep to this muscle. The sensory rootlets of the cervical plexus will be divided as this dissection transitions anterior to the trapezius, and these rootlets and the node-bearing specimen are then elevated off of the levator scapulae and splenius capitis muscles. While advancing the specimen superomedially, the sensory rootlets of the cervical plexus are divided distally in order to preserve their contributions to the phrenic nerve. The Penrose drains are then pulled posteriorly and secured to provide optimal exposure to the carotid sheath structures and more anterior neck (Fig. 8.3B). The neck dissection specimen is then dissected on to and off of the carotid sheath contents. The hypoglossal nerve is identified and preserved throughout its course, and the specimen is dissected up to the lateral aspect of the omohyoid muscle and released. Hemostasis is then provided using bipolar cautery. The wound is irrigated with sterile saline solution and the wound inspected again for signs of bleeding.

Wound Closure and Drain Placement

Two 7-mm Blake (Ethicon) flat suction drains are placed in the depth of wound through a separate stab incision and are secured with a suture of 2-0 nylon or 2-0 silk. Care must be taken to avoid placing the drain in the inferior aspect of the neck posterior to the jugular vein, as this can contribute to development of a chylous fistula. The wound is closed in layers with 3-0 Vicryl for the subcutaneous and platysmal layers with skin staples or 5-0 nylon being used to approximate the skin edges.

Specimens

The neck dissection specimen should be divided into levels II, III, IV, and V and the postauricular and suboccipital regions and sent for permanent section analysis.

POSTOPERATIVE CARE

The drain is connected to a closed bulb suction and is removed when the total drainage is <30 mL for 24 hours. Sutures or staples are removed 6 to 10 days after surgery. Patients who undergo a posterolateral neck dissection are typically admitted for 24-hour observation in the hospital.

COMPLICATIONS

Complications of the posterolateral neck dissection include all of the complications associated within the standard neck dissection including chyle leak, bleeding, and neural injury. Due to the extensive posterior–inferior and inferior dissections, the risk of injury to the spinal accessory nerve and/or brachial plexus is greater than in more standard neck dissections. The surgical misadventures involving these neural structures can best be avoided by careful dissection of these nerves under direct visualization.

RESULTS

A case series review of 55 patients treated over a 10 year period from 1982 through 1991 with surgery including a posterolateral neck dissection who had a minimum of 3 years of follow up at MD Anderson Cancer Center included 35 patients with melanoma, 10 with squamous cell carcinoma and 10 of other histologic types. In this series, the primary tumor was controlled in 89% of patients (94% of patients with melanoma) and regional metastasis was controlled in 93% of patients (89% of patients with melanoma).

PEARLS

- Identification and preservation of the spinal accessory nerve in the posterior triangle of the neck is a high priority.
- Exposure of the posterior and anterior neck during dissection will allow for thorough removal of lymph nodes.
- Identification of the phrenic nerve, spinal accessory nerve and the brachial plexus will preserve these important structures.

PITFALLS

- Chylous fistula may occur if the thoracic duct is accidentally avulsed.
- Spinal accessory nerve injury may occur unless the nerve is identified, carefully dissected, and preserved throughout its entire course.
- Brachial plexus injury can be prevented by early identification and careful dissection.
- Disinsertion of the SCM muscle from the mastoid can be prevented by prior delineation of the SCM.

INSTRUMENTS TO HAVE AVAILABLE

- Cautery for the skin incision and dissection
- Bipolar cautery for bleeders on the muscles and around the carotid sheath
- Allis clamps for nerve and specimen retraction
- 7-0 Blake suction drain

SUGGESTED READING

Rochlin DB. Posterolateral neck dissection for malignant neoplasms. *Surg Gynecol Obstet* 1962;115:369–373.
Goepfert H, Jesse RH, Ballantyne AJ. Posterolateral neck dissection. *Arch Otolaryngol* 1980;106(10):618–620.
De Langen ZJ, Vermey A. Posterolateral neck dissection. *Head Neck Surg* 1988;10(4):252–256.
Plukker JT, Vermey A, Roodenburg JL. Posterolateral neck dissection: technique and results. *Br J Surg* 1993;80(9): 1127–1129.
Diaz EM Jr, Austin JR, Burke LI, et al. The posterolateral neck dissection. Technique and results. *Arch Otolaryngol Head Neck Surg* 1996;122(5):477–480.

9 MANAGEMENT OF THE UNKNOWN PRIMARY CARCINOMA OF THE HEAD AND NECK

Umamaheswar Duvvuri

INTRODUCTION

Many patients with squamous cell carcinoma of the head and neck (SCCHN) present with metastasis to the cervical lymph nodes. Of these, patients with metastatic carcinoma in the cervical lymph nodes, generally excluding the supraclavicular region without an identifiable primary cancer, are defined as patients who harbor a squamous cell carcinoma of the head and neck of unknown primary origin (SCCHNUP). Patients with isolated supraclavicular metastatic carcinoma usually have a primary source from the skin or infraclavicular areas (breast, lung, esophagus, and ovary), entities that are not described here. Retrospective studies suggest that SCCHNUP is a relatively rare disease, affecting between 1% and 3% of new cases of SCCHN. These patients provide a particularly challenging clinical problem to the head and neck surgeon, and thorough physical examination and evaluation are necessary to identify the site of the primary tumor.

Patients who present with SCCHNUP can be treated either with surgery, followed by adjuvant treatment, or with primary nonsurgical therapy. However, the identification of a primary site is enormously helpful in better defining the targeted areas for radiation therapy and provide more accurate staging and prognostic information for these patients. This chapter delineates the evaluation and management of patients with squamous cell carcinoma (SCC) metastatic to the neck from an unknown primary and provides new insights into the application of transoral robotic technologies for the treatment and diagnosis of patients with SCCHN of unknown primary of the head and neck.

HISTORY

The classic history for patients with SCCHN of unknown primary is that of a heavy smoker and/or drinker, typically a pack-a-day of cigarettes for more than 10 years with varying degrees of alcohol intake. However, in the recent past, the history has shifted to include a larger number of patients who report never having been smokers or who have stopped smoking in the distant past and have a minimal history of alcohol intake. It is possible that these patients may have a tumor that is related to the human papillomavirus (HPV), an etiologic factor contributing to the development of their cancer. Thus, it is important to take a thorough history on all patients with an emphasis on alcohol and tobacco consumption, and it is also important to question whether these patients have engaged in high-risk sexual behaviors, as this may also contribute to the diagnosis of an HPV-related malignancy. Female patients should be questioned about their gynecologic history and specifically a history of abnormal Pap smear. It is also important to ascertain whether these patients have complaints of hoarseness, dysphasia, odynophagia, or otalgia, all of which may point to a site of primary tumor. A dermatologic history is also relevant, and patients should be questioned about prior skin surgery or head and neck cutaneous SCC.

PHYSICAL EXAMINATION

A thorough examination of the head and neck is mandatory in all patients who present with occult lymph node metastasis. The physical examination should include palpation of the neck to determine whether the lymph nodes are fixed to underlying structures or if it is freely mobile. Palpation should also include examination of the thyroid and tracheal regions, as well as the nodal lymphatic basins of levels I through VI. Many cases of SCCHNUP are initially diagnosed by excision of a mass in the neck, which is ultimately confirmed to be SCCHN. In these patients, the physical examination can be challenging, since postsurgical scarring and induration can impact palpation and examination of the residual cervical lymph nodes. An examination of the oral cavity and oropharynx should be performed, ideally with indirect mirror laryngoscopy to examine the base of tongue (BOT) and tonsil fossae. Bimanual palpation of the BOT and tonsil fossae is also required. The physical examination should also include a careful evaluation of the cutaneous structures of the head and neck, since previously treated primary malignancies of the skin can present with isolated metastatic SCC. It should be noted that a prior history of skin cancer or skin excisions should also be included, and physical stigmata of prior skin resections, such as scars or liquid nitrogen-induced cryoablation, should also be documented.

Once this portion of the physical examination is concluded, these patients should all be examined with a flexible fiberoptic nasopharyngolaryngoscopy. This provides a better view of the BOT, tonsil fossae, glottis, hypopharynx, and supraglottic structures. It is important to evaluate the mobility of the vocal fold and look for areas of salivary pooling or submucosal masses in the postcricoid area. The nasopharynx should also be examined to exclude the possibility of a nasopharyngeal carcinoma.

INDICATIONS

Patients who present with a diagnosis of SCCHNUP are candidates for this procedure of robotic excision of the BOT. The diagnosis of SCCHNUP should be established on the basis of pathologic evaluation of enlarged cervical lymph node(s).

CONTRAINDICATIONS

There are no contraindications to surgery based on anatomic factors. However, patients who have significant medical comorbidities that may preclude the administration of general anesthesia may not be candidates for surgery. Those patients who have a demonstrable primary cancer that appears deeply invasive on preoperative imaging do not require robotic surgery to identify the primary cancer.

PREOPERATIVE PLANNING

Radiographic Imaging

Computed tomography (CT) and/or magnetic resonance imaging (MRI) with contrast is generally considered to be the first-line imaging for patients with SCCHN metastatic to the neck from an unknown primary. If the CT and MRI do not identify the primary tumor, a positron emission tomography with integrated CT (PET/CT) may be useful. If a PET/CT scan is performed it should be performed before panendoscopy, since the biopsies or surgical interventions may in fact induce FDG (18-Flouro-DeoxyGlucose) avidity on the PET/CT scan, which could be a false positive. PET/CT scanning has been shown to identify approximately 25% of cancers that were not detected after an evaluation that did not include PET.

Laboratory Studies

Even with an extensive investigation and thorough physical examination, a primary cancer may not be found. New diagnostic procedures can potentially aid in the identification of the primary cancer or at least suggest a subsite from which the primary cancer could have arisen. Detection of HPV or Epstein-Barr virus (EBV) in the fine needle aspiration from a metastatic lymph node may be useful and may provide prognostic information.

The majority of primary cancers that are identified among patients with SCCHN of unknown primary are located within the oropharynx. Furthermore, recent studies suggest that a large percentage (up to 70%) of SCCs of the oropharynx are HPV related, and only a small percentage of cancers from nonoropharyngeal head and neck sites are HPV related. Therefore, histologic detection of HPV within tissue biopsies from the lymph node strongly suggests that the oropharynx is the source of the primary cancer. Immunohistochemical analysis of p16 is a valuable biomarker and can identify those cancers that are associated with HPV infection. HPV in situ hybridization also provides confirmatory data that validate HPV etiology.

EBV is also a sensitive marker for carcinoma of the nasopharynx, and positivity on lymph node aspirates for EBV strongly suggests the nasopharynx as the source. It should be noted that nasopharyngeal carcinomas typically metastasize to the posterior neck, level 5; and isolated level 5 nodal metastases in a patient should raise the index of suspicion for an occult primary NPC. However, it should be noted that despite the relatively high frequency of HPV- and EBV-positive cancers of the oropharynx and nasopharynx, respectively, a negative result does not necessary exclude the oropharynx or nasopharynx as the source of the primary cancer. Therefore, a complete physical examination is still mandated for all patients with SCCHNUP.

SURGICAL TECHNIQUE

Patients in whom the unknown primary cancer remains occult despite having a tonsillectomy and directed biopsies of the BOT may benefit from a robotic BOT resection to identify the primary cancer. It should be noted that these patients typically have HPV-related cancers, and the surgeon should have a high index of suspicion for a primary cancer in the oropharynx. The overall goal of the robotic BOT resection procedure is to use an en bloc resection approach under high magnification to remove all lingual tonsil tissue from the inferior portion of Waldeyer ring in order to identify the primary cancer.

A direct laryngoscopy and examination should be performed under anesthesia to evaluate the oral cavity, oropharynx, larynx, and hypopharynx. An esophagoscopy should also be performed. I recommend bimanual palpation of the mucosal surfaces of the BOT and tonsil while the patient is under anesthesia to obtain a better evaluation of these areas and potentially discover the occult source of the primary cancer. Directed biopsies to the areas of clinical suspicion of the BOT should be performed, to try to identify the occult primary cancer.

I also recommend that a bilateral palatine tonsillectomy should be performed in patients with adequate lymphoid tonsil tissues that are in fact palatine tonsils, as part of the initial evaluation. It has been suggested that approximately 10% of cancers of the tonsil will have contralateral cervical lymph node metastases, and thus I recommend a prophylactic bilateral palatine tonsillectomy for these patients. In those patients in whom the radiographic imaging and initial operative endoscopy do not reveal the primary cancer, additional evaluation is warranted.

Surgical management of the patient with SCCHNUP requires operative endoscopy. This operative endoscopy is performed with the patient supine on the operating table and intubated transorally ideally with a relatively small endotracheal tube such as a 6-0. The table should be turned 180 degrees and the upper and lower teeth protected with custom-made splints. I then place a suture in the midline of the tongue, which is a half mattress to allow for traction to be placed on the tongue. Both arms are then tucked for the patient (Fig. 9.1). Surgery is begun by examining the oral cavity and oropharynx with bimanual palpation to evaluate the potential source of the primary cancer. Direct laryngoscopy and endoscopy are then performed using standard laryngoscope blades. If this fails to reveal the site of the primary cancer, operative intervention is undertaken by performing palatine tonsillectomies. I find that intraoperative consultation with the pathologist for the evaluation of palatine tonsils to be of limited value, since many cancers of unknown primary origin tend to be very small in size. Therefore, I prefer to send the palatine tonsils for permanent section evaluation. If preoperative evaluation of the patient's neck metastasis demonstrates HPV-related disease, then there is a high likelihood that the occult primary cancer is to be found somewhere within the oropharynx. Therefore,

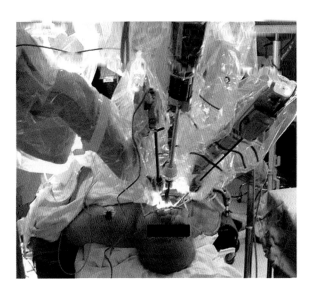

FIGURE 9.1 Depiction of the placement of robotic instruments in the TORS approach for BOT resection. The patient's mouth is retracted using a Dingman retractor with a flat blade. The daVinci robot is then docked with instruments in the patient's mouth.

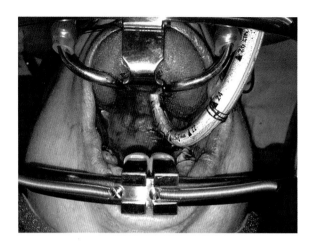

FIGURE 9.2
The exposure of the oropharynx is obtained using a Dingman mouth retractor with a flat blade. The endotracheal tube is sutured to one side. The lateral pharyngeal walls and the circumvallate papillae are exposed.

I undertake robotic-assisted lingual tonsillectomy in these patients at the same sitting as the performance of the palatine tonsillectomies.

In order to perform the robotic-assisted lingual tonsillectomy, the patient's mouth is opened using a Dingman mouth gag with the flat retractor blade, and the endotracheal tube is sutured off to the side opposite to the entry of the surgical robot. After opening the mouth and exposing the BOT, the surgical robot is brought into the field. It should be noted that the exposure obtained should demonstrate the circumvallate papillae and the lateral pharyngeal walls (Fig. 9.2). Once this exposure is obtained with a combination of flat blade retraction as well as other maneuvers that may be necessary, the mouth gag is then suspended on a Mayo stand. The arms of the surgical robot are then brought into position and are introduced into the patient's mouth for a transoral robotic surgery (TORS) approach. I use a 5-mm Maryland and a 5-mm cautery Bovie to perform the dissection.

The initial incision is made along the circumvallate papillae from the left to right side. The lingual tonsil is then bisected in the midline, and surgery begins by performing a lingual tonsillectomy on one side (Video 9.1). The dissection plane is to the level of the musculature of the BOT. Since this is a diagnostic procedure as well as a resection of a relatively small cancer, *we do not resect the muscle of the BOT*. This also avoids excessive entry into the lingual artery or unwanted blood loss. The dissection is then carried from midline to lateral taking care to transect the glossotonsillar fold and remove any tonsil tissue that is present in the glossotonsillar sulcus. It should be noted that leaving lymphoid tissue at the area of the glossotonsillar sulcus can result in a missed diagnosis, since the occult primary cancer can be quite small (on the order of a few millimeters in size). The dissection is then carried inferiorly to the level of the vallecula. The area of the vallecula is easily identified by the appearance of minor salivary glands, which appear as small white lobular tissue, at the area of the vallecula. It should be noted that in this area there are often small blood vessels, which supply the mucosa, which are controlled with electrocautery. Care must be taken not to transect the epiglottis or inadvertently injure the supraglottic structures (Fig. 9.3). Once the dissection is completed on one side, a similar procedure is performed on the contralateral BOT.

A suture is then placed at a specific site in the specimen to orient the tissue for consultation and frozen section diagnosis (Fig. 9.4).

I prefer to start the dissection by performing ipsilateral resection of the BOT in the initial setting. The site operated is ipsilateral to the site of the neck metastasis. However, it is known that cancer of the BOT can have bilateral metastasis. I have an approximately 8% rate of lymph node metastasis from an occult cancer of the BOT. For this reason, I prefer to offer bilateral lingual tonsillectomy for patients with metastatic carcinoma from an unknown primary.

POSTOPERATIVE CARE

Patients who have undergone TORS for an unknown primary cancer are extubated in the operating room or upon transfer to the postoperative recovery unit. The patients are then managed in the hospital overnight with intravenous pain medication as well as gastroesophageal reflux disorder prophylaxis with proton pump inhibitors and H_2-blocker for reflex precautions. I also treat patients with sucralfate to minimize gastric acid reflux to the open wound at the BOT. The patients are usually allowed to have a diet of soft foods, which are able to be swallowed with relative ease on the first postoperative day. It should be noted that clear liquids are most difficult to swallow in this immediate postoperative period. I do not routinely place a nasogastric feeding tube in these patients since I have not found a need to do so. Patients are then free to follow any diet they can tolerate as soon as they are able to have their pain under good control. Patients are usually discharged from the hospital on the first postoperative day.

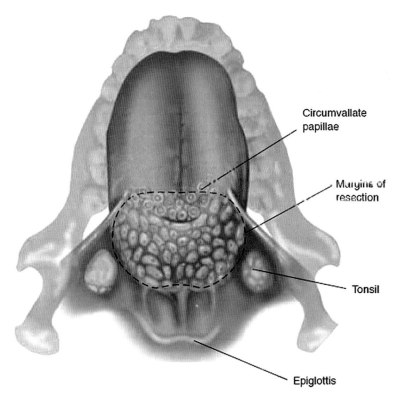

Circumvallate
papillae

Margins of
resection

Tonsil

Epiglottis

FIGURE 9.3
Structures of the supraglottis
and oropharynx.

COMPLICATIONS

The risks and type of complications observed with transoral robotic resection of the BOT for an unknown primary cancer are similar to those seen with other transoral approaches for resection of the BOT. There is a potential risk of injury to the lingual artery, which can result in significant bleeding. However, the robotic lingual tonsillectomy procedure does not resect a significant portion of intrinsic tongue musculature, and therefore the lingual artery is not at significant risk in many of these cases. There is, however, the possibility of experiencing some postoperative bleeding when the eschar that covers the surgical defect sloughs off. Most bleeding can be managed with observation, or if it bleeds from a more anterior portion of the BOT, topical cautery can be used. However, more active bleeding or bleeding from a deeper portion of the surgical wound may require control of the bleeding in the operating room. I have not had any patients have significant bleeding as a consequence of having a resection of the BOT for an unknown primary cancer.

RESULTS

Patients typically experience pain and dysphagia after robotic-assisted surgery of the BOT. The pain lasts for 2 days through 2 weeks as the wound heals and granulates (Fig. 9.5). Most patients do have dysphagia but are able to tolerate oral intake as early as postoperative day 1 to 2. Patients typically work with a speech

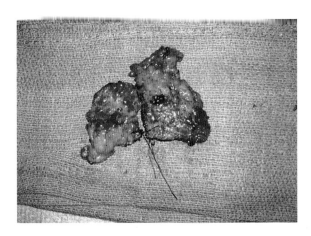

FIGURE 9.4 A typical resection specimen is shown. The entire extent of the BOT is resected from the left glossotonsillar sulcus to the right glossotonsillar sulcus and inferiorly to the valleculae.

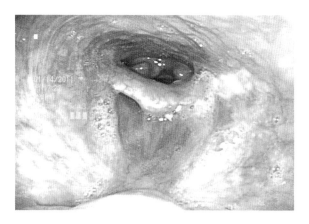

FIGURE 9.5

The appearance of the tongue base 2 months after robotic-assisted resection. This is the appearance prior to initiation of radiation therapy. The vallecula is preserved, and the tongue base is well healed.

pathologist with some basic swallowing exercises to facilitate early resumption of swallowing. The long-term risk of feeding tube dependence is highly correlated with the modality that is used to complete the definitive treatment of these patients. Those patients who undergo extensive chemoradiotherapy for the management of the disease tend to have a higher rate of feeding tube dependence.

Patients who have a small-volume primary cancer can often be treated with surgery alone, by definitively resecting the primary cancer with clear margins and a neck dissection. However, I typically postpone the neck dissection for 1 to 2 weeks after the primary TORS procedure. The neck dissection can be performed at the same time as TORS surgery; however, I prefer to have the final pathology reports so that if a close margin is identified, then further resection of the primary site can be performed at the time of the neck dissection. I have been able to identify the site of the primary cancer in approximately 90% of patients who have undergone the robotic-assisted lingual tonsillectomy for patients with SCCHN metastatic to the neck from with an unknown primary. The average size of the cancer is approximately 5 to 6 mm, and the vast majority of these lesions are indeed HPV related.

In those patients who present with a low-volume primary cancer, it is possible to perform a robotic-assisted resection of the BOT to achieve negative margins and subsequently clear the neck without having to subject the patients to additional adjuvant therapy. In my experience, patients treated in this fashion have excellent oncologic and functional results and return to work quickly without suffering from the long-term problems associated with chemoradiation. However, those patients who present with a large volume cancer may in fact require adjuvant or definitive therapy with chemoradiation, but the identification of the primary site of the cancer allows for accurate staging of the patient and potentially improves the radiation fields that can be delivered to the patient to control the cancer.

For patients who have large volume metastatic cancer in the neck, the TORS lingual tonsillectomy affords the opportunity to obtain a definitive diagnosis and to identify the primary cancer. However, I still offer these patients definitive chemoradiotherapy in the absence of lymph node dissection to avert the need for additional surgical therapy, when chemoradiation cannot be avoided. Even in these groups of patients, I tend to see improved functional results since the radiation field can be tailored to the appropriate subsite of the oropharynx, and radiation to the entire Waldeyer ring could be avoided.

My experience has shown that the TORS procedure is a safe and effective way of managing patients with SCCHN from an unknown primary provided that the key surgical steps and oncologic principles are adhered too. The use of minimally invasive surgeries facilitates the identification of the unknown primary cancer, provides patients with prognostic information, and allows for patients to be stratified to clinical trial protocols. It is also possible to definitively resect the primary cancer and to remove all active cancer from the neck and to avoid adjuvant therapy in select patients. The long-term sequelae of dysphagia may be reduced in those patients who can be treated with an adjuvant dose of radiation after surgical therapy.

PEARLS

- Proper history taking and physical examination are critical for assessing the patient's risk factor(s) for harboring an HPV-related cancer.
- Careful radiographic evaluation including CT or PET/CT scan is critical for demonstrating the subsite in which the primary tumor may be located. In addition, it provides important information regarding the extent of lymph node metastasis or distant metastasis.
- Extensive resection of the lingual tonsil tissues has surprisingly little effect on long-term swallowing function, but there is acute dysphagia that is noted with this. I have not had any patients experience persistent problems or permanently rely on gastrostomy tube feeding.
- A bilateral robotic lingual tonsillectomy is the preferred method for removing tissue in order to diagnose patients with SCC of an unknown primary and whom the primary has not been found by a standard examination under anesthesia.

PITFALLS

- Not removing tissue from the glossotonsillar sulcus can lead to inadequate tissue removal and missing the chance to diagnose the site of an unknown primary cancer.
- Inadvertent removal of tongue musculature leads to possible injury to the lingual artery and excessive bleeding.
- Dysphagia and pain are the most common temporary side effects associated with this procedure and can be managed with narcotic pain medications, as well as swallowing therapy.
- There is a small risk of postoperative hemorrhage as a consequence of this procedure, but it should be recognized early, and appropriate management is required, including potential operative control of hemorrhage.

INSTRUMENTS TO HAVE AVAILABLE

- Operative headlight
- Tooth guard
- Dingman retractor with various-sized flat tongue retractor blades
- daVinci Robotic System, Intuitive Surgical
- 5-mm spatula tip monopolar cautery
- 5-mm Maryland dissector
- 2-0 silk suture

SUGGESTED READING

Haas I, Hoffmann TK, Engers R, et al. Diagnostic strategies in cervical carcinoma of an unknown primary (CUP). *Eur Arch Otorhinolaryngol* 2002;259:325–333.

Begum S, Gillison ML, Nicol TL, et al. Detection of human papillomavirus-16 in fine-needle aspirates to determine tumor origin in patients with metastatic squamous cell carcinoma of the head and neck. *Clin Cancer Res* 2007;13:1186–1191.

Waltonen J, Ozer E, Hall N, et al. Metastatic carcinoma of the neck of unknown primary origin: evolution and efficacy of the modern workup. *Arch Otolaryngol Head Neck Surg* 2009;135:1024–1029.

Balaker AE, Abemayor E, Elashoff D, et al. Cancer of unknown primary: does treatment modality make a difference? *Laryngoscope* 2012;122(6):1279–1282.

Mehta V, Johnson P, Tassler A, et al. A new paradigm for the diagnosis and management of unknown primary tumors of the head and neck. *Laryngoscope* 2013;123:146–151.

10 TECHNIQUE FOR EXCISION OF CERVICAL SCHWANNOMA

Seiji Kishimoto

INTRODUCTION

Schwannomas are benign tumors of the neural sheath with approximately 25% to 40% of extracranial schwannomas occurring in the head and neck region. Cervical schwannomas usually involve cranial nerves IX, X, XI, or XII, the cervical sympathetic chain, phrenic nerve, or cervical or brachial plexus (Table 10.1).

The diagnosis of cervical schwannoma begins with an accurate history and physical examination. The symptoms and signs are variable and depend primarily on the origin and location of the tumor. However, most patients are asymptomatic and only present with a mass in the neck. Schwannomas are frequently difficult to characterize by fine needle aspiration biopsy (FNAB). Clinical history, physical examination, and imaging studies, particularly magnetic resonance imaging (MRI), suggest the diagnosis. The best treatment is surgical resection. However, as schwannoma is a benign tumor without neurologic dysfunction, postoperative nerve paralysis can have a major impact on quality of life. Enucleation or tumor removal while preserving the involved nerve should thus be attempted if possible.

HISTORY

The initial complaint is usually a solitary asymptomatic cervical mass that slowly enlarges at a rate of 2.5 to 3 mm/year. However, when the mass extends from the parapharyngeal space to the neural foramena of the skull base (jugular foramen or hypoglossal canal), symptoms related to neurologic deficits, such as hoarseness, dysphagia, aspiration, dysarthria, or shoulder drop, can appear depending on the nerve involved. When the mass extends into a spinal foramen, paresthesia, weakness, and muscle atrophy of the upper limb and pain or paresthesia of the neck may be present.

PHYSICAL EXAMINATION

The mass is usually roughly spherical, with a smooth surface. In some cases, the tumor is fusiform in shape along the course of the involved nerve. Such a mass is usually mobile about an axis perpendicular to the long axis of the involved nerve, but with no mobility along the long axis of the involved nerve.

Sometimes, pulsation is palpable in the tumor. Discriminating pulsation from the carotid artery itself from a pulsatile tumor (carotid body tumor or paraganglioma) is important. If the carotid artery runs along the surface of the tumor, this indicates the possibility of schwannoma of the cervical sympathetic chain. However, if the carotid artery is displaced medially to the tumor, schwannoma of the vagus nerve (VN) may be suggested.

In the case of schwannoma of the cervical or brachial plexus, compression of the mass may cause pain or numbness of the neck, shoulder, or upper limb.

TABLE 10.1   Nerve of Origin for Cervical Schwannomas
• Vagus nerve
• Accessory nerve
• Hypoglossal nerve
• Cervical sympathetic chain
• Phrenic nerve
• Cervical plexus
• Brachial plexus

INDICATIONS

The indications for surgical excision of schwannoma depend on the involved nerve, symptoms, size and location of the lesion, and risk of surgical intervention. Surgical excision should be considered to prevent progressive neurologic deficits due to an enlarging mass. Relatively small tumors usually involve only one nerve, but multiple nerves may come to be involved as the tumor enlarges. The disability resulting from dysfunction of multiple nerves is significant, and early surgical intervention should therefore be considered.

CONTRAINDICATIONS

The most important factor in determining indications for surgical excision is the age of the patient, since these tumors grow very slowly. In general, surgical intervention is not recommended for patients over 60 years old.

PREOPERATIVE PLANNING

Imaging Studies

Characteristic findings on computed tomography (CT) include a well-circumscribed, heterogeneously enhancing mass with or without central necrosis (Fig. 10.1). MRI reveals signal isointensity on T1-weighted imaging (Fig. 10.2), and a "target sign" is sometimes apparent after the administration of a contrast agent (Fig. 10.3).

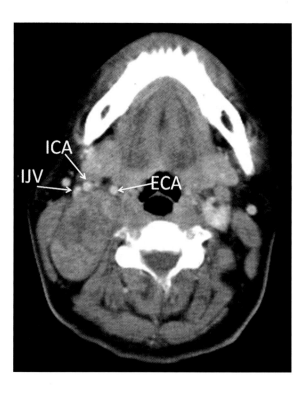

FIGURE 10.1
Schwannoma of the right cervical sympathetic chain. Contrast-enhanced axial CT scan shows a well-circumscribed, heterogeneously enhancing mass with central necrosis. IJV, internal jugular vein; ICA, internal carotid artery; ECA, external carotid artery.

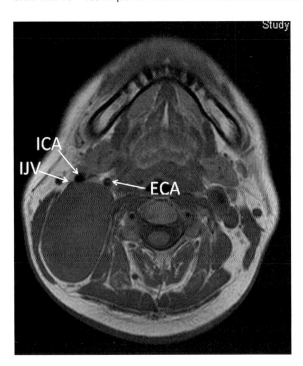

FIGURE 10.2 The mass appears signal isointense on T1-weighted axial MRI scan. IJV, internal jugular vein; ICA, internal carotid artery; ECA, external carotid artery.

T2-weighted imaging reveals a mass with heterogeneous signal hyperintensity (Fig. 10.4). These findings suggest the diagnosis of schwannoma. Neither CT nor MRI demonstrates active irregular invasion to the surrounding tissue, as would be seen in malignant schwannoma.

Imaging diagnostic modalities such as ultrasonography, CT, and MRI offer great help in identifying the tumor and its positional relations to surrounding vessels and nerves. In cases with schwannoma of the VN, the tumor grows between the common/internal carotid artery and the internal jugular vein (IJV), increasing the distance between and separating the artery and vein (Fig. 10.5). In cases with schwannoma of the cervical sympathetic chain, no separation is observed between the IJV and common/internal carotid artery (Figs. 10.1 to 10.4).

Paraganglioma arising from the VN or carotid body should be differentiated from schwannoma using diagnostic imaging modalities. Paraganglioma is classically isodense when compared to muscle on precontrast CT, with more reliable homogeneous enhancement postcontrast. Post–gadolinium MRI sequences of paraganglioma show extremely bright contrast enhancement in a characteristic "salt-and-pepper" pattern, representing the low signal intensity of vascular flow voids.

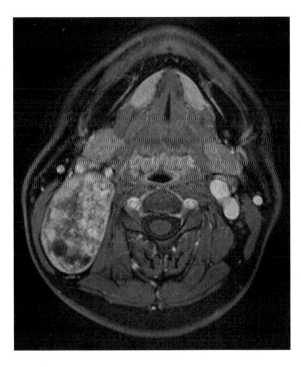

FIGURE 10.3 After administration of contrast agent, a "target sign" is apparent.

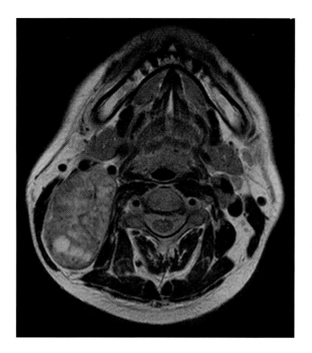

FIGURE 10.4
T2-weighted axial MRI scan reveals a mass with heterogeneous signal hyperintensity.

Fine Needle Aspiration Biopsy

Schwannomas are frequently difficult to characterize on FNAB, which often reveals only hypocellular, nondiagnostic specimens due to the presence of either significant cystic degeneration or a dense stromal component. In addition, FNAB may injure the vessels and cause adherent injury unfavorable to the operation. FNAB of a neck mass that is clinically suspected as a schwannoma is therefore not recommended and is used to eliminate the possibility of malignancy, rather than to confirm a diagnosis of schwannoma.

SURGICAL TECHNIQUE

The most important point is preservation of VN function. To identify the VN and avoid harmful manipulations, intraoperative monitoring with a NIM electromyographic endotracheal tube is very useful. The probe of the nerve monitor is placed on the identified structure, and a positive response is elicited. Other nerves (e.g., accessory nerve, hypoglossal nerve, and ansa cervicalis) can be identified by contraction of innervated muscles when

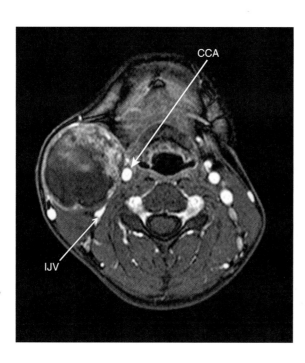

FIGURE 10.5
Schwannoma of the right VN. Gadolinium-enhanced, T1-weighted axial MRI scan shows that the tumor is growing between the common/internal carotid artery and the IJV, increasing the distance between the artery and vein (*separation*). IJV, internal jugular vein; CCA, common carotid artery.

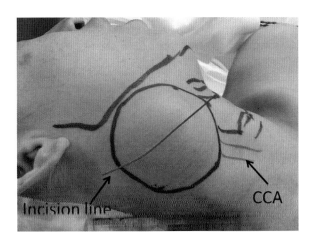

FIGURE 10.6 A depiction of schwannoma of the VN (6 × 5 cm). The common carotid artery (CCA) runs deep to the tumor. The *red line* indicates the line of the transverse skin incision along a skin crease overlying the mass.

the probe is placed. To obtain a clear response, administration of muscle relaxant should be discontinued after induction of anesthesia.

By careful palpation or Doppler ultrasonography, the location of the carotid artery and the IJV should be confirmed before starting any operation.

SURGICAL TECHNIQUE

As most cervical schwannomas originate from the VN or cervical sympathetic chain, surgical techniques for schwannomas in these two locations are described.

Schwannoma of the Vagus Nerve (Video 10.1)

The tumor is located between the common carotid artery (CCA) and IJV, and these two vessels are displaced posteromedially by the tumor (Fig. 10.5).

A transcervical approach is employed. A transverse skin incision is made along a skin crease overlying the mass (Fig. 10.6). The resulting skin flap is elevated in the subplatysmal layer, and the fascia of the sterno-cleidomastoid muscle is exposed and retracted posteriorly. If the carotid artery and IJV are superficial to the tumor, careful dissection and retraction of these structures are necessary to achieve wide exposure of the lateral surface of the tumor (Fig. 10.7).

However, if these vessels run behind the tumor, the tumor can be widely exposed without dissection of the vessels. Using the probe of the nerve monitor, a positive response of the VN is elicited at the caudal portion of the tumor.

By carefully identifying the VN on the capsule of the tumor, an entry line through the tumor capsule is determined without harm to the VN (Fig. 10.8). As the tumor capsule contains multiple layers, meticulous and gentle layer-by-layer exposure down to the level of the innermost layer of the capsule is necessary (Figs. 10.9 and 10.10). After the innermost layer of the capsule is exposed, a dissection between the outer layers (pseudocapsule) and

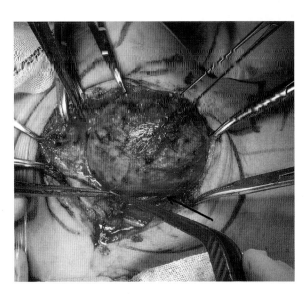

FIGURE 10.7 The IJV (*arrow*) is dissected free from the tumor and mobilized laterally. The capsule of the tumor is widely exposed.

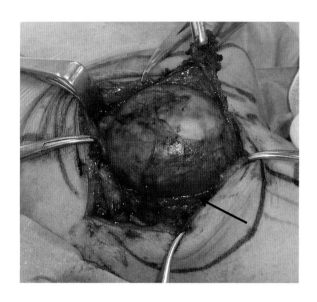

FIGURE 10.8

The nerve monitor probe is placed on the surface of the capsule. After confirming negative response of the VN, the outermost layer of the capsule is incised longitudinally, grasped with fine forceps and unfolded. *Arrow*, IJV.

FIGURE 10.9

Schematic drawing of the schwannoma. The capsule of the tumor contains multiple layers. The nerve bundle runs between the layers of the capsule. (Modified from Hashimoto S. Functional preservation by means of inter-capsular resection for cervical schwannoma [in Japanese]. *JOHNS* 2004;20:591–593.)

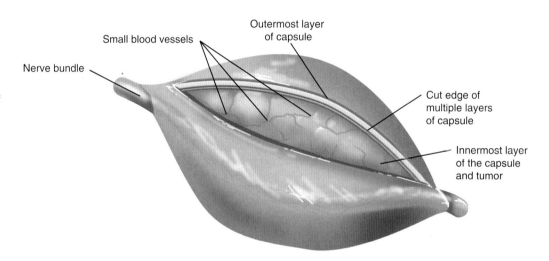

FIGURE 10.10

Meticulous and gentle layer-by-layer incision (*arrows*) of the capsule and exposure down to the level of the innermost layer of the capsule are important.

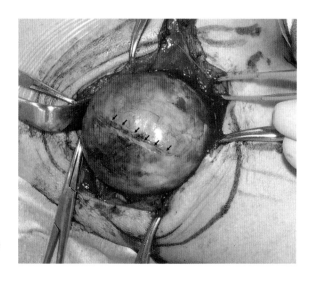

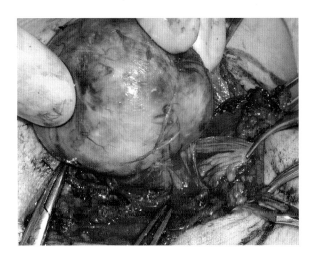

FIGURE 10.11 After exposure of the innermost layer of the capsule, complete enucleation of the tumor with this layer is performed.

the innermost layer (true capsule) begins. The edges of the dissected layer are grasped with fine toothless forceps in several places, and the entire tumor is elevated with the capsule. This manipulation facilitates dissection of the layer behind the tumor. Complete enucleation of the tumor including the innermost capsule is thus performed (Fig. 10.11). This is important to prevent tumor recurrence.

When the tumor is too large, circumferential dissection becomes difficult, and in such cases, debulking of the central part of the tumor with the aid of an ultrasonic aspirator facilitates circumferential dissection.

Bleeding from the inner surface of the capsule should be carefully controlled using bipolar electrocautery. Finally, the tip of the drainage tube is placed inside the preserved capsule to control bleeding.

Using these techniques, function of the VN is preserved (Fig. 10.12).

Schwannoma of the Cervical Sympathetic Chain

The IJV and internal and external carotid arteries are displaced anteriorly by the tumor, but with no separation between the vein and arteries (Figs. 10.1 to 10.4 and 10.13). These findings suggest that the tumor originates from the cervical sympathetic chain. After elevation of the subplatysmal cervical skin flap, the internal and external carotid artery, IJV, and vagus, accessory, and hypoglossal nerves are identified. Extirpation of enlarged lymph nodes is important to obtain good exposure of the surgical field (Fig. 10.14).

The VN is confirmed using the probe of the nerve monitor, by eliciting a positive response from this nerve. The outermost layer of the tumor capsule is incised in a cephalocaudal direction between the IJV and accessory nerve. Cut edges on both sides of the outermost layer of the capsule are grasped with fine toothless forceps and pulled. This manipulation enables elevation of the important nerves and vessels without harm (Fig. 10.15).

A network of small vessels is present on the surface of the capsule. After coagulation of these vessels using the bipolar coagulator, multiple layers of the capsule are incised one by one (Fig. 10.16). It should be kept in mind that, in most cases, the parenchyma of the tumor is directly continuous with the ganglion of the sympathetic chain (Fig. 10.17). The sympathetic chain is therefore transected proximal and distal to the tumor, and a postoperative sequela of this operation is the development of Horner syndrome.

Finally, the innermost layer of the capsule is preserved, and enucleation of the tumor, including this layer, is completed (Fig. 10.18). Using this technique, unnecessary exposure of the superior laryngeal nerve and glossopharyngeal nerve can be avoided.

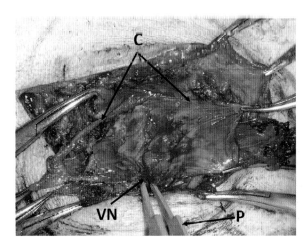

FIGURE 10.12 After complete enucleation of the tumor, positive response of the vagus nerve (VN) in the capsule (C) is confirmed using the probe (P) of the nerve monitor.

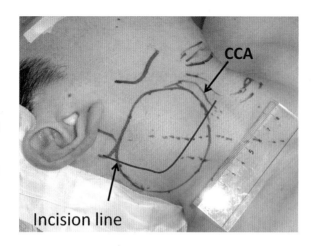

FIGURE 10.13

Depiction of the schwannoma in the cervical sympathetic chain (7 × 6 cm). The common carotid artery (CCA) is displaced anteriorly by the tumor. The transverse skin incision line is extended in a cephalic direction.

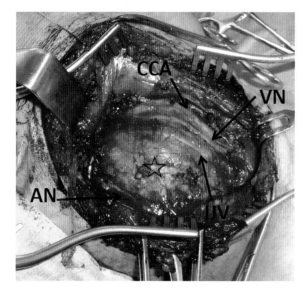

FIGURE 10.14

Exposure of nerves and vessels on the surface of the tumor (*star*). CCA, common carotid artery; IJV, internal jugular vein; VN, vagus nerve; AN, accessory nerve.

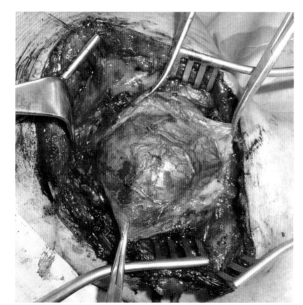

FIGURE 10.15

The outermost layer of the tumor capsule is incised in cephalocaudal directions between the IJV and accessory nerve. Cut edges on both sides of the outermost layer of the capsule are grasped with fine toothless forceps and pulled.

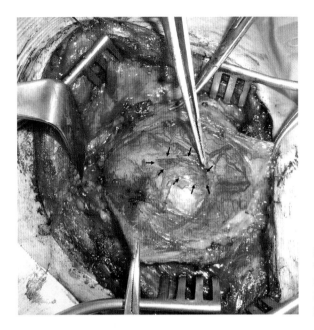

FIGURE 10.16 After careful coagulation of the vessels on the surface of the capsule, the deeper layer of the capsule is incised and unfolded (*arrows*). This manipulation is repeated several times until the innermost layer is exposed.

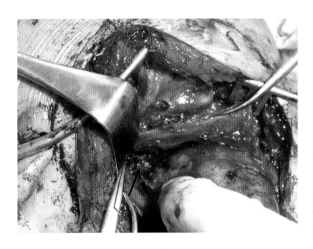

FIGURE 10.17 *Arrow* indicates direct connection of the cephalic end of the tumor and the ganglion of the sympathetic chain.

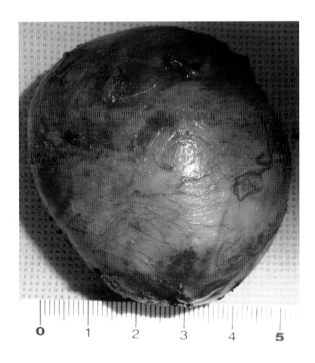

FIGURE 10.18 Enucleated tumor with the intact innermost layer of the capsule.

POSTOPERATIVE CARE

A suction tube is inserted into the wound and retained until the daily volume of drainage fluid decreases to <10 mL. Pressure dressings are removed on the first postoperative day.

Edema of the upper respiratory tract should be checked endoscopically once or twice a day on the first 2 postoperative days.

COMPLICATIONS

Hematoma: If the capsule is preserved, bleeding from the inner surface can cause hematoma. However, hematoma is usually absorbed spontaneously without treatment.

Neurologic Deficits

Schwannoma of the Vagus Nerve
Usually, both superior and inferior laryngeal nerves are involved. Therefore, in addition to hoarseness, severe aspiration can become problematic in some cases. If rehabilitation activities for phonation and swallowing are not effective within 6 months, surgical restoration of those functions should be planned.

Schwannoma of the Cervical Sympathetic Chain
When the sympathetic chain is transected, Horner syndrome will appear. However, symptoms of this syndrome do not affect quality of life.

In some cases, first bite syndrome can appear.

Schwannoma of Other Nerves
Resection of a schwannoma of the cervical plexus leads to anesthesia of the skin in the territory of the affected nerve or paralysis of the diaphragm.

Injury of the brachial plexus will cause motor or sensory dysfunction of the shoulder and upper limb.

RESULTS

En bloc tumor and nerve resection or tumor enucleation seems not to alter the recurrence rate. However, incomplete resection results in slow local recurrence over a period of months to years.

The preservation rate of neurologic functions following intracapsular enucleation is 30% to 80% in cases with schwannoma of the VN. However, in most reported cases with schwannoma of the cervical sympathetic chain, Horner syndrome results after the operation.

PEARLS

- As schwannoma is a benign and slowly growing tumor without serious symptoms, strict surgical indications should be applied.
- Precise subcapsular layer-by-layer dissection is desirable to preserve neurologic function.
- Information on anatomical relationships between the tumor and vessels from imaging studies is important to differentiate schwannomas of the VN and cervical sympathetic chain.
- Intraoperative monitoring with the NIM electromyographic endotracheal tube is very useful to detect the VN and prevent damage.
- In cases involving a large schwannoma, debulking of the mass using ultrasonic aspiration facilitates further dissection.

PITFALLS

- Damage to the superior laryngeal nerve causes severe aspiration.
- Excessive traction on the nerve causes severe damage and dysfunction.

INSTRUMENTS TO HAVE AVAILABLE

- NIM Electromyographic Endotracheal Tube with Nerve Monitoring Systems (Medtronic, Minneapolis, MN)
- CUSA Ultrasonic Aspirator (INTEGRA, Plainsboro, NJ)

SUGGESTED READING

Furukawa M, Furukawa MK, Katoh K, et al. Differentiation between schwannoma of the vagus nerve and schwannoma of the sympathetic chain by imaging diagnosis. *Laryngoscope* 1996;106:1548–1552.

de Araujo CE, Ramos DM, Moyses RA, et al. Neck nerve trunk schwannomas: clinical features and postoperative neurologic outcome. *Laryngoscope* 2008;118:1579–1582.

Kawashima K, Sumi T, Sugimoto T, et al. First-bite syndrome: a review of 29 patients with parapharyngeal space tumor. *Auris Nasus Larynx* 2008;35:109–113.

Tomita T, Ozawa H, Sakamoto K, et al. Diagnosis and management of cervical sympathetic chain schwannoma: a review of 9 cases. *Acta Otolaryngol* 2009;129:324–329.

Gibber M, Zevallos JP, Urken ML. Enucleation of vagal nerve schwannoma using intraoperative nerve monitoring. *Laryngoscope* 2012;122:790–792.

11

TECHNIQUE FOR THE SURGICAL EXCISION OF CAROTID BODY TUMORS

James L. Netterville

INTRODUCTION

The carotid body tumor (CBT) is the most common paraganglioma arising within the head and neck region. Paragangliomas are tumors that arise from the branchiomeric paraganglia, which are distributed from the skull base down to the aortic arch. These neoplasms may also arise from paraganglia of the middle ear (tympanic paraganglioma), the jugular bulb, the vagus nerve at the skull base or in the neck, and the sympathetic trunk. Less frequently, these tumors may arise in the larynx, thyroid gland, and intrathoracic region around the aortic arch.

Our institution and others have established in the literature that resection of these tumors is not only technically feasible but can be done on a routine basis with low morbidity. Cranial nerve injury still remains the most common sequela of surgical treatment of CBTs. First bite syndrome, described as intense preauricular pain (periparotid) with initial bites of each meal, is also seen frequently after the resection of these tumors. Baroreceptor failure, which can rarely occur in a transient fashion after unilateral resection, can be a severe and debilitating sequela after bilateral tumor resection, related to the loss of carotid sinus feedback.

The management of CBTs has evolved over the last several decades. Significant changes in the evaluation and treatment include (1) decreased use of diagnostic angiography secondary to improvements in computed tomography (CT) and magnetic resonance imaging (MRI); (2) increased incidence in nonoperative observation in asymptomatic older patients; (3) greater emphasis on preservation of the cranial nerves during resection; and (4) limited targeted use of preoperative embolization for massive complex CBT.

HISTORY

Patients commonly present within one of three subgroups: (1) an asymptomatic mass in the neck; (2) an incidental finding discovered on a CT or MRI scan, performed for evaluation of a separate problem; and (3) as members of family with inherited paraganglioma syndrome. In the past, the majority of these patients presented with an asymptomatic mass in the neck. However, with the significant increase in the use of imaging of the head and neck over the last two decades, more than half of the patients now present with a less obvious tumor incidentally noted on CT or MRI. A CBT <2.5 cm is difficult to palpate unless it presents in a very thin individual. If one is diligent in evaluating the history of patients with CBTs, other family members are commonly discovered with paragangliomas. Although it is commonly cited that <10% of patients have familial tumors, I have noted that 32% of the CBT patients in my series have familial paraganglioma syndrome.

The vast majority of these patients are asymptomatic with no deficits in adjacent cranial nerve function. A small number of patients with tumors >5 cm present with complaints of weak voice and dysphagia secondary to deficits in function of the vagus and hypoglossal nerves. In patients with CBT presenting with preoperative cranial nerve deficits one must rule out an occult vagal or jugular paraganglioma which is far more likely to cause nerve damage.

PHYSICAL EXAMINATION

During the physical examination for evaluation of a potential CBT, the surgeon should define the characteristics of the tumor, the function of the adjacent cranial nerves, examine the neck for the rare potential of metastatic lymph nodes and finally look for evidence of other head and neck paragangliomas.

Initially the neck is palpated to assess the size and location of the tumor and to discover other distinct masses. Classic teaching notes that one can move the CBT back and forth in the horizontal plane, but it has very little mobility to up and down pressure, resulting in little movement in the vertical plane. This finding is often very subtle and not a reliable indication to differentiate the CBT from other masses in the neck. Often one can feel the pulsation from the tumor, but this can also occur with metastatic nodes lying adjacent to the carotid artery. The contralateral neck is also carefully examined to ensure that other occult tumors are not overlooked.

Cranial nerves VII, IX, X, XI, and XII and the sympathetic trunk are evaluated for any deficits in function. If significant dysfunction of the cranial nerves is noted, it is often an indication of an occult vagal or jugular paraganglioma. A careful examination of the eyes must be performed to rule out Horner's syndrome, which would indicate a primary tumor of the sympathetic trunk. One must also undertake a complete examination of the external auditory canal, the tympanic membrane, and the middle ear to rule out occult tympanic, jugular, or vagal tumors.

INDICATIONS

1. A resectable CBT in a young healthy patient
2. A small resectable contralateral CBT with multiple tumors putting the ipsilateral vagal and hypoglossal nerves at risk
3. CBT with suspected or proven malignant growth
4. Significant cervical mass effect in the otherwise asymptomatic patient
5. Patient preference with obvious tumor show in a thin neck

CONTRAINDICATIONS

1. An asymptomatic, slow-growing tumor in an older patient. This age cutoff is quite relative depending on the patient's overall health and performance status.
2. Previous contralateral loss of vagal and or hypoglossal function
3. Patient preference in a stable or very slowly enlarging tumor

PREOPERATIVE PLANNING

With improvement in the quality of MRI, CT, and CT angiography, the need for preoperative arteriogram is now limited to the few larger tumors that undergo preoperative embolization. The most frequently used initial form of imaging to study the CBT is MRI. MRI/magnetic resonance angiography (MRA) has been shown to be very effective in identifying and evaluating paragangliomas of the head and neck. The ability of MRI/MRA to identify local recurrence as well as new primary lesions makes it the preferred imaging modality both in initial evaluation and for long-term follow-up.

It is rare for a CBT to present as a secreting tumor, with only 3% exhibiting neuroendocrine activity producing vasoactive amines (i.e., catecholamines and dopamine). However, most patients undergo a 24-hour urine evaluation for catecholamine secretion to rule out a vasoactive tumor.

Although many articles extol the benefits of preoperative embolization, it is a very invasive, expensive procedure that is often performed under monitored anesthesia. Avoiding the use of embolization for smaller tumors significantly reduces the length of hospital stay by 1 to 2 days, thereby reducing costs. For an experienced surgical team, it adds little benefit in tumors <5 cm.

Preoperative counseling is recommended for patients to better understand their postoperative clinical course. A thorough discussion is held with the patient and the family to explain baroreflex failure, first bite syndrome, the potential for cranial nerve deficits, and the rare chance of vascular complications. If tumor banking services are available, it is recommended to sign up the patients to participate in this valuable data collection process that will allow for further molecular and genetic evaluation. Finally a preoperative consultation is obtained with the vascular surgery team to be on standby to perform resection of the carotid and reconstruction as needed.

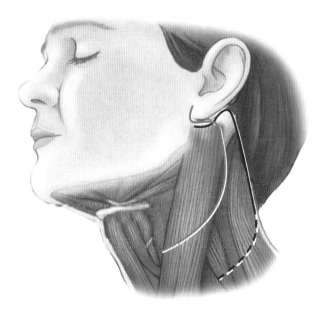

FIGURE 11.1 A central neck incision is outlined that may extend in the preauricular crease as needed to gain further access to the parapharyngeal space. In younger females, an extended hairline incision will give good exposure as well. Each incision must provide access to the carotid artery above and below the tumor dissection.

SURGICAL TECHNIQUE

The major emphasis of this surgical procedure is neural preservation. Often during discussions on this topic, the emphasis is placed on the technical dissection of the carotid artery, with little attention paid to the cranial nerves. The main point to remember is that the carotid artery can be successfully grafted; however, significant injury to the vagus and hypoglossal nerves results in lifelong functional deficits in speech and swallowing. Early mobilization of these nerves away from the surface of the tumor, along with control of intraoperative bleeding, will prevent the vast majority of injuries that occur to these nerves. Although nerve monitoring of vagal function is gaining in popularity for tumors requiring dissection of the vagus and recurrent laryngeal nerves, it is rarely needed for the primary CBTs with no previous surgical dissection. It can be helpful in the dissection of recurrent tumors or those rare CBTs that have significant superior extension compressing the nerves as they exit the skull base.

A transcervical incision is placed in a cervical crease line as seen in Figure 11.1. To aid in the resection of tumors with high parapharyngeal extension, the incision is curved up under the lobule and extended along the preauricular regions as needed to mobilize over the parotid. In females, placement of the incision has evolved to incorporate a more aesthetically pleasing orientation. It is outlined with a short preauricular limb that then courses posteriorly under the lobule to extend into the hairline and then inferiorly within the hair-bearing scalp approximately 6 to 12 cm as needed (Fig. 11.2). For larger tumors or for more inferior vascular control, the incision can be extended forward in an inferior cervical skin crease. Flaps are elevated in a subplatysmal fashion. The great auricular nerve is dissected and preserved. However, if the nerve is in an unfavorable position, it is divided with a scalpel and a neurorrhaphy is performed during the closure to reapproximate the ends of the nerve. Both techniques have resulted in return of auricular sensation postoperatively.

A selective nodal dissection of levels IIA and III is the initial step in this procedure. This allows for sampling of the lymph nodes at risk for malignant spread and yields excellent exposure of the CBT with the

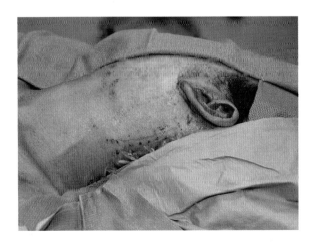

FIGURE 11.2 Outline of an extended hairline incision after 2 cm of hair was removed to allow the incision to be positioned within the hair-bearing scalp. The cervical extension is rarely needed but may be extended into a skin crease in the inferior aspect of the neck.

FIGURE 11.3
After a regional dissection of levels II-III nodes, the first step of tumor removal is isolating and dissecting the vagus nerve (VN) and the hypoglossal nerve (HN) from within the venous vascular envelope, which surrounds the tumor. CCA, common carotid artery; ICA, internal carotid artery; T, tumor; IJV, internal jugular vein.

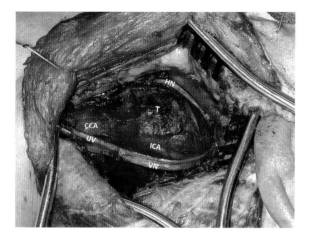

surrounding cranial nerves lying in the hypervascular venous envelope. The anterior border of the sternocleido-mastoid muscle is dissected from the mastoid to the omohyoid. The digastric muscle is dissected and mobilized, leading to exposure and ligation of the proximal occipital artery. This vessel often provides partial vascular supply to the superior aspect of the tumor. At this point, a selective dissection is performed of level IIA to expose the spinal accessory nerve. If no nodes are positive, this is the superior extent of the dissection. The nodes of levels IIA and III are then dissected skeletonizing the internal jugular vein and it branches. If suspicious nodes are identified, they are sent for frozen section evaluation. Branches of the jugular vein are divided as needed to allow retraction of the vein yielding a wide exposure of the carotid artery, and the tumor surrounded by the hypoglossal and vagal nerves (Fig. 11.3). The vascular envelope that surrounds the tumor extends along the carotid system beyond the surface of the tumor. Dividing the vascular envelope caudally and cephalad exposes the proximal common carotid artery and distal internal carotid artery. The hypoglossal nerve (XII) is dissected off of the lateral surface of the tumor (Fig. 11.4). The ansa cervicalis can be dissected off the surface of the tumor if it is uninvolved, or it can be divided several centimeter below its attachment to the XII nerve at this time. Dissecting anteriorly and posteriorly along the XII nerve will allow for identification of the union of the hypoglossal and vagus nerves. At this point, both nerves interlink fibers. The union of these two nerves is left undisturbed, in order to avoid inadvertent vocal cord paralysis. The vagus nerve is then dissected away from the tumor and the internal carotid artery to a level below the bifurcation of the carotid artery (Fig. 11.5).

After exposure of the carotid artery beyond the edges of the tumor, vascular control is obtained by dissection around the common carotid artery inferior to the tumor, and then a tunnel is dissected around both the internal and external carotids distal to tumor involvement. The plane of dissection between the tumor and the distal internal carotid artery is established first. The vast majority of the time, it is not necessary to dissect in the subadventitial plane, as is commonly recommended. If the adventitia has not been invaded by tumor, the dissection may proceed outside of this layer allowing for preservation of a thicker artery wall. Generous use of the bipolar cautery will aid in this dissection and minimize blood loss. The tumor is dissected off of the lateral surface of the internal carotid artery as dissection proceeds inferior toward the bifurcation (Fig. 11.6). The tumor is then dissected off of the external carotid and its branches as necessary prior to dissection of the carotid bifurcation. Frequently the ascending pharyngeal artery is clipped at the medial surface of the external carotid.

The tumor is dissected away from the lateral surface of the bifurcation (Fig. 11.7). At this point, the tumor and the internal carotid artery are rotated anteriorly to expose the posterior deep extension of the tumor

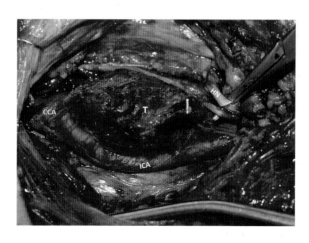

FIGURE 11.4
The hypoglossal nerve is found within the vascular envelope on the anterior superior surface of the tumor. T, tumor; CCA, common carotid artery; ICA, internal carotid artery; HN, hypoglossal nerve.

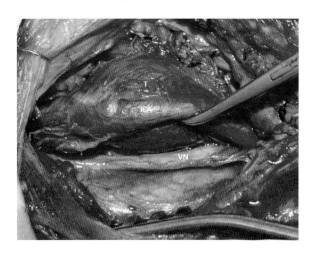

FIGURE 11.5 The vagus nerve is dissected away from where it was tethered to the posterior lateral surface of the tumor and the internal carotid artery. T, tumor; VN, vagus nerve; ICA, internal carotid artery.

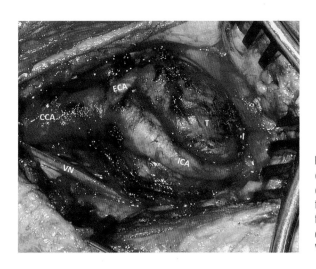

FIGURE 11.6 With the cranial nerves under careful observation, vascular control is obtained by dissection of the common carotid inferior to the tumor as well as the internal and external carotid branches superior to tumor involvement. ECA, external carotid artery; CCA, common carotid artery; ICA, internal carotid artery; VN, vagus nerve; T, tumor.

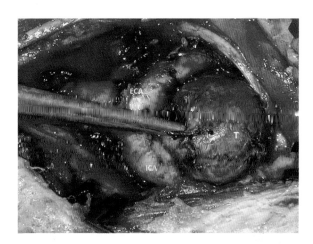

FIGURE 11.7 Dissection progresses from superior to inferior along the well visualized tumor–internal carotid interface. With retraction of the tumor away from the artery, this fibrous vascular interface is cauterized with an irrigating or "ISOCOOL" tips bipolar cautery and sharply divided with vascular dissection scissors. The region of the bifurcation is dissected after the majority of the tumor is freed from the arteries. T, tumor; ICA, internal carotid artery; ECA, external carotid artery.

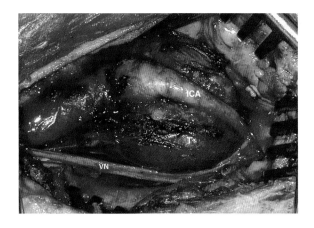

FIGURE 11.8

The artery is rotated medially to allow dissection of the posterior aspect of the bifurcation. It is often easier to deliver the tumor mass off the posterior surface of the carotid. T, tumor; VN, vagus nerve; ICA, internal carotid artery.

(Fig. 11.8). Usually one can see the superior laryngeal nerve stretched across the deep surface of the tumor. It is dissected free, with good postoperative function in most cases (Fig. 11.9). Finally the deep extension of the tumor is dissected away from the medial aspect of the bifurcation. Rarely there is a small artery extending out from the bifurcation into the tumor. If the length of this artery is insufficient to hold a clip, then a 4-0 Prolene is used to oversew the region of the stump of the vessel at the carotid bifurcation. The tumor is finally delivered away from the deep surface of the carotid artery and the region of the bifurcation. After completion of the resection, the carotid is inspected for areas of injury, and the cranial nerves are redraped in their normal positions. The intact superior laryngeal nerve can be seen deep to the bifurcation of the carotid artery (Fig. 11.10).

When more exposure is needed, the digastric and stylohyoid muscles are released from the mastoid and the styloid. In order to prevent injury to the glossopharyngeal nerve, it is identified on the undersurface of the stylopharyngeus muscle and dissected away from the internal carotid artery. Further superior exposure is then achieved by removing the styloid process, effectively releasing the stylomandibular ligament, which allows access to the entire infratemporal fossa.

When tumor invades the artery, or the integrity of the internal carotid artery wall is in question after complete tumor resection, it is wise to use the saphenous vein to perform bypass grafting of the internal carotid artery. Our colleagues in vascular surgery perform this bypass graft. Rarely the vagus and or hypoglossal nerves are grossly involved by tumor. The preoperative discussion with the patient determines whether these nerves are resected to clear the tumor or left intact with a small amount of tumor on the external fascia of the nerve.

After extensive irrigation, a closed suction drain is placed, the platysma layer is closed with 3-0 Vicryl, and the subcutaneous layer is closed with 4-0 subcuticular suture, with Steri-strips placed over the incision line (Fig. 11.11).

POSTOPERATIVE MANAGEMENT

For the initial unilateral resection, the patients are observed in a monitored bed for the first 24 hours to treat the mild baroreflex failure, which rarely occurs transiently after a unilateral resection. If the surgery is for resection of the second side CBT, the patient is observed in the surgical ICU to allow for treatment as necessary for early onset of baroreflex failure. The patient is asked to return to the office for a checkup in 6 weeks, as no sutures need to be removed in the early postoperative period (Fig. 11.12).

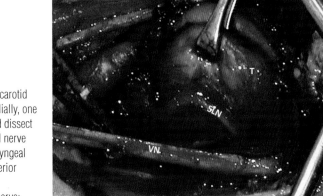

FIGURE 11.9

As the tumor and the carotid artery are rotated medially, one begins to look for and dissect the superior laryngeal nerve along with other pharyngeal branches off the posterior surface of the tumor.
T, tumor; VN, vagus nerve; SLN, superior laryngeal nerve.

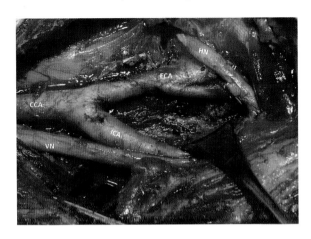

FIGURE 11.10 After the completion of the tumor dissection, the superior laryngeal nerve is visualized deep to and between the intact internal and external carotid arteries. The hypoglossal and the vagus nerves are intact framing the dissection. HN, hypoglossal nerve; ECA, external carotid artery; CCA, common carotid artery; ICA, internal carotid artery; VN, vagus nerve.

RESULTS

In a recent review of our patients, a total of 154 patients with 215 CBTs were identified. The average age at presentation was 45 years, with an age range of 14 to 88 years. Sixty-six patients (43%) were male and 88 (57%) female.

A family history was present in 50 (32%) of patients. In patients with a positive family history, 37 (74%) had bilateral CBTs, 11 (22%) had an associated jugular paraganglioma, 19 (38%) had an associated vagal paraganglioma, and 8 (26%) had another form of paraganglioma. In contrast, in those patients without a family history, 23 (22%) had bilateral CBTs, 18 (17%) had a jugular paraganglioma, 14 (13%) had a vagal paraganglioma, and 7 (7%) had some other paraganglioma. There were 124 patients who underwent surgical resection of a CBT, 25 of which had bilateral CBT resection, making for 149 total CBTs resected. Thirty-seven (30%) of CBTs underwent preoperative embolization. Carotid repair was performed in 23 (19%) of tumors resected.

COMPLICATIONS

In patients with bilateral CBT resection, baroreceptor failure occurred in 20 (80%) patients. First bite syndrome was documented in 34 surgical patients (27%). Eleven patients underwent a secondary surgical procedure to address cranial nerve deficits. One palatal adhesion, six vocal fold injections, and four medialization laryngoplasties were performed.

Metastatic tumor was discovered in five patients (3.25%). All of these patients had metastatic tumor in the regional lymph nodes. One of the five patients had metastases to the vertebra, and one patient had metastasis to the vertebra and liver.

PEARLS

- The carotid artery can be successfully grafted; however, significant injury to the vagus and hypoglossal nerves results in lifelong functional deficits in speech and swallowing.
- Selective nodal dissection of levels IIA and III is the initial step.

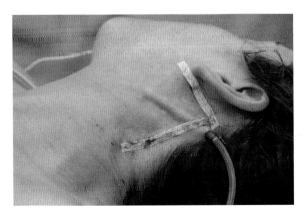

FIGURE 11.11 The incision is closed with 3-0 Vicryl in the deep layers and 4-0 Vicryl to close the subcuticular layers, with Steri-strips to seal the wound.

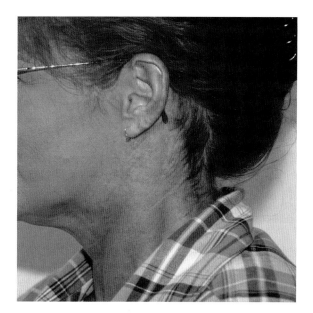

FIGURE 11.12

The patient seen at 8 weeks postoperatively demonstrates excellent early hearing with minimal cervical edema. The early hair regrowth begins to cover the location of the incision within the hair-bearing inferior cervical region.

- Early mobilization of the vagus and the hypoglossal nerves away from the tumor surface
- Meticulous control of intraoperative bleeding
- The vast majority of the time, it is not necessary to dissect in the subadventitial plane.

PITFALLS

- Failure to involve a multidisciplinary team
- Failure to have vascular surgery on standby
- Failure to prepare for baroreflex failure
- Attempting surgical treatment of CBT with little previous experience

INSTRUMENTS TO HAVE AVAILABLE

- Standard head and neck tray

SUGGESTED READING

Hallet JW, Nora JD, Hollier LH, et al. Trends in neurovascular complications of surgical management for carotid body and cervical paragangliomas. A fifty year experience with 153 tumors. *J Vasc Surg* 1988;7:284–289.

Netterville JL, Civantos FJ. Rehabilitation of cranial nerve deficits after neurologic skull base surgery. *Laryngoscope* 1993;103(11 pt 2 suppl 60):45–54.

Robertson D, Hollister AS, Biaggioni I, et al. The diagnosis and treatment of baroreflex failure. *New Engl J Med* 1993; 329:1449–1455.

Netterville JL, Reilly KM, Robertson D, et al. Carotid body tumors: a review of 30 patients with 46 tumors. *Laryngoscope* 1995;105:115–126.

Boedeker CC, Ridder GJ, Schipper J. Paragangliomas of the head and neck: diagnosis and treatment. *Fam Cancer* 2005; 4:55–59.

Langerman A, Athavale S, Rangarajan S, et al. Natural history of cervical paragangliomas. *Arch Otolaryngol Head Neck Surg* 2012;138(4):341–345.

12

VAGAL PARAGANGLIOMAS

Mark S. Persky

INTRODUCTION

Paragangliomas represent highly vascular neoplasms embryologically arising from the paraganglia of neural crest origin and most commonly occur in the head and neck region. Paraganglia are part of the diffuse neuroendocrine system, previously known as the amine precursor decarboxylate system, and have the potential to secrete neuropeptides and catecholamines. Vagal paraganglia are normal structures that are intimately associated with the perineurium of the vagus nerve. While they may occur anywhere along the course of the vagus nerve, they are most often located within or just below the nodose (inferior) ganglion, which is just inferior to the skull base at the jugular foramen, and less often within the middle and jugular (superior) ganglion. Its location in this area predisposes vagal paragangliomas to early involvement of the other lower cranial nerves, including the glossopharyngeal, accessory, and hypoglossal nerves, and dysfunction of these multiple lower cranial nerves may be apparent with larger or long-standing tumors. Multicentric paragangliomas are common in familial cases (78% to 87%) but also occur in 10% of sporadic tumors, and appropriate studies should be performed to identify the presence of additional paragangliomas. Malignant vagal paragangliomas are uncommon, and their diagnosis can only be confirmed by the presence of metastatic tumor, usually within regional lymph nodes. There are no strict histologic criteria within the primary tumor that can differentiate between benign and malignant paragangliomas. Paragangliomas are highly vascular, and they characteristically demonstrate early neural involvement in addition to skull base and potential intracranial extension. These factors all contribute to the challenging nature of effectively treating these tumors. Traditionally, surgery has been the preferred method of treatment, especially with the evolution of more sophisticated cervical and skull base approaches. Postoperative cranial nerve dysfunction may be anticipated in patients with larger tumors and skull base involvement; therefore, a focus on rehabilitation efforts is necessary.

Approximately 1% to 3% of paragangliomas secrete catecholamines. A fivefold increase in catecholamines is sufficient to produce symptoms. Symptoms consistent with a functioning tumor are tachycardia, excessive sweating, weight loss, and hypertension. Secreting paragangliomas account for approximately 2% of all instances of secondary hypertension. Twenty-four–hour urine collection in these patients will show elevated levels of the catecholamine metabolites, metanephrine and vanillylmandelic acid. Serum catecholamines will show elevated levels of norepinephrine in functioning extra-adrenal paragangliomas. Elevated serum epinephrine is indicative of a concurrent pheochromocytoma. Paraganglioma familial syndrome subtypes 1 and 4 (PGL1 and PGL4) are associated with a higher incidence of concurrent pheochromocytoma. Conversely, multiple endocrine neoplasia type IIA (pheochromocytoma, medullary thyroid carcinoma, and parathyroid hyperplasia) and type IIB (pheochromocytoma, medullary thyroid carcinoma, parathyroid hyperplasia, and mucosal neuroma) are associated with head and neck paragangliomas.

HISTORY

Vagal paragangliomas are slow growing with a female:male preponderance of 2:1 to 3:1 and a mean duration of symptoms of 2 to 3 years before presentation. The most common symptom is a slowly growing, asymptomatic mass in the superior aspect of the neck. As the tumor enlarges, it encroaches upon the lower cranial nerves and the adjacent sympathetic chain. Approximately 33% to 50% of patients have cranial nerve neuropathy at presentation involving, in decreasing frequency, the vagal, hypoglossal, spinal accessory, and sympathetic plexus nerves. Signs and symptoms include unilateral vocal cord paralysis, hoarseness, dysphagia, nasal regurgitation, atrophy of the hemitongue, shoulder weakness, and Horner syndrome. The initial presence of vocal cord paralysis with or without hoarseness helps to differentiate vagal paragangliomas from carotid body tumors.

Vagal paragangliomas account for up to 5% of all head and neck paragangliomas. While they arise most commonly from the nodose (inferior) ganglion, vagal paragangliomas can originate from the middle and superior ganglion and less frequently anywhere along the course of the vagus nerve. Compared to the discrete carotid body, vagal paraganglia are distributed more diffusely within the nerve or perineurium. Vagus nerve fibers fan out or "splay over" the surface of the vagal paraganglioma or, early in their development, enter the substance of the tumor, and therefore, preservation of the vagus nerve is usually not possible with complete tumor resection.

Vagal paragangliomas are ovoid- or spindle-shaped tumors and most commonly present as an asymptomatic mass in the superior aspect of the neck, typically more cephalad than carotid body tumors. Since most vagal paragangliomas originate at the inferior (nodose) ganglion, the tumor tends to spread inferiorly into the poststyloid parapharyngeal area. Extension superiorly toward the skull base in the area of the jugular foramen results in early involvement of the internal jugular vein, adjacent cranial nerves (IX, XI, XII) (Fig. 12.1), and internal carotid artery, manifesting the typical anterior/medial displacement of this artery (Fig. 12.2). The vagus nerve is located in the poststyloid compartment of the parapharyngeal space (Fig. 12.3).

PHYSICAL EXAMINATION

Vagal paragangliomas present as slowly growing, firm masses in level II of the neck. Although these represent vascular tumors, they generally do not present as pulsatile masses although there may be associated bruits. The mobility of the tumor to palpation reveals that it is fixed in a vertical direction due to its intimate involvement with the vagus nerve. Medial parapharyngeal extension may cause a bulge of the lateral wall of the oropharynx and medial displacement of the tonsil. With enlargement of the tumor, both the vagus and adjacent cranial nerves are involved. The vagus nerve is affected most commonly, followed by the hypoglossal and spinal accessory nerves; therefore, ipsilateral vocal cord paresis/paralysis, weakness of the tongue, and atrophy of the sternocleidomastoid and trapezius muscles may be presenting findings. Involvement of the sympathetic plexus may cause Horner syndrome.

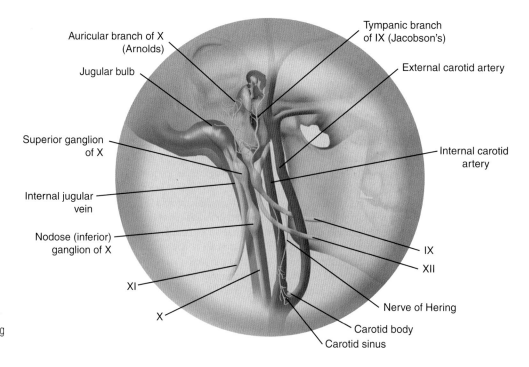

FIGURE 12.1

Illustration of the anatomy of the superior aspect of the vagus nerve with adjacent structures at risk for involvement with an enlarging vagal paraganglioma.

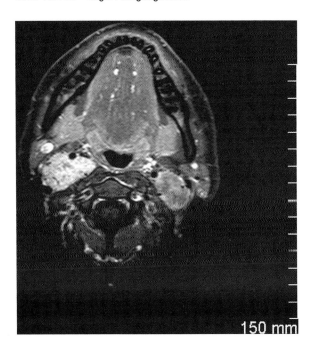

FIGURE 12.2 MRI of a patient with bilateral vagal paragangliomas and typical anterior–medial displacement of the internal carotid arteries.

INDICATIONS

Surgery is indicated for patients presenting with paresis/paralysis of the vagus nerve assuming that advanced age, physical disabilities, and comorbidities are not contraindications. One should assume that total dysfunction of the vagus nerve will result and that adjacent cranial nerve dysfunction will possibly be a sequela. One must realize that paragangliomas are radiosensitive and that doses of 45 Gy delivered over 5 weeks can prevent tumor growth and cranial nerve dysfunction in over 90% of patients. Documentation of a malignant vagal paraganglioma by imaging studies and subsequent needle aspiration biopsy will require primary tumor resection, modified neck dissection, and adjuvant radiation therapy.

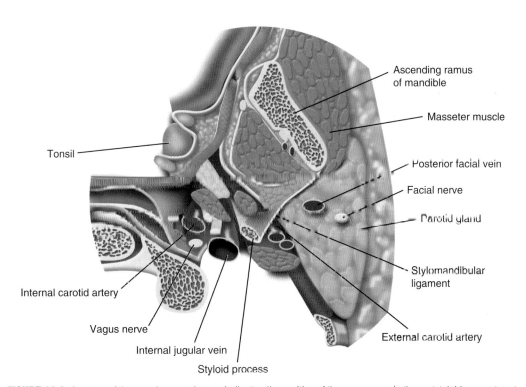

FIGURE 12.3 Anatomy of the parapharyngeal space indicating the position of the vagus nerve in the poststyloid compartment.

CONTRAINDICATIONS

Traditionally, surgical resection has been the mainstay of treatment for these tumors, but the outcome is dependent on many factors that may influence the ideal result of total tumor removal while minimizing postoperative complications. Older patients do not adapt well to acute neural deficits that may define the course of postoperative vagal paraganglioma patients. Even with existing pretreatment cranial nerve dysfunction, patients may not easily tolerate postoperative total cranial nerve paralysis with absolute loss of cranial nerve function, especially if more than one nerve is affected or if there are preexisting contralateral cranial nerve deficits. Relative contraindications to surgery include extensive skull base or intracranial involvement, advanced age, medical comorbidities, and bilateral or multiple paragangliomas, which may result in unacceptable postoperative morbidity such as bilateral lower cranial nerve palsies. Paragangliomas are very slowly growing tumors that may not result in cranial nerve dysfunction for long periods of time. In appropriate cases, observation with magnetic resonance imaging (MRI) surveillance may be the most appropriate choice of "treatment."

PREOPERATIVE PLANNING

Computed tomography (CT) is an excellent imaging technique to identify paragangliomas and to document the extent of tumor with precise evaluation of possible bone invasion. The classical CT findings of paragangliomas include a homogenous mass with intense enhancement following intravenous contrast administration. Tumor location, displacement of major vessels, and patterns of involvement or invasion of surrounding structures aid in differentiating the various types of paragangliomas. Vagal paragangliomas may be differentiated from carotid body tumors with CT because they tend to displace both the internal and external carotid arteries anteriorly.

MRI provides meticulous soft tissue detail and defines neural involvement and possible skull base involvement, especially with gadolinium enhancement. Augmented by its ability to image in multiple planes, MRI is superior to CT in defining the relationship of the vagal paragangliomas to adjacent vascular structures. MRI studies of vagal paragangliomas demonstrate a background tumor matrix of intermediate-intensity signal on T1- and proton density–weighted images and moderately high-intensity signal on T2-weighted images along with scattered areas of focal signal voids, reflecting high-flow blood vessels. Intense homogenous contrast enhancement is displayed. On T2-weighted images, the classical MRI "salt and pepper" appearance reflects signal voids mixed with regions of focally high signal intensity. MRI is more effective than CT in identifying small synchronous paragangliomas, especially those tumors smaller than 5 mm. More recent studies have disclosed that unenhanced and contrast-enhanced three-dimension time-of-flight (3D TOF) angiography may be

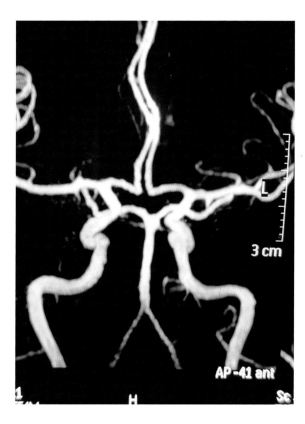

FIGURE 12.4

MRA demonstrating an intact circle of Willis with excellent bilateral cerebral circulation.

even more effective than T1-weighted, dual T2-weighted, and fat-suppressed MRI imaging in detecting small paragangliomas. The imaging studies are also of great importance in ruling out the presence of a vagal paraganglioma on the contralateral side. Bilateral vagal body tumors may be synchronous or metachronous, and this information is critical in formulating a plan of management.

Magnetic resonance angiography (MRA) provides excellent visualization of the major head and neck vasculature and can demonstrate vessel displacement, gross tumor involvement, and possible compromised blood flow to the contralateral brain during surgical injury if there is an incomplete circle of Willis (Fig. 12.4).

Radioisotope scintigraphy provides a noninvasive imaging modality that is particularly useful as a screening method for families with a family history of paragangliomas. Additionally, these studies can aid in the identification of infrequently occurring metastatic disease. Vagal paragangliomas have a high density of somatostatin type 2 receptors on their cell surface. Octreotide is a somatostatin analog that, when coupled to the radioisotope indium [111], creates a scintigraphic image of tumors expressing somatostatin type 2 receptors. [111] Indium pentetreotide (Octreoscan) scintigraphy demonstrates a high accuracy in tumor detection. Octreotide scanning has also been reported to be effective in defining postoperative tumor recurrence with a resolution of up to 1 cm, especially when scarring may make CT or MRI interpretation more difficult. More recently, ^{18}F-DOPA positron emission tomography has proven to be a useful and sensitive tool for the detection of vagal paragangliomas. The study can visualize tumors as small as 1 cm. A variety of additional imaging techniques exist including ^{123}I-metaiodobenzylguanidine (MIBG), ^{18}F-fluorodopamine (^{18}F-FDA-PET), and ^{18}F-fluoro-2-deoxyglucose (^{18}F-FDG-PET).

Angiography plays an important role in the evaluation of vagal paragangliomas if surgery is contemplated. Preoperative evaluation of extensive paragangliomas requires a thorough investigation of the blood supply of the tumor (and possible anastomoses), displacement of vessels, potential compromise of the vessels by tumor invasion, and adequacy of intracranial circulation if sacrifice of the internal carotid artery becomes necessary. Superselective angiography, if necessary for larger tumors, also allows safe preoperative embolization of the tumor vasculature, hopefully avoiding proximal vessel occlusion and unexpected migration of embolization material into the cerebral or systemic circulation.

Although these are vascular tumors, fine needle aspiration biopsy can be safely performed to establish a definitive diagnosis. However, imaging studies with the classical findings of paragangliomas are usually sufficient to render the diagnosis.

SURGICAL TECHNIQUE

Preoperative embolization is performed for large or highly vascular vagal paragangliomas. Although not uniformly accepted, there are major advantages in using combined endovascular embolization and subsequent surgery including a decrease in tumor size associated with interruption of the vascular supply, decreased intraoperative blood loss, and improved visualization of the surrounding anatomy.

Surgery is performed within 2 days of angiography and embolization in order to avoid recruitment of collateral tumor blood supply and prior to the onset of significant postinflammatory effect. Steroids are administered on a short-term basis if there is concern about edema that may compromise dissection. The anesthesiologist must be prepared to counteract the alpha- and beta-adrenergic catecholamine cardiovascular effect when dealing with "secreting" tumors.

There is no substitute for adequate surgical exposure and identification and preservation, if possible, of normal anatomical structures before beginning the tumor resection. This can almost always be accomplished by a transcervical approach. Proximal and distal control of the carotid arteries and the internal jugular vein, especially in dealing with large paragangliomas, insure additional safety.

The extent of skull base or intracranial involvement can vary in vagal paragangliomas. Most vagal paragangliomas originate in the nodose (inferior) ganglion, approximately 2 cm below the jugular foramen. When these tumors grow, they tend to extend to the skull base as well as involve the poststyloid parapharyngeal space. As with all paragangliomas, complete radiographic evaluation with contrast-enhanced MRI and CT studies will define the extent of involvement.

Description of Technique

The patient is placed on the table in a supine position. After the satisfactory induction of general endotracheal anesthesia with a vocal cord motion monitoring tube, the patient's head is turned to the opposite side and the neck is prepped and draped, allowing visualization of the ipsilateral face. A modified Blair incision is outlined extending in the preauricular crease extending toward the mastoid tip and then along the anterior border of the sternomastoid muscle and curving anteriorly below the mandible. This is infiltrated with 1% Xylocaine with 1:100,000 epinephrine. The incision is performed, and skin flaps are elevated anteriorly deep to the platysma muscle and superficial to the parotid fascia. Hemostasis throughout the procedure is accomplished with electrocautery, bipolar cautery, and Harmonic scalpel. The external jugular vein crossing the sternomastoid muscle is ligated, and the greater auricular nerve is sharply transected to provide exposure. The inferior posterior portion of the parotid salivary gland is then separated off the anterior border of the sternomastoid muscle superior to its insertion on the mastoid process. The posterior belly of the digastric muscle and the stylohyoid muscle are then identified deep to the parotid gland. These muscles are mobilized and retracted superiorly. Care is taken not to traumatize the soft tissue of the parotid gland, which is directly superior to the posterior belly of the digastric muscle, since the facial nerve may be just adjacent to the muscle, especially posteriorly. At this point, the contents of the carotid sheath are individually isolated and identified. The internal carotid artery and the internal jugular vein are carefully dissected off of the tumor toward the skull base. The vagal paraganglioma is apparent at this time. Before starting the tumor resection, additional exposure is necessary. The accessory and hypoglossal nerves are identified. The accessory nerve, if possible, should be dissected off of the tumor and retracted posterolaterally. The same should be done with the hypoglossal nerve and retracted superiorly. It should also be noted if these nerves are involved by the paraganglioma, which would require their sacrifice. This would certainly be the situation if there was dysfunction noted preoperatively. Isolation and control of the carotid sheath contents at the level of the hyoid bone will require ligation of the common facial vein. Vessel loops should be placed around the carotid arteries and internal jugular vein. At this time, care is taken that the internal carotid artery flow is not compromised. To obtain proper visualization of the poststyloid parapharyngeal space, total removal of the styloid process is necessary (Fig. 12.5). To accomplish this, a small periosteal elevator should strip all soft tissue off the styloid process. The three muscles attached to the styloid process should be transected at their origin. Using a small bone cutter, the styloid process should then be transected at its attachment to the undersurface of the petrous bone. This will provide much needed increased exposure to the poststyloid area. Additional exposure of this area will result by anterior dislocation of the mandible out of the glenoid fossa. The vagal paraganglioma can then be surgically resected. In uncommon circumstances, the vagus nerve can be preserved and use of the monitoring vocal cord endotracheal tube can help to guide your resection with possible preservation of vocal fold function. Almost always, the vagus nerve requires sacrifice, and with adequate exposure of the skull base, a complete resection can be accomplished. Tumor involvement of the adjacent lower cranial nerves (CNs IX, XII, XII) may require their sacrifice.

After resection, the wound is copiously irrigated with saline, and any bleeding points are controlled with bipolar cautery. A suction drain is then inserted, and the wound is then closed with subcutaneous 4-0 Vicryl and 5-0 Monocryl subcuticular closure.

POSTOPERATIVE MANAGEMENT

The result of vagal dysfunction is quite variable, and the disability is frequently related to the age and general medical condition of the patient. Resection of the vagus nerve results in supraglottic hypesthesia and vocal cord paralysis, and permanent medialization of the vocal cord is therefore necessary. Postoperatively, early

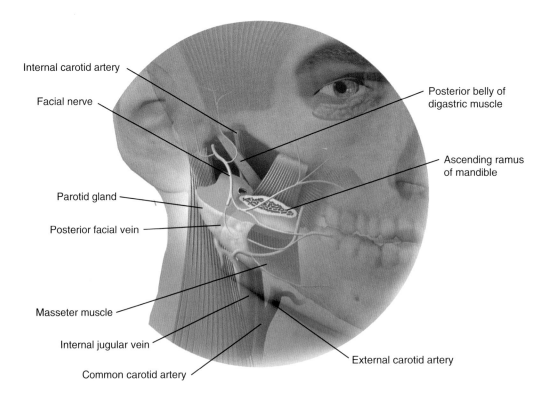

FIGURE 12.5

Illustration of the transcervical approach to the parapharyngeal space with partial cutaway of parotid and mandible for better perspective.

swallowing therapy will help control aspiration. If the vagus nerve has not been sacrificed but is not functioning due to neuropraxia, then temporary vocal cord medialization is indicated to potentiate swallowing and improving voice quality. If there are continuing problems with oral intake and handling secretions, a gastrostomy and possible tracheostomy may be appropriate for proper care. The oropharyngeal hypesthesia resulting from possible sacrifice of the glossopharyngeal nerve is best managed with swallowing therapy, especially with attempts at directing the food bolus to the contralateral side. Dysfunction of the accessory nerve with paralysis of the sternomastoid and trapezius muscles requires physical rehabilitation with active and passive range-of-motion exercises to improve shoulder function.

Hypoglossal nerve dysfunction requires speech and swallowing therapy to rehabilitate the ipsilateral tongue paralysis. If there is an associated vagal and/or glossopharyngeal nerve dysfunction, intensive swallowing therapy assumes an important role in preventing life-threatening aspiration.

Possible Postoperative Rehabilitation

Aspiration and hoarseness (CN X)
  Vocal cord medialization
  Swallowing therapy
Tongue dysfunction (CN XII)
  Speech therapy
Pharyngeal sensation (CN IX)
  Swallowing therapy
Shoulder weakness (CN XI)
  Physical therapy

COMPLICATIONS

In addition to some of the obvious complications such as hematoma/seroma or infection, there are other complications specific to vagal paraganglioma surgery, and these can be grouped into nerve injuries and vascular injuries.

Nerve Injury

Paraganglioma surgery should anticipate postoperative nerve dysfunction, and familiarity with rehabilitation techniques is necessary for proper patient care. If tumor resection results in nerve resection, cable grafts using greater auricular or sural nerve are an option, especially with the accessory and hypoglossal nerves. Rehabilitation for patients with postoperative nerve dysfunction is dependent on the functional deficit and may require additional surgical intervention including transoral hemipalatal adhesion for palatal insufficiency and vocal cord for medialization procedures to potentiate swallowing and improving voice quality.

Dissection in the parapharyngeal space often results in "first bite syndrome," which is characterized by intense pain with the first bite of food at a meal. The pain may be quite severe but subsides as the patient continues the meal. This syndrome develops as a result of sympathetic denervation of the myoepithelial cells of the parotid salivary gland. This problem improves gradually and spontaneously in most patients.

Vascular Injury

The incidence of intraoperative or postoperative stroke has dropped dramatically as surgical and anesthetic techniques have improved. This improvement has been attributed to multiple factors including detailed preoperative imaging and angiographic evaluation to determine vessel involvement by tumor, carotid occlusion testing, and advancements in surgical arterial revascularization techniques. The presence of a vascular surgeon should be anticipated if internal carotid artery involvement is indicated by imaging studies. Vagal paragangliomas are usually not intimately associated with the great vessels, thereby making vascular injury less likely.

PEARLS

- Careful evaluation of imaging studies will provide invaluable information in predicting the ease of surgical exposure and relationship to adjacent vascular and neural structures.
- Focusing on exposure of the tumor and visualization/mobilization of normal vascular and neural structures will allow optimal tumor resection.
- Intraoperative vessel loop control of the major vessels will insure a safer resection, especially if vessel reconstruction is necessary.

- Inclusion of voice and swallowing therapists and physical rehabilitation early in the patient's postoperative course will result in more effective recovery of function.
- Communication with the patient and family concerning postoperative expectations for potential functional problems will set the stage for better addressing these issues if they occur.

PITFALLS

- Identify all normal structures first since the tumor will displace normal anatomy.
- Use care when transecting the base of the styloid process to avoid injury to the facial nerve.
- Identify, dissect, and mobilize the superior extent of the internal carotid artery to avoid injury during mobilization of the tumor.
- Careful hemostasis will allow for better identification and preservation of vascular and neural structures.

INSTRUMENTS TO HAVE AVAILABLE

- Nerve stimulator
- Facial nerve monitor
- Nerve monitoring endotracheal tube
- Hemostatic agents—for example, oxidized cellulose, collagen, fibrin sealants, and polysaccharide hemostatics
- Bipolar cautery
- Vessel loops for retracting nerves and blood vessels

SUGGESTED READING

1   Netterville JL, Jackson CG, Miller FR, et al. Vagal paraganglioma: a review of 46 patients treated during a 20-year period. *Arch Otolaryngol Head Neck Surg* 1998;124:1133–1140.
2   Sniezek JC, Netterville JL, Sabri AN. Vagal paragangliomas. *Otolaryngol Clin North Am* 2001;34(5):925–939.
3   Persky MS, Setton A, Niimi Y, et al. Combined endovascular and surgical treatment of head and neck paragangliomas—a team approach. *Head Neck* 2002;24:423–431.
4   Persky MS, Hu K. Paragangliomas of the head and neck. In: Harrison LB, Sessions RB, Hong WK, et al., eds. *Head and Neck Cancer: A Multidisciplinary Approach*. Philadelphia, PA: Lippincott Williams & Wilkins, 2009:655–687.

13 INTRAOPERATIVE MEDIALIZATION LARYNGOPLASTY (THYROPLASTY TYPE I)

Ricardo L. Carrau

INTRODUCTION

A paralyzed true vocal fold (TVF) affects all the basic laryngeal functions, decreasing its ability to protect the tracheobronchial airways during swallowing, reducing the efficiency and strength of the cough, eliminating the natural positive pressure on expiration (that aids with inflation of the lungs), and causing varied degrees of dysphonia and vocal fatigue. In addition, a TVF palsy decreases the efficiency of a Valsalva maneuver; thus, patients may exhibit problems lifting significant weight or forcing a bowel movement. Medialization of a paralyzed cord does not restore all these functions, but it facilitates neuromuscular compensation by the unaffected contralateral side.

A medialization laryngoplasty or thyroplasty type I involves the medialization of a paralyzed or paretic TVF by the insertion of a paraglottic implant. Silicone and polytetrafluoroethylene (Gortex; W.L. Gore and Associates, Newark, DE) are the most commonly implanted, but others, such as titanium, hydroxyapatite, cartilage, fascia, acellular dermis, and an adjustable balloon, have been reported.

Most surgeons prefer to complete this procedure under local anesthesia and sedation to observe the function of the vocal fold (VF) and adjust the implant according to changes in the patient's voice, cough, and airway. In select patients, however, such as those undergoing elective sacrifice due to oncologic surgery, or in patients who suffer iatrogenic or penetrating trauma to the neck with injury to the recurrent laryngeal or vagus nerve, an immediate thyroplasty (i.e., done at the same stage as the oncologic resection or exploratory surgery) may correct a potential glottic gap before symptoms arise.

HISTORY

Medialization laryngoplasty or thyroplasty type I was first described and later popularized by Isshiki during the 1970s. In 1993, Netterville reported on the immediate medialization of the TVF following skull base or head and neck surgeries involving the sacrifice of the vagus or recurrent laryngeal nerves. He demonstrated the safety and efficacy of the technique, thus improving the expediency of the rehabilitation of patients with a vagal or recurrent nerve injury.

PHYSICAL EXAMINATION

A preoperative or intraoperative cervical examination ascertains the presence of masses, scars, or excessive subcutaneous adipose tissue, which may interfere with the exposure or alter the plan of surgery. In patients undergoing elective surgery, a preoperative flexible fiberoptic laryngoscopy offers unparalleled advantages to ascertain the functions of the larynx, namely, airway, swallowing, voice, and cough. Special consideration is taken to ascertain the position of the VFs and arytenoids (horizontal and vertical planes) during normal and forced ventilation, vocalization, and cough, as well as the VFs tone, bulk, and mucosal integrity. However, due to the indications and nature of an immediate thyroplasty I, the surgeon cannot ascertain the functional position of the VF and arytenoid after the vagus or recurrent laryngeal nerve has been injured or sacrificed. Some patients, however, may have presented preoperative paresis associated with hoarseness, shortness of breath, or dysphagia. These symptoms should be assessed preoperatively as they are assumed to worsen postoperatively. A functional assessment of all cranial nerves is fundamental, as it has implications regarding the outcome of voice/speech and swallowing and possibly the extent of the resection.

INDICATIONS

An immediate thyroplasty is indicated in patients undergoing elective sacrifice of the vagus or recurrent laryngeal nerve due to oncologic surgery or in patients who suffer iatrogenic or penetrating trauma to the neck with injury to either of these nerves.

CONTRAINDICATIONS

A contraindication to an immediate thyroplasty is the presence, or suspicion, of glottic airway stenosis due to edema or abductor paralysis or paresis of the contralateral TVF. A relative contraindication is the presence of a coagulopathy, congenital or acquired. This situation, however, is rare in patients undergoing elective surgery, although it might be encountered in patients with trauma to the neck.

PREOPERATIVE PLANNING

Whenever possible, an informed consent (from the patient or relatives) should be obtained clarifying goals, expectations, and risks. This is important, as an immediate thyroplasty is associated with a greater need for revision (for misplacement and under- or overcorrection).

An immediate thyroplasty type I requires no other preparation other than that indicated by the clinical examination and flexible fiberoptic laryngoscopy. I empirically use broad-spectrum perioperative prophylactic antibiotics and systemic corticosteroids.

TECHNIQUE

Positioning of the neck and placement of the incision are often dictated by the requirements of the oncologic surgery and/or the need to control the great vessels of the neck. If possible, however, the neck is positioned in neutral or slightly extended position. Similarly, the best placement for the incision is a skin crease near the level of the inferior edge of the thyroid cartilage. In many instances, however, the thyroplasty type I is completed through the incision for the primary surgery or an extension.

The laryngotracheal complex should be stabilized using a single- or double-hook retractor lodged at the inferior or superior border of the thyroid cartilage. It can also be used to retract and rotate the thyroid cartilage to facilitate visualization. The strap muscles and perichondrium are retracted with a blunt Senn retractor to expose the cartilage of the thyroid ala (Fig. 13.1). Posteroinferiorly, the insertion of the sternothyroid muscle is transected using a bipolar electrocautery, thus exposing the inferior border of the thyroid ala. This exposure is similar to that of a vertical hemilaryngectomy.

A window is then made in the thyroid ala in order to insert a prosthesis. The dimensions of the window differ according to the dimensions of the thyroid ala (vary with height, gender, and age). Most windows range between 4×8 mm and 5×10 mm and are placed 3 to 4 mm above the inferior border of the ala and 5 mm (i.e., women) to 10 mm (i.e., men) posterior to midline (Fig. 13.2). A high-speed drill with a 2-mm coarse diamond or hybrid burr is most commonly used, since most adults have undergone some ossification of the inferior aspect of the thyroid ala. Typically, the window is drilled down until the inner cortex of the thyroid ala has been thinned enough to be removed with 1- to 2-mm bone curette. Care is taken to drill out the window at perpendicular angles (avoiding "saucerization"), especially at the inferior aspect. Thinning of the lower strut may lead to fracturing, which will cause difficulty in stabilizing the implant. After exposure of the inner perichondrium, a bone curette, Cottle, or duckbill elevator is inserted between the alar cartilage and the inner perichondrium to widen this space. Alternatively, in patients whose cartilage has not ossified, the margins of the window can be cut using a no. 67 Beaver blade and the cartilage elevated with a middle ear spatula or Cottle elevator.

The inner perichondrium is initially preserved during the window elevation or drilling; however, once the dissection is completed, I prefer to incise it following the long axis of the window. This maneuver allows the implant to medialize only the muscle corresponding to this area instead of medializing the entire inner perichondrium (paraglottic space) (Fig. 13.3). A small artery will usually be encountered at the most posterior aspect of the incision and can be obliterated with the bipolar electrocautery. Others have reported the

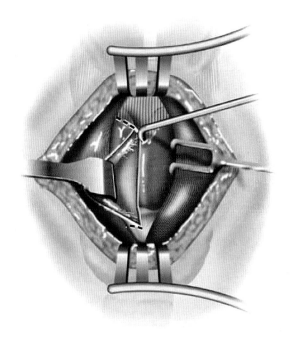

FIGURE 13.1 The thyroid cartilage is exposed through a transcervical horizontal incision close to the level of the inferior edge of the thyroid ala. Alternatively it can be exposed through the same incision (or extension of the incision) used for an oncologic resection or cervical exploration. Elevate subplatysmal flaps, divide strap muscles and perichondrium in the midline, and elevate them from the thyroid ala en bloc. Stabilization of the larynx with a single or double hook greatly facilitates this dissection and opening of the window.

use of polytetrafluoroethylene or premade silicone prosthesis; however, I prefer to carve an implant from a medium-density medical-quality silicone block. Despite the "extra" work involved, this allows better customization of the implant, does not undergo reorganization like the polytetrafluoroethylene strip, and is more cost-effective. The implant is carved to be wider and longer than the window and to have a "peg" that will protrude through the window (Fig. 13.3). The former avoids extrusion of the implant through the window, and the latter prevents migration in the coronal or sagittal planes. In fact, the prosthesis extends 4 to 6 mm posterior to the window to place the point of maximal medialization (4 to 5 mm deep) as far back as possible. This helps to avoid and sometimes corrects an anterior subluxation of the arytenoid cartilage.

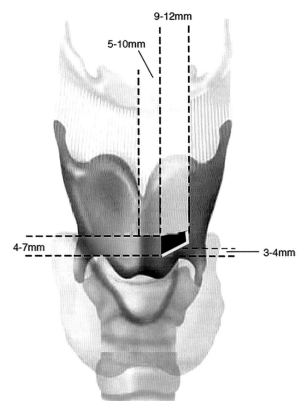

FIGURE 13.2 Approximate dimensions and position of the thyroplasty window. During an immediate thyroplasty, the window is opened as close to the inferior edge of the thyroid ala as possible while still preserving an inferior strut.

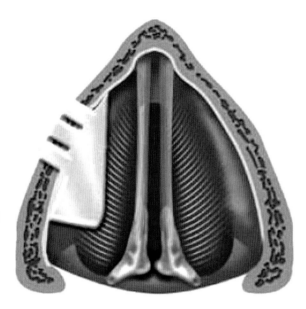

FIGURE 13.3
Paraglottic silicone implant medializing the vocal process and VF. The implant adds bulk to the VF and, in some cases, displaces the arytenoid posteriorly. The implant is adjustable, is partially reversible, and is associated with a relatively low degree of technical difficulty and low morbidity. In addition, it does not interfere with neural recovery.

Transverse incisions through the coronal plane of the "peg," and extending halfway into the implant allow the surgeon to bend the silicone implant, which facilitates its insertion (Fig. 13.3). Once the implant is inserted and stabilized, the strap muscles and perichondrium are reapproximated with absorbable sutures. The skin is closed using a multilayer technique.

POSTOPERATIVE MANAGEMENT

Patients are advised to rest their voice for 72 hours and to avoid activities that may require a Valsalva maneuver. Antitussive medications and humidified air can be provided as needed. Corticosteroids may be continued empirically.

COMPLICATIONS

The most common complication of an immediate thyroplasty type I is failure to correct the glottic gap due to over- or undermedicalization of the VF. Inadequate placement of the implant, either too cephalad into the ventricle (or false cord) or too caudal into the subglottis, or too anterior causing early anterior contact, is also relatively common. Extrusion of the implant into the ventricle, infection, and airway compromise are possible but rare complications.

RESULTS

Overall, the results after an immediate thyroplasty are satisfactory. The great majority of the patients will be able to protect the tracheobronchial tree against aspiration and will be satisfied with their voice. Nonetheless, a professional voice user may require revision of the prosthesis or adjunctive procedures such as arytenoid repositioning to reach an optimal result.

PEARLS

- Stabilization of the laryngotracheal complex with a single- or double-hook retractor greatly facilitates the exposure and opening of the thyroid ala window, as well as the insertion of the implant.
- Window and implant are placed as inferior as possible on the thyroid ala.
- A high-speed burr with a 2-mm burr is the safest way of opening the thyroid ala window.
- Incise the inner perichondrium to avoid medializing the entire hemilarynx.
- The point of maximal medialization should be as far posterior as possible. This helps to avoid the anterior displacement of the arytenoid cartilage.
- Be fastidious with hemostasis.

PITFALLS

- An immediate thyroplasty is based on empirical medialization of the TVF as the true functional deficit cannot be assessed reliably in the vast majority of patients; thus, the need for revision is higher than a thyroplasty performed under sedation.
- Beware of fracturing the inferior cartilagenous strut. If fractured, it can be repaired using wire or a 1.5-mm titanium adaptation plate.
- Beware of an artery medial to the inner perichondrium close to the posterior aspect of the window.

INSTRUMENTS TO HAVE AVAILABLE

- Flexible fiberoptic laryngoscope
- Bovie electrocautery with insulated tip
- Bipolar electrocautery and insulated bayonet
- Double-hook retractor
- Single-hook retractor
- Senn retractor (dull)
- High-speed drill
- 2-mm hybrid burr
- Bone curette 1 and 2 mm
- Cottle elevator
- Middle ear duckbill elevator
- Medium-density medical silicone block
- 0.4-mm thick Gore-Tex patch (alternate)

SUGGESTED READING

Netterville JL, Jackson CG, Civantos F. Thyroplasty in the functional rehabilitation of neurotologic skull base surgery patients. *Am J Otol* 1993;14(5):460–464.

Carrau R, Herlich A, Rosen C. Visualization of the glottis through a laryngeal mask during medialization laryngoplasty. How I do it. *Laryngoscope* 1998;108(5):769–771.

Carrau R, Pou A, Eibling D, et al. Laryngeal framework surgery for the treatment of aspiration. *Oper Tech Otolaryngol Head Neck Surg* 1998;9:126–134.

Pou A, Carrau R, Eibling D, et al. Laryngeal framework surgery for the management of aspiration in high vagal lesions. *Am J Otolaryngol* 1998;19:1–7.

Carrau R, Pou A, Eibling D, et al. Laryngeal framework surgery for the management of aspiration. *Head Neck* 1999;21(2):139–145.

Jalisi S, Netterville JL. Rehabilitation after cranial base surgery. *Otolaryngol Clin North Am* 2009;42(1):49–56, viii.

Young VN, Zullo TG, Rosen CA. Analysis of laryngeal framework surgery: 10-year follow-up to a national survey. *Laryngoscope* 2010;120(8):1602–1608.

14

OPEN THYROIDECTOMY

Jeremy L. Freeman

INTRODUCTION

The traditional approach for surgery of the thyroid gland is through the open technique. There has been a recent movement in some centers toward minimally invasive procedures, which include the minimally invasive video-assisted thyroidectomy innovated by the Italian surgeons and transaxillary robotic procedures made popular by the Korean group. I limit my remarks to the open technique.

Thyroidectomy is performed for structural and functional problems of the thyroid. The structural issues that require surgical consideration are tumors or other masses that compress adjacent organs (larynx, trachea, esophagus), tumors that are or are thought to be malignant, or large unsightly tumors. The vast majority of functional problems requiring thyroidectomy are hyperthyroid states.

Thyroidectomy has been performed in one form or another since the 12th century. Up until the late 19th century, it had been looked upon as a "dangerous" operation not to be taken lightly with the mortality being exceedingly high. Then, on to the surgical scene came Theodor Kocher, who was Chair of Surgery at the University of Bern, Switzerland. He refined the technique, bringing operative morbidity and mortality to an acceptable level; he was able to teach his methods to a host of surgeons from around the world, including William Halstead and Charles Mayo. Kocher won the Nobel Prize for thyroid surgery and left a legacy of technical skill so that surgeons around the world can now perform this procedure with safety and efficiency.

A brief discussion of the pathology of thyroid neoplasms is provided below in a separate section. In general, the broad classification of thyroid neoplasms includes benign tumors, well-differentiated malignant tumors, poorly differentiated malignant tumors, and medullary thyroid cancer. The incidence of thyroid cancer is increasing at a staggering rate—according to the American Cancer Society, the incidence has almost quadrupled in the last 20 years. However, the mortality rate has remained constant—this suggests that the true incidence is probably not rising but our detection rate, usually of tiny lesions, is. This increase in incidence is probably due to the increased use of ultrasonography of the neck, which is highly sensitive and detects masses in the thyroid that would not have been discovered by clinical examination, and if malignant, these masses may have never become clinically significant. In addition, there is an increased awareness by pathologists of the fine nuances of pathologic diagnosis of cancer of the thyroid, and perhaps the criteria applied recently would not have been in the past.

It must be borne in mind that a large segment of the population harbors asymptomatic microscopic cancer of the thyroid. Reports vary in autopsy and surgical studies; the highest incidence of cancer of the thyroid found in autopsies is in the Japanese and Finnish population (>30%). This fact should be considered when making decisions regarding management of microscopic disease detected by ultrasonography.

Several organizations such as the American Thyroid Association, National Comprehensive Cancer Network, and the British Thyroid Association have gone to great lengths to establish guidelines for the management of thyroid masses.

Benign masses in the thyroid gland can be disorders of colloid metabolism (i.e., colloid nodules), inflammatory conditions (i.e., various forms of thyroiditis such as Hashimoto's), and benign neoplasms such as follicular adenoma. Malignant tumors of follicular cell origin are either well or poorly differentiated. Tumors of parafollicular or C cells are medullary cancers of the thyroid.

The most common, well-differentiated thyroid malignancy is papillary carcinoma of the thyroid (PTC). There are now well-documented criteria for making the diagnosis. There are morphologic criteria, which consist of the identification of papillary formation, but it is necessary to detect nuclear and cytoplasmic criteria as well. The latter includes washed out nuclei (Orphan Annie nuclei), nuclear grooves, nuclear inclusions, micronucleoli, powdery chromatin, cellular overlapping and crowding, psammoma bodies, and atypical cells.

There exists a spectrum of pathologic appearances of PTC, which correlates with biologic aggressiveness of the cancer and ultimately outcome—these next three variants are the poorly differentiated types. Next in aggressive activity to the common PTC described above is the tall cell variant in which >50% of the lesion is comprised of cells where the height to width ratio is >3:1. Prognosis is poorer in this cancer than the more common PTC. Further along the spectrum is insular carcinoma in which the malignant-appearing cells tend to form little distinct islands or "insulae." This is a particularly aggressive cancer. The final type of the PTC group is anaplastic carcinoma, which may demonstrate all of the characteristics of lesions mentioned above but has a highly malignant appearance with many bizarre cells, mitoses, and invasive behavior. This is one of the most aggressive cancers in the body, and the outcome is universally fatal. PTC is characterized by a significant propensity for regional metastatic spread to the central compartment lymph nodes and less frequently to the lateral neck.

The second common well-differentiated malignancy is follicular carcinoma. This cancer is characterized by vascular and/or capsular invasion. It should be noted that often the cells appear benign, but the aforementioned criteria qualify this tumor as malignant. Follicular carcinoma can metastasize to distant sites, most commonly to the lungs, by hematogenous routes. Results of treatment of this cancer are generally somewhat worse than the more common PTC. The third type of follicular-derived malignancy is the Hurthle cell carcinoma. This is a cancer comprised predominantly of "Hurthle cells" (also known as Ashkenazy cells or oncocytes) and is thought to be a variant of follicular cells. These cells are cuboidal and contain granular, eosinophilic cytoplasm. They are rich in mitochondria. These cancers may also demonstrate, as with follicular carcinoma, vascular and/or capsular invasion.

Medullary carcinoma of the thyroid, in contrast to the follicular cell–derived cancers, originates from parafollicular or C cells, which embryologically are neural crest derivatives. The cancer is comprised of spindle-shaped cells in varying degrees of organization. One of the hallmarks of this cancer is the presence of amyloid detected by Congo red staining. This cancer can occur in a hereditary fashion, sporadically or with multiple endocrine neoplasia (MEN) syndromes. This cancer displays varying tendencies to aggressive behavior but has a marked propensity for lymph node metastases. The cancer secretes calcitonin and carcinoembryonic antigen so that immunohistochemical staining of these substances can make the diagnosis pathologically. Diagnosis and surveillance are also aided by serum determinations of both of these markers. Detection can also be made of the hereditary types in many cases by the determination of ret oncogene in the blood—this oncogene allows identification of suspected cases via umbilical cord blood in the newborn and in suspected family members in known kindreds facilitating early management of potentially lethal cases. The pathology in patients with hyperthyroid states demonstrate hyperplastic and convoluted papillae with a background of an inflammatory picture consistent with an autoimmune condition.

HISTORY

The usual presentation is a mass in the thyroid. In the era before the widespread use of ultrasonography, most masses were detected by palpation. Now most masses are detected by ultrasound and to a lesser extent computed tomography (CT), magnetic resonance imaging (MRI), or positron emission tomography, and in a large number of cases, these masses are incidental findings on imaging done for reasons other than suspicion of a thyroid problem. Some patients present with compressive symptoms such as dysphagia or airway compromise either acute or chronic due to a large mass in the thyroid or diffuse enlargement due to colloid goiter, thyroiditis or malignancy. A small number of patients with cancer may present with evidence of metastatic spread usually to the lateral neck before the primary in the thyroid has been discovered. It is rare for patients to have distant metastases at the time of their first presentation.

The history of medullary cancer of the thyroid may be similar to PTC; however, with the advent of advanced biochemical and molecular testing, patients with this disease may be detected by elevated calcitonin and/or increase in serum ret oncogene determination. In infants with a known genetic predisposition, analysis of umbilical cord blood for ret oncogene can make the diagnosis at birth thereby allowing early intervention. Elucidation of a family history is important as this may give a clue as to the genetics and the need to manage family members. In addition, patients should be asked about symptoms as they pertain to multiple endocrine neoplasia type 2 (MEN 2).

Patients with a hyper- or hypofunctioning gland present with systemic symptoms consistent with metabolic hyper or hypoactivity. Thus, patients with hyperthyroidism may complain of nervousness, anxiety, heat intolerance, weight loss, tachycardia, tremors, and inability to focus, concentrate, or sleep. Patients with Graves disease have exophthalmos. Patients with hypofunction complain of fatigue, weight gain, and sluggishness. The primary management of hyperfunction is medical with surgery reserved for those patients who fail medical

TABLE 14.1 Risk Factors		
Patient Factors	**Tumor Factors**	**Imaging Factors**
• Age	• Dysphagia	• Invasive lesion
• Elevated serum calcitonin	• Firm/fixed nodule	• Metastatic nodes
• Ethnicity	• Lymphadenopathy	• Stippled calcification
• Family history (syndrome)	• Rapid increase in size	
• Place of birth	• Size >4 cm	
• Radiation exposure	• Suspicious/atypical/positive cytology	
	• Vocal cord paresis	

Source: Mt. Sinai Hospital/University of Toronto.

management. It is still not known specifically what the hormonal effect of pregnancy is on thyroid masses, but at times women will present with a thyroid mass or malignancy during pregnancy. This brings up a management dilemma. Surgery is deferred until term unless the tumor is causing significant compression or the malignancy is high grade or demonstrating aggressive behavior. Hyperfunctioning glands in pregnancy sometimes require surgical management if symptoms and biochemistry are not controlled by medical management.

It is important, in patients in whom follicular cell–derived malignancy is suspected, that a thorough history be obtained for patient- or tumor-related risk factors (see Table 14.1). Clarification of these factors significantly affects decision making for surgical intervention.

Patients should be questioned about how they perceive their body image with large cosmetically obtrusive masses. Certainly a patient's own desires regarding the removal of a mass should be considered in making a decision for intervention or not.

PHYSICAL EXAMINATION

Most tumors are palpable and often visible when the patient presents with a mass that has been detected clinically. In patients whose tumors have been discovered by imaging, the mass is usually not palpable. Careful documentation of the characteristics of the mass should be performed as clues that may help facilitate diagnosis and surgical approach may be established (e.g., retrosternal goiter focuses attention to an approach to the mediastinum and a fixed hard mass may suggest malignancy). Those patients who present with lymph node metastasis present with palpable adenopathy in the lateral neck compartment(s).

Examination of the larynx is mandatory in any patient with a mass in the thyroid. The presence of impairment of vocal cord mobility in the presence of a mass in the thyroid is a strong predictor of an invasive malignancy.

Patients with hyperthyroidism should have a thorough system review for the documentation of signs of metabolic abnormalities.

INDICATIONS

Total Thyroidectomy

1. Patients with FNA proven follicular cell–derived cancer
2. Patients with a high risk for cancer (e.g., 70-year-old man from the Philippines with 6-cm nodule, stippled calcification on ultrasound, and suspicious cytology)
3. Patients with medullary carcinoma of the thyroid
4. Patients with compressive symptoms and diffuse thyroid disease
5. Patients with large, unsightly, or symptomatic goiters
6. Patients with hyperthyroidism

Subtotal Thyroidectomy

1. Patients with unilateral, solitary masses with a low index of suspicion for malignancy (e.g., 25-year-old white female with a 2-cm nodule with benign or indeterminate cytology)
2. Patients with compressive symptoms and a unilateral mass

CONTRAINDICATIONS

1. Patient with a diagnosis of anaplastic carcinoma with massive locally invasive tumor
2. A systemically infirm patient with severe organ failure (e.g., severe cardiac compromise, dementia, and renal disease)

It may be efficacious to remove primary follicular cell cancers of the thyroid in the face of distant metastases to facilitate the administration of radioactive iodine.

PREOPERATIVE PLANNING

The patient with a mass in the thyroid gland should have a serum thyroid stimulating hormone level, an ultrasound, and a fine needle aspiration (FNA) biopsy. FNA is an extremely useful diagnostic modality, but the sensitivity and specificity are still not high enough that clinicians can put a great deal of confidence in the results, unless malignancy is reported; this cytologic diagnosis can be relied upon. There are myriad reporting systems according to country, institution, and individuals. A major attempt has been made to standardize reporting of FNA results by the National Institutes of Health, which is referred to as the "Bethesda Classification."

Based on the history, physical examination, imaging, and FNA result, the patient can be classified as being low or high risk for malignancy. While there is no formula using the above parameters, there are risk factors that are noteworthy to predict for malignancy (Table 14.1). From a patient perspective they include ethnicity (Filipinos have a very high incidence of thyroid cancer) or exposure to ionizing radiation remotely. Tumor factors include rapid enlargement or evidence of regional metastases. An imaging finding that is highly predictive of cancer is stippled calcification on ultrasound or CT/MRI. Malignant, suspicious, or atypical cytology on FNA is highly predictive of cancer. The whole of the clinical and investigatory picture should be analyzed to determine a risk category.

Those patients with a large retrosternal goiter, compressive symptoms, suspected regional metastases, or invasive tumors should have cross-sectional imaging to demonstrate extent of disease. This study is helpful in decision making for approaching the thyroid through transcervical versus sternotomy access.

Patients in whom medullary carcinoma of the thyroid is suspected should have certain studies including serum calcitonin, carcinoembryonic antigen, as well as ultrasound of the thyroid and cross-sectional imaging of the neck, thorax, and abdomen (looking for metastatic disease). Ret oncogene determination is done for suspected family members in hereditary and syndromic situations.

Patients with hyperthyroidism usually have been thoroughly evaluated by an endocrinologist by the time they are referred to a surgeon. They will have had thyroid function studies, uptake radioactive scanning, and imaging. As mentioned above, these individuals have usually failed medical management from a biochemical or symptomatic point of view; they may have been intolerant to the medication or their symptoms are so severe that surgical intervention is mandatory.

Patients with hyperthyroidism are given a 1-week preoperative course of potassium iodide to assist in minimizing vascularity of the gland. It is mandatory that beta blockade be continued pre- and postoperatively to mitigate against a thyroid storm.

SURGICAL TECHNIQUE

There are two basic surgical procedures for open thyroidectomy; total or subtotal. Since total thyroidectomy is actually a bilateral subtotal procedure, only a subtotal procedure will be described.

The surgery is performed under general anesthesia; local anesthesia is possible in those rare cases where a patient has a major aversion to general. There is, however, no compelling advantage for a local anesthetic. Patients are placed in the prone position with a bolster under the shoulders to extend the neck. Care should be taken in patients with cervical spine disease. Some surgeons prefer not to place a bolster, claiming that this maneuver distorts the anatomy of the recurrent laryngeal nerve.

The incision is planned midway between the cricoid cartilage and the sternal notch (Fig. 14.1). It is preferable to place the incision more superiorly in pliable neck skin rather than inferiorly toward the clavicles; this mitigates against migration of the incision caudad and unsightly scarring. The breadth of the incision is usually from the medial borders of the sternomastoid muscles. In the patient with a short neck in which the cricoid cartilage almost touches the sternal notch, it is necessary to place the incision on the cricoid. If a uni- or bilateral neck dissection is necessary, the incision is extended toward the mastoid tip on one or both sides.

Superior and inferior flaps are elevated using blended cutting and coagulation cautery. Appropriate elevation is performed for the neck dissection if required through the extended incision. Securing of the flaps is maintained by suturing the skin edge to the drapes. I have tried a number of securing techniques including self-retaining retractors and dural hooks but has found that simple suturing with 1-0 silk works best.

The midline raphe is then divided from the sternal notch to as close to the thyroid notch as possible in order to facilitate exposure of the gland. I then gently place my finger between the sternothyroid muscle and

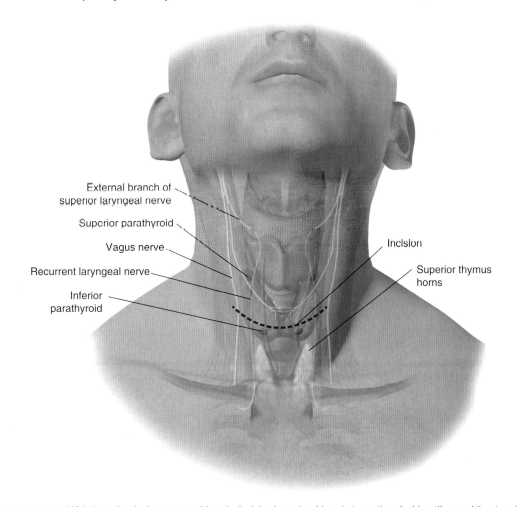

FIGURE 14.1 With the patient in the prone position, the incision is made midway between the cricoid cartilage and the sternal notch. Incisions placed more superiorly are more cosmetic than those approaching the sternal notch.

The labels in the figure read: External branch of superior laryngeal nerve; Superior parathyroid; Vagus nerve; Recurrent laryngeal nerve; Inferior parathyroid; Incision; Superior thymus horns.

the sternohyoid muscle (on both sides if total thyroidectomy is performed) to bluntly develop the intervening plane. With a Jackson retractor gently retracting the sternohyoid, the deep strap sternothyroid is demonstrated. This latter broad-banded muscle is then divided horizontally with cautery to facilitate exposure of the thyroid. This has been decried by some surgeons with the assertion that it compromises phonation; since there is no compelling evidence supporting this and I have not personally seen this occur; I have therefore continued to employ division of the muscle. With gentle blunt dissection using a "peanut dissector," the divided ends of the sternohyoid muscle are reflected superiorly and inferiorly off the gland. The entire lobe of the thyroid should be exposed at this point.

Identification of the recurrent laryngeal nerve and the inferior parathyroid glands is the next step. With the entire lobe exposed, it is prudent to identify the trachea for landmark purposes. I use a "pinch burn technique" using bipolar cautery. The ophthalmic bipolar cautery can be used as a precision cutting and coagulation instrument by holding the tissue, gently bringing the tips together, holding the tissue while current is applied, gently squeezing the tissue, and, while the current is still on, sliding the tips off. Using this technique, the central compartment tissue abutting the inferior border of the isthmus of the thyroid is dissected free thereby exposing the airway.

Attention is now directed to the lateral aspect of the lobe to be resected. The surgeon's thumb of the non–instrument-bearing hand applies traction to the trachea, pushing it to the opposite side. A Jackson retractor applies gentle traction on the cut end of the inferior sternohyoid muscle hooking it at a 45-degree angle to the airway and pulling it inferolaterally. This maneuver exposes the triangle bounded by the carotid artery, the lateral border of the trachea, and the inferior border of the thyroid lobe. The recurrent laryngeal nerve will almost always be found in this triangle. A "peanut" dissector in this triangle in the direction of the excursion of the nerve will find the structure easily. At times the nerve will not be found here but will be in the vicinity. Sweeping the adjacent soft tissue from superior to inferior in the direction of the nerve will expose it when it is not in the triangle. Some surgeons locate and confirm the physiologic integrity of the nerve using nerve monitors. I feel that this is not a substitute for a sound surgical anatomical knowledge of the nerve position; atraumatic surgical technique ensures the electrophysiologic well-being of the nerve.

If one is resecting the right lobe and difficulty is encountered identifying the right recurrent nerve, consideration should be given that a "nonrecurrent laryngeal nerve" is present. This occurs in about 1% of nerves. Attention should then be given to the superior aspect of the lobe looking for the nerve coming directly from the carotid sheath coursing to the posterior aspect of the cricothyroid joint.

In removing a very large mass with a significant mediastinal component, blunt finger dissection along the surface of the gland is usually effective in delivering the mass from the mediastinum into the neck, allowing for identification of the nerve and parathyroid glands. Most large mediastinal masses can be removed by a transcervical method. Sternotomy is not usually necessary but may have to be done for deeply plunging tumors, malignancies thought to invade the great vessels in the mediastinum, tumors that descend behind the innominate artery and vena cava, or in patients who are short and squat making transcervical removal technically difficult.

Once the position of the nerve is confirmed visually, the inferior parathyroid gland should be identified. It is usually found as a 2 × 3-mm caramel-colored ellipsoid structure at the superior horn of the thymus gland in the lateral axis of the thyroid and thymus. However, the position can be quite variable and identification is made visually. The parathyroid gland at times may be buried within the substance of the thymus or in the superior mediastinum, making easy identification through the standard neck approach difficult. Larger inferior thyroid vessels can be ligated with sutures or clips; smaller ones are managed with bipolar cautery.

Attention is now turned to the superior aspect of the lobe. A small Jackson retractor is placed under the sternohyoid muscle to expose the lobe that is covered by the superior cut end of the sternothyroid muscle. Bipolar cautery dissects the muscle in a cephalad direction off the superior lobe.

With a large mass or a mass that has a significant mediastinal component, it may be necessary to release the upper pole as described below in order to facilitate identification of the inferior parathyroid gland and the recurrent nerve inferiorly. The space between the medial aspect of the upper lobe and the cricothyroid muscle is then identified (Joll space). A "peanut" dissector then is used to apply a gentle sweeping motion to the medial aspect of the lobe thereby separating it from the cricothyroid muscle and exposing the Joll space. The small wisp of the external branch of the superior laryngeal nerve (EBSLN) is then seen coursing from lateral to medial lying on the surface of the muscle usually under a serosal layer.

Once the EBSLN has been secured, an Allis clamp is applied to the superior lobe and it is pulled in an inferior direction. The superior thyroid vascular axis is then identified and the vessels are ligated separately with either cautery or suture ligation.

A larger Jackson retractor is then placed so that the sternohyoid muscle is retracted laterally perpendicular to the airway. The interface between the investing fascia and the gland proper is then identified, and the fascia is then dissected free of the gland laterally approximately halfway along the lateral border. The superior parathyroid gland that looks similar to the inferior one is usually seen along this lateral border and can safely be swept laterally on its blood supply. This superior gland derives its major blood supply from the inferior thyroid axis along the thyrothymic axis, but contributions are also from the superior thyroid vascular axis. It is essential to ensure that the entire superior aspect of the thyroid is included in the specimen. A common error is to leave thyroid tissue in the bed by ligating the superior vessels low on the gland (Fig. 14.2).

Once all the above are completed, the previously identified recurrent laryngeal nerve is then traced to its entrance into the posterior aspect of the cricothyroid joint. The technique employed is spreading the tissue above and just medial to the nerve with a fine hemostat and coagulating this tissue with bipolar cautery. At times thyroid tissue can abut the nerve just as it is entering the joint. It may be necessary to

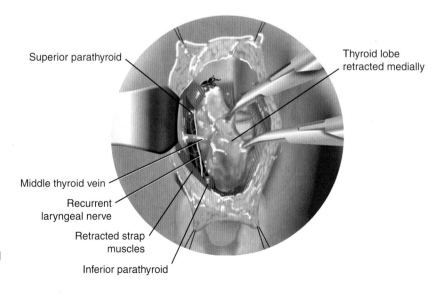

FIGURE 14.2

The recurrent laryngeal nerve and superior/inferior parathyroid glands are displayed with the thyroid lobe retracted medially on the trachea.

Superior parathyroid

Thyroid lobe retracted medially

Middle thyroid vein

Recurrent laryngeal nerve

Retracted strap muscles

Inferior parathyroid

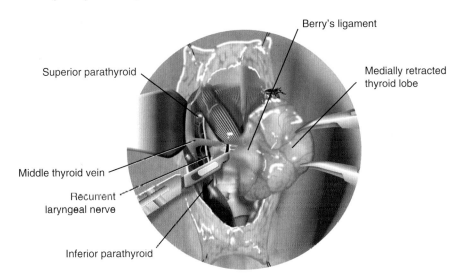

FIGURE 14.3 All relevant anatomy is displayed. Note the EBSLN is shown as it enters the cricothyroid muscle (this nerve should be identifiable in the majority of cases). Sharp dissection is this case (or bipolar cautery dissection) is used to divide the thyrotracheal (Berry) ligament to release the lobe from the airway.

use scalpel dissection to separate the thyroid from the nerve. This is another common area to inadvertently leave thyroid tissue. The suspensory ligament of Berry that attaches the fascia investing the gland to the cricoid and trachea is located just medial to the nerve as it enters the larynx; the cephalocaudad length varies between patients. Usually sharp dissection or bipolar cautery is necessary to separate the gland from the trachea at this point (Figs. 14.3 and 14.4). Pinch burning with bipolar cautery then precisely allows removal of the underside of the gland from the underlying tracheal cartilage. This is performed until the gland is about 1 cm from the nerve and then monopolar cautery can be used. It should be ensured that the pyramidal lobe is identified and followed superiorly as much as technically possible to be included in the specimen. This latter maneuver allows maximum removal of thyroid tissue if radioactive iodine administration is contemplated.

If a total thyroidectomy is to be performed, the same procedure is carried out on the opposite side. If a subtotal procedure is done, then a Kelly clamp is applied vertically across the contralateral lobe and the lobe in question is resected and sent to pathology. It is preferable to perform as extensive a procedure that allows exposure of the trachea so that, in the event of a postoperative hematoma that requires emergency airway establishment, the trachea is in full view no longer covered by the thyroid.

If cancer is proven or suspected, a thorough search for lymphadenopathy by inspection and palpation is conducted in the central compartment, the paratracheal area, the superior mediastinum, and level 4. If suspicious nodes are encountered, they are removed in as much of an en bloc fashion as possible.

The surgical field is then copiously irrigated and any bleeding is managed using bipolar cautery. The anesthetist is then asked to apply positive pressure (Valsalva maneuver) looking for any bleeding. Sometimes annoying oozing occurs at the point of entry of the recurrent nerve into the larynx. If there is reticence to apply

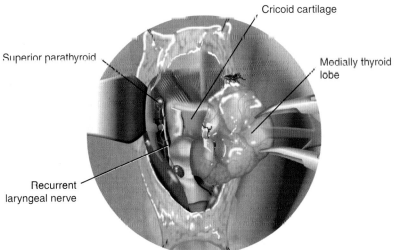

FIGURE 14.4
With the Berry ligament divided and relevant anatomy displayed, the lobe is dissected from the airway.

cautery to this area, I have found that a small pedicle of sternothyroid or a free piece of sternothyroid muscle applied to the bleeding area can act as a promoter of coagulation.

Suction drainage is not generally used for any thyroidectomy unless there has been troublesome bleeding intraoperatively or there remains a large "dead space" as a result of a large mass.

No attempt is made to approximate the sternothyroid muscles. The sternohyoid muscles are approximated in the midline using continuous absorbable 3-0 suture. A 1-cm dehiscent area is deliberately left at the inferior aspect of this closure so that, in the event of a hematoma, this allows drainage under the skin rather than allowing the blood to occlude the airway. The platysma is approximated by a continuous 4-0 absorbable suture, and the skin is then reapproximated using a 4-0 subcuticular absorbable suture. Steri-Strips are then applied to the incision, and no other dressing is employed.

POSTOPERATIVE MANAGEMENT

Patients are closely monitored in the recovery room for bleeding and airway compromise. If the patient's condition is stable for 2 hours, they are transferred to the ward where they are closely monitored for at least 12 hours. A serum parathyroid hormone (PTH) level is done 1 hour postoperatively. Serum calcium is performed at 12 hourly intervals. Observation for the development of Trousseau and/or Chvostek sign is done every 4 hours; the presence of either one of these signs triggers a calcium measurement. It has been shown that PTH level is highly predictive of parathyroid insufficiency. When levels fall below a critical level (1.1 pmol/L), patients are placed on prophylactic oral calcium and vitamin D; this allows for early discharge. Monitoring and weaning are performed as an outpatient. Asymptomatic patients above 1.6 can safely be discharged on the first postoperative day. Patients in between these levels are monitored closely. Patients whose calcium and PTH plummet or in those who become symptomatic, intravenous calcium may be necessary until the serum calcium has stabilized. Patients who have undergone total thyroidectomy are given thyroid hormone replacement on discharge.

If drains are used, the Jackson Pratt variety are preferred and they are attached to suction "grenades." They are usually removed in 48 hours or when effluent is scant (<25 mL/24 hours). Steri-Strips are removed in 7 days. As skin sutures are absorbable, no removal is necessary. All patients undergoing thyroid surgery should have an examination of the larynx in the postoperative period.

Postoperatively all patients are monitored in conjunction with the Endocrinology Service. Decisions regarding application of radioactive iodine for malignant tumors are made in a multidisciplinary fashion. Currently there is a tendency, using various guidelines (American Thyroid Association, Thyroglobulin-based evidence, Mayo Clinic Guidelines using MACIS scoring), to less usage of radioactive iodine since the evidence is increasing that there is no value added in giving radioactive iodine to early well-differentiated cancer or cancers with favorable pathology.

COMPLICATIONS

The complications and incidence of open thyroidectomy in our institution are as follows:

1. Hematoma <1%
2. Permanent injury to the recurrent laryngeal nerve 0.01%
3. Permanent bilateral vocal cord paralysis 0%
4. Permanent hypoparathyroidism 4%
5. Permanent injury to the EBSLN?
6. Seroma <1%
7. Wound infection <1%

These potential complications should be discussed openly with the patients who are to undergo open thyroidectomy as part of the consenting process.

Hematoma requires emergency drainage and identification and management of the bleeding source under general anesthetic since a hematoma may cause tracheal compression with loss of airway. A large rapidly expanding hematoma may need to have the incision opened on the nursing unit, the strap muscle sutures cut and the hematoma evacuated in order to restore the airway. The patient must then be transferred to the operating room where the wound should be explored, hemostasis obtained, and the wound irrigated and then closed as in the original surgery.

Permanent injury to the recurrent laryngeal nerve results in unilateral vocal cord paralysis. This is usually the result of intraoperative blunt trauma, trauma from cautery, or inadvertent sectioning of the nerve. Many of these paralyzed vocal cords while not regaining movement are compensated by the mobile cord gradually moving across the midline to oppose the paralyzed one and thereby reinstating almost normal phonation. Those patients who do not attain a normal voice within 6 to 8 months may undergo a vocal cord medialization procedure with Isshiki laryngoplasty type I being the most popular technique. Alternatively, recently good voice results have been obtained with the Miyauchi procedure whereby one of the descending branches of the ansa cervicalis is anastomosed to the severed end of the recurrent nerve before it enters the larynx. Permanent bilateral cord paralysis as a result of bilateral recurrent nerve injury fortunately is rare but devastating. Tracheostomy is the treatment of choice, although occasionally a patient with both vocal cords paralyzed in the paramedian position will have an adequate airway for phonation and breathing with little exertion. Very good results have been reported in the treatment of bilateral vocal cord paralysis using laser arytenoidectomy or cordotomy.

The true incidence of injury to the EBSLN is not known with certainty since the only accurate way to diagnose this is by cricopharyngeal electromyography, which is not widely available. Occasionally patients will complain of a dysphonia postoperatively, but there is no obvious laryngeal finding. These patients may have an injury to the EBSLN. These injuries may be crippling in patients who rely on their voice for livelihood.

Transient hypoparathyroidism is managed as described above. Permanent hypoparathyroidism is managed with oral calcium and vitamin D.

Seromas are rare events but resolve well with serial needle aspiration of the fluid. Usually resolution occurs with three or four aspirations.

Wound infections are rare following this surgery but, when they occur, are adequately treated with appropriate antibiotics as an outpatient. Rarely does an abscess occur requiring wound exploration through the incision and drainage.

RESULTS

Total thyroidectomy in experienced hands is a safe and effective operation. The results in terms of survival and recurrence for early follicular cell cancers approach 100% and 0%, respectively. The results are not as good with advanced stage cancer.

The results of treatment of medullary cancer of the thyroid vary with stage of presentation and whether it is familial, associated with MEN 2A, sporadic, or associated with MEN 2B (increasing aggressive biology).

Results of treatment of benign conditions, compressive tumors, and cosmetically obtrusive tumors are excellent. Results of treatment of hyperthyroidism with total thyroidectomy is excellent in returning the patient to a biochemically euthyroid state and significantly improving symptoms.

PEARLS

- Open thyroidectomy is performed for structural and functional problems.
- Structural problems include suspicion of malignancy, compressive symptoms, and cosmetically unsightly goiters.
- Functional problems are usually hyperthyroid states, and surgery is performed in the majority of instances for failure of medical management.
- The incidence of follicular cell–derived thyroid cancer has increased at a staggering rate probably as a result of widespread use of ultrasonography and more awareness of pathologic criteria.
- All patients with thyroid nodules or functional problems require a history, physical examination (including visualization of the larynx), thyroid function studies, ultrasonography, and FNA of any significant nodules.
- Surgery for suspicion of cancer is performed for patients in the significant risk strata.
- Open thyroidectomy that is done after careful evaluation and preoperative planning following the strategic approach as outlined above is a safe and rewarding operation.
- Wide exposure of the gland is mandatory.
- Removal of the lobe should be done only after both parathyroids (not always possible), the recurrent laryngeal nerve, and the EBSLN have been identified.
- Results of treatment for all groups is highly successful.

PITFALLS

- Failure to adhere to strict risk stratification indications will result in needless surgery.
- Failure to have a strategic and careful stepwise approach to open thyroidectomy as outlined above will result in poor outcomes.

INSTRUMENTS TO HAVE AVAILABLE

- A basic head and neck—thyroidectomy pack

SUGGESTED READING

Cushing S, Palme C, Odett N, et al. Prognostic factors in well-differentiated thyroid carcinoma. *Laryngoscope* 2004;
       114(12):2110–2115.
Vescan A, Witterick I, Freeman J. Parathyroid hormone as a predictor of hypocalcemia after thyroidectomy. *Laryngoscope*
       2005;115:2105.
Cibas ES, Ali SZ. The Bethesda system for reporting thyroid cytopathology. *Thyroid* 2009;19(11):1159–1165.
Cooper DS, Doherty GM, Haugen BR, et al. Revised American Thyroid Association Management Guidelines for patients
       with thyroid nodules and differentiated thyroid cancer. *Thyroid* 2009;19(11):1167–1214.
Randolph GW. *Surgery of the Thyroid and Parathyroid Glands*. Philadelphia, PA: Saunders/Elsevier, 2013.

15 ROBOTIC THYROIDECTOMY FOR THYROID CANCER; USING A GASLESS, TRANSAXILLARY APPROACH

Woong Youn Chung

INTRODUCTION

Over the last decade, improved socioeconomic status has increased interest in health and quality of life. This trend has greatly influenced the so-called doctor–patient relationship and treatment planning. Previously, patients' attitudes to therapy were somewhat passive, and patients usually followed doctors' recommendations. However, nowadays, patients study their diseases using the Internet or specialty publications and seek advice about their disease statuses and treatment options from various experts. Subsequently, they actively participate in therapeutic decision making with their doctors. Accordingly, many medical and surgical therapies had been modified based on quality of life associated factors, such as postoperative pain, morbidity, length of hospitalization, cosmesis, and return to full activity. In accord with these concepts, minimally invasive surgery has rapidly developed in various surgical fields.

Minimally invasive and endoscopic surgical techniques have only recently been used in the head and neck area, due to the spatial and anatomical limitations imposed by a lack of preexisting working space, the hypervascularities of target organs, and the fact that these organs are surrounded by critical nerves and major vessels.

After the first report was issued on endoscopic thyroidectomy by Hüscher et al. in 1997, various types of minimally invasive and endoscopic surgical techniques were introduced for the thyroid gland. However, endoscopic thyroidectomy had some limitations: (1) the operative view is unstable because surgeons tend to rely on assistants (rotating residents, interns) to hold scopes; (2) it is difficult to perform sharp dissection around the recurrent laryngeal nerve (RLN) or in the Berry's ligament region with endoscopic instruments; and (3) the straight and relatively unsophisticated design of endoscopic instruments makes it difficult to perform meticulous lymph node dissection in deep, narrow areas or regions with an angled approach.

In the late 20th century, dexterous robotic technology with computer-enhanced, master–slave telemanipulator systems was introduced to the surgical field. The use of surgical robotic systems has enabled surgeons to overcome the above mentioned shortcomings of endoscopic thyroidectomy by providing three-dimensional images in magnified view and allowing greater dexterity and more accurate instrument movements, for example, by hand-tremor filtering, by motion scaling, and by enabling fine movements. Furthermore, the camera and instruments are completely controlled by the surgeon. These advantages are particularly useful when the operative field is deep and narrow and when sharp dissection is needed.

In 2007, the surgical safety and feasibility of robotic thyroid surgery using a gasless, transaxillary approach was first introduced by surgeons in Korea, and since then, many studies have been performed concerning the technical aspects and functional or surgical outcomes of robotic thyroid surgery. Currently, robotic thyroid surgery is viewed as a promising method in the minimally invasive surgical armamentarium for the thyroid gland.

In this chapter, the detailed method of robotic thyroidectomy for the management of well-differentiated thyroid cancer is described.

HISTORY

In 1909, Theodor Kocher won the Novel prize for performing the first successful total thyroidectomy using an aseptic technique, and for a century, conventional open thyroidectomy was considered the safest and most effective method and the standard operative approach to the thyroid gland. However, the conventional open method requires a long skin incision and a wide skin flap in the anterior neck area, which can lead to prominent hypertrophic scars or keloids and discomfort in the anterior neck due to fibrosis and adhesions.

The minimally invasive approach to thyroid surgery was introduced by Gagner et al. in 1996, who issued the first report on endoscopic subtotal parathyroidectomy for secondary hyperparathyroidism. Subsequently, Hüscher et al. reported the successful performance of endoscopic right thyroid lobectomy for a thyroid nodule, and in 1997, Yeung et al., described endoscopic thyroid and parathyroid surgery.

In 1998, Shimizu introduced video-assisted neck surgery using a gasless technique, and in 2000, Ikeda described an axillary approach and Ohgami using a breast approach. To improve cosmetic results, endoscopic thyroidectomies based on various approaching routes have been described, such as cervical (minimally invasive video-assisted thyroidectomy), anterior chest wall, breast, axillary, axillo-bilateral-breast, bilateral axillary, unilateral axillo-breast, and bilateral axillo-breast approach and postauricular and axillary approach. To create working space, continuous CO_2 insufflation method and a gasless method using an external retractor have been applied. These various approach routes and methods for sustaining working space have their own advantages and pitfalls, and thus, currently no one technique can be described as better or optimal. Nevertheless, more comfortable, less demanding, and efficient methods are favored and widely used by beginner surgeons.

During the transaxillary approach, which was introduced by Ikeda, the surgeon approaches the lateral aspect of the thyroid, from which he can easily manipulate the superior and inferior poles of the thyroid and identify the parathyroid and RLN. Ikeda used continuous CO_2 insufflation to create working space, but when this method is used, the field of view can easily be disturbed by smoke or fumes created during electrical cautery and or by a Harmonic scalpel. To solve these problems, I developed a gasless endoscopic operation method using an external retractor and a transaxillary approach in 2001. The gasless endoscopic method presents no risks of complications, such as hypercapnia, respiratory acidosis, tachycardia, subcutaneous emphysema, or air embolism, and is based on the use of an external retractor which I designed which can be connected to a continuous suction line by a channel in the midline of the retractor blade.

Our operative technique takes advantage of the gasless method and the transaxillary approach. The most remarkable benefits of this method were realized while performing central compartment neck dissection (CCND) on malignant tumors from the carotid artery to substernal notch and prelaryngeal area, including paraesophageal lymph nodes. Other additional benefits of this lateral approach are that the anterior surfaces of the sternocleidomastoid (SCM) (sternal head) and strap muscle are not dissected, which enables the surgeon to preserve the sensory nerves around the anterior neck area, and thus, to avoid any postoperative hyperesthesia in its region.

Nevertheless, endoscopic surgery has its limitations due to the technical complexities associated with managing nonflexible endoscopic instruments given a two-dimensional (2D), flat operative view. However, the da Vinci surgical robotic system (Intuitive, Inc., Sunnyvale, CA) substantially overcomes the haptic (nontactile sense), optic (2D representation), and instrumental limitations of conventional endoscopic procedures and facilitates minimally invasive surgery. In 2007, we used the dexterity of this robotic system (the da Vinci S system) to perform the first successful robotic thyroidectomy using a gasless, transaxillary approach in patients with cancer of the thyroid, and since, the technical safety, feasibility, functional benefits, and surgical outcomes of this approach have been serially described.

PHYSICAL EXAMINATION

A complete examination of the head and neck must be performed. The size and mobility of the primary tumor are important. It is also critical to note fixation to the skin or underlying structures since this may be a contraindication to this procedure. The identification of the enlarged lymph nodes in the central neck as well as the lateral neck greatly influences the decision making with regard to the extent and type of surgery to be performed.

INDICATIONS

I had performed 650 gasless endoscopic thyroidectomies using a transaxillary approach from 2001 before performing the first robotic thyroidectomy. Based on the feasibility and safety of endoscopic thyroidectomy for papillary thyroid microcarcinoma, initial cases treated by robotic thyroidectomy were limited to well-differentiated thyroid carcinoma (WDTC) with a tumor size of ≤2 cm without definite extrathyroidal tumor invasion (T1 lesion) or to follicular neoplasm with a tumor size of ≤5 cm. Lesions located in the thyroid dorsal area, especially adjacent to the tracheoesophageal groove, were considered ineligible due to the possibility of injuring the trachea, esophagus, or RLN during robotic thyroidectomy. However, as robotic experience accumulated, I was able to manage unexpectedly encountered advanced cases, such as cases with definite adjacent muscle invasion or multiple nodal metastasis, successfully without open conversion. Currently, the indications for robotic thyroidectomy have been expanded to include patients with T3 or larger size lesions.

All patients are preoperatively diagnosed and histologically confirmed by ultrasonography-guided fine-needle aspiration biopsy. Staging neck ultrasonography and neck CT scan can be used to evaluate preoperative clinical stages. The eligibility criteria for robotic thyroidectomy are as follows: (1) WDTC, (2) a primary tumor size of ≤ 4 cm, and (3) minimal invasion by primary tumor into the anterior thyroid capsule and strap muscle.

CONTRAINDICATIONS

The exclusion criteria that should be applied are (1) definite tumor invasion of an adjacent organ such as the RLN, esophagus, major vessels, or trachea; (2) metastasis to multiple lymph nodes in multilevels of the lateral neck; or (3) perinodal infiltration at a metastatic lymph node.

SURGICAL TECHNIQUE

With the patient placed in the supine position under general anesthesia, the neck is extended slightly, and the lesion-side arm is raised and fixed to provide the shortest distance from the axilla to the anterior neck. A 5- to 6-cm vertical skin incision is then made along the lateral border of the pectoralis major muscle in the axilla (Fig. 15.1). A subplatysmal skin flap from the axilla to the anterior neck area is then dissected over the anterior surface of the pectoralis major muscle and clavicle by electric cautery under direct vision. After exposing the medial border of the SCM muscle, the dissection is approached through the avascular space between the sternal and clavicular heads of the SCM and beneath the strap muscle until the contralateral lobe of the thyroid is exposed (Fig. 15.2). Next, an external retractor is inserted through the skin incision in the axilla and raised to maintain the working field (Video 15.1). According to this method, robotic arms are inserted through a single incision in the axilla (Fig. 15.3). To prevent interference between robotic arms, the placement of the ProGrasp forceps and the angle and interarm distances of the robotic arms are extremely important. For the approach from the right-side, a 12-mm trocar for the camera and a dual-channel endoscope with 30-degree down view are located in the center of the axillary incision. The camera should be placed in the lowest part of the incision and its tip directed upward. An 8-mm trocar for the ProGrasp forceps is then positioned on the right of the camera parallel with the suction tube of the retractor blade. At this point, the ProGrasp forceps must be located as close as possible to the retractor blade. The 5-mm trocar of a Maryland dissector is then positioned on the left of the camera, and the 5-mm trocar of a Harmonic curved shears on the right side of the camera. The Maryland dissector and the Harmonic curved shears should be as far apart as possible (Fig. 15.4; Video 15.2). The Harmonic curved shears is used for all dissections and ligations of vessels. After traction of the upper pole of the thyroid in the medial–inferior direction with the ProGrasp forceps, the superior thyroid artery is divided (Fig. 15.5). The ProGrasp forceps is used to draw the upper pole of the thyroid steadily and is repeatedly repositioned during the gradual dissection. By peeling the thyroid gland off of the cricothyroid muscle, the superior parathyroid gland is identified and preserved (Fig. 15.6). The dissection is performed carefully so as not to injure the RLN insertion site. Central lymph node dissection is performed after dissection of the superior pole. Before central lymph node dissection, the RLN should be identified and only then should node dissection be performed (Fig. 15.7). After tracing the path of the nerve, the thyroid gland is completely detached from the trachea. Caution should be taken not to injure the RLN by thermal damage caused by direct contact with the Harmonic curved shears or by exposure to its energy (Fig. 15.8). After the right thyroid lobectomy, the contralateral lobectomy is performed via subcapsular dissection while preserving both parathyroid glands and the RLN (Figs. 14.9 and 14.10; Video 15.3). In some cases, to improve contralateral tracheoesophageal groove exposure, the operating table can be tilted to 10 to 15 degrees right side up. After extracting the specimen, I irrigate the operative fields. Finally, a Jackson-Pratt suction drain is inserted through a separate skin incision under the axillary skin incision, and the wound is closed cosmetically (Fig. 15.11).

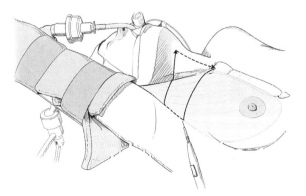

FIGURE 15.1 Positioning of the patient.

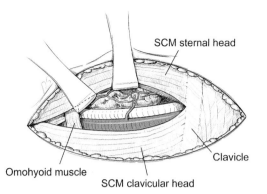

FIGURE 15.2
Approaching route (the space between two branches of SCM).

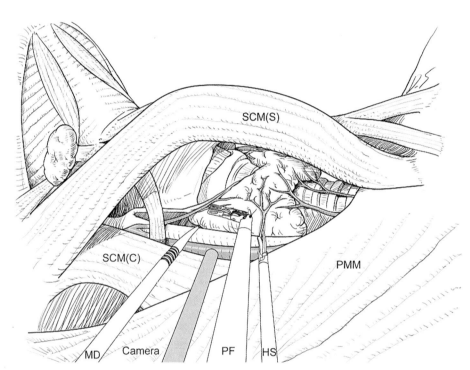

FIGURE 15.3
Insertion of robotic instruments. SCM (S), sternal head of sternocleidomastoid muscle; SCM (C), clavicular head of sternocleidomastoid muscle; MD, Maryland dissector; PF, ProGrasp forceps; HS, Harmonic curved shears; PMM, pectoralis major muscle.

FIGURE 15.4
Docking and instrumentation. The camera should be placed in the center of the axillary incision, and the camera tip should be directed upward. The ProGrasp forceps (*first arm*) should be located as close as possible to the ceiling of the working space. Maryland dissector (*second arm*) and Harmonic curved shears (*third arm*) should be as far apart as possible.

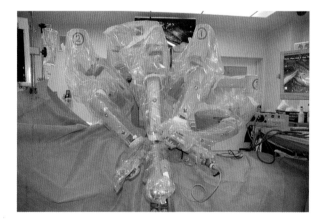

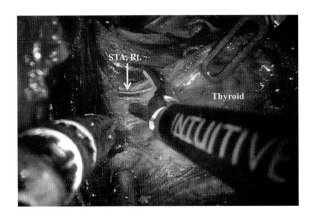

FIGURE 15.5 The ligation of the superior thyroid vessels (STA). Drawing the upper pole of the thyroid in the medial–inferior direction with the ProGrasp forceps, the STA are divided. STA, Rt., right superior thyroid artery.

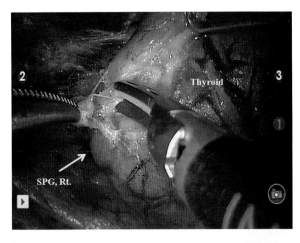

FIGURE 15.6 The identification of the superior parathyroid gland. The superior parathyroid gland is identified and preserved by peeling the thyroid gland off of the cricothyroid muscle. SPG, Rt., right superior parathyroid gland.

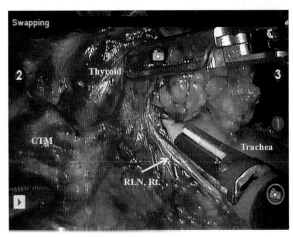

FIGURE 15.7 Ipsilateral identification of the RLN. After tracing the course of the RLN, the thyroid can be completely detached from the trachea. CTM, cricothyroid muscle; RLN, Rt., right recurrent laryngeal nerve.

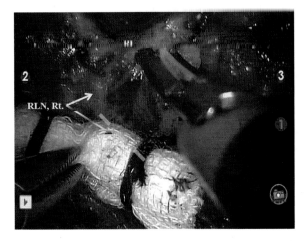

FIGURE 15.8 In the area of the Berry's ligament, great caution should be taken to prevent direct or indirect thermal injury of the RLN by the Harmonic curved shears. BL, Berry ligament; RLN, Rt., right recurrent laryngeal nerve. *Yellow dot line* is the course of RLN covered by rolled gauze.

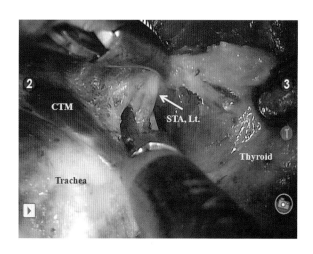

FIGURE 15.9

Ligation of the contralateral upper pole of the thyroid gland. After drawing the contralateral thyroid gland anteriorly with the ProGrasp forceps, the STA are divided. CTM, cricothyroid muscle; STA, Lt., left superior thyroid artery.

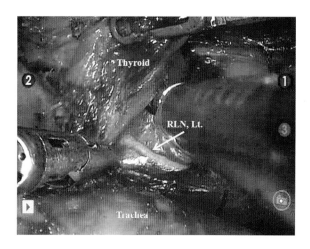

FIGURE 15.10

Identification of contralateral RLN. Contralateral thyroidectomy usually proceeds with subcapsular dissection to preserve the parathyroid gland and RLN. RLN, Lt., left recurrent laryngeal nerve.

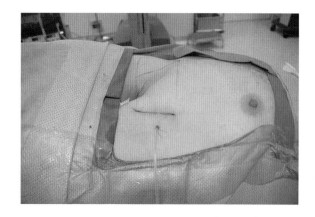

FIGURE 15.11

Postoperative wound after drain insertion and skin closure.

POSTOPERATIVE MANAGEMENT

Postoperative pain can be controlled by the usual postoperative medication regimen.

The routine period of drain placement after the operation is usually different from each surgeon according to their own experience and preference. However, if the drainage amount is <50 mL/day, the drain can be safely removed without any risk of postoperative seroma.

Discharge and outpatient hospital follow-up plan is based on the surgeon's experience and preference.

COMPLICATIONS

The complications of robotic thyroidectomy are similar to those of conventional open or endoscopic thyroidectomy (Table 15.1). Hypoparathyroidism (transient/permanent), recurrent (inferior) laryngeal nerve injury, superior laryngeal nerve injury, hemorrhage/seroma, and wound infection can occur after CCND regardless of the surgical methods. However, tracheal injury and ipsilateral arm paralysis are method-specific complications of robotic thyroidectomy. Because the surgeon might not have tactile sensation during the robotic operation, the tracheal wall might be injured, especially around the Berry's ligament, when due caution is not taken. We have also experienced several cases of transient ipsilateral arm paralysis due to the use of an incorrect patient position; this complication is believed to have resulted from overtraction of the shoulder. Nevertheless, arm movements recovered in all cases within the first postoperative month.

RESULTS

The application of robotic technology to thyroid carcinoma provides greater functional benefits (with acceptable surgical outcomes) than the conventional open procedure. I anticipate that further developments of the robotic technique will expand the indications of robotic thyroidectomy and improve its surgical outcomes.

PEARLS

- Surgeons should be experienced at open thyroid gland surgery before conducting a robotic procedure on the thyroid gland.
- Surgeons should receive sufficient education and training (in animals or cadavers) regarding the manipulations of robotic instruments before conducting actual operations in patients.
- One of the most important points for successful robotic thyroid surgery is the development of adequate working space.
- During a surgeon's initial experiences with robotic surgery, stepwise extensions of the surgical procedure increase the likelihood of successful treatment.
- This surgical procedure requires many steps, which include patient positioning and preparation, creating the surgical working space, docking the robot, using the robot to remove the thyroid, and wound closure. In addition to mastering the technical aspects of the robotic surgical system, a team approach and a consistency of team members, including operating room staff and anesthesia personnel, are more important than for conventional open and endoscopic thyroid surgery.

PITFALLS

- Despite its excellence, robotic thyroidectomy has its limitations. Robotic gasless transaxillary thyroidectomy is more invasive because of the wide dissection required from the axilla to the anterior neck and more time consuming than the conventional open method.

TABLE 15.1   Perioperative Complications Following Robotic Thyroidectomy for Thyroid Cancer
Hemorrhage/seroma
Hypoparathyroidism (transient/permanent)
Ipsilateral arm paralysis (transient)
Recurrent (inferior) laryngeal nerve injury
Superior laryngeal nerve injury
Tracheal injury
Wound infection

- It is not easy for beginner surgeons to approach the contralateral upper pole of the thyroid using this method. For contralateral upper pole dissection, all instruments should cross over the trachea, and the approach should be deep and narrow area while the trachea is pushed down. This awkward procedure is sometimes very difficult when the trachea is prominent, especially for beginner surgeons.
- Some regions in deep and narrow working spaces may be inaccessible if a nonarticulating Harmonic curved shears is used during robotic thyroidectomy. Although Harmonic curved shears result in minimal thermal spread as compared with other energy sources, some limitations exist when the shears is applied in taxing cases, such as in those with RLN nerve or tracheal invasion. To overcome such limitations, many instrumental experiments have been tried, and more appropriate energy devices will be developed soon.

INSTRUMENTS TO HAVE AVAILABLE

- Patient position: arm board, soft pillow
- Development of working space
  - Electrocautery with regular and extended sized tip
  - Vascular Debakey or Russian forceps (extended length)
  - Army Navy retractor × 2
  - Right-angled retractors × 2
  - Breast-lighted retractor × 2
- Maintenance of working space
  - Chung retractor
  - Table mount and suspension device (BioRobotics Seoul, Korea, or Marina Medical, Sunrise, FL)
- Robotic procedure
  - 5-mm Maryland dissector
  - 8-mm ProGrasp forceps
  - 5-mm Harmonic curved shears
  - Dual-channel 30-degree endoscope (used in the rotated down position)
  - Endoscopic graspers and forceps
  - Endoscopic suction irrigator

ACKNOWLEDGMENT

Sources of financial support: No external funding was provided for this study.

SUGGESTED READING

Kang SW, Jeong JJ, Nam KH, et al. Robot-assisted endoscopic thyroidectomy for thyroid malignancies using a gasless transaxillary approach. *J Am Coll Surg* 2009;209(2);e1–e7.

Kang SW, Jeong JJ, Yun JS, et al. Robot-assisted endoscopic surgery for thyroid cancer: experience with the first 100 patients. *Surg Endosc* 2009;23(11);2399–2406.

Kang SW, Lee SC, Lee SH, et al. Robotic thyroid surgery using a gasless, transaxillary approach and the da Vinci S system: the operative outcomes of 338 consecutive patients. *Surgery* 2009;146(6);1048–1055.

Lewis CM, Chung WY, Holsinger FC. Feasibility and surgical approach of transaxillary robotic thyroidectomy without CO(2) insufflation. *Head Neck* 2010;32(1);121–126.

Ryu HR, Kang SW, Lee SH, et al. Feasibility and safety of a new robotic thyroidectomy through a gasless, transaxillary single-incision approach. *J Am Coll Surg* 2010;211(3);e13–e19.

16 GOITER SURGERY

Gregory W. Randolph

INTRODUCTION

Halsted wrote, "The extirpation of the thyroid gland for goiter perhaps typifies better than any other operation, the supreme triumph of the surgeons art." The normal complex anatomy of the base of the neck can be distorted in sometimes predictable but sometimes unpredictable patterns by goiter. Size, vascularity, distortion of the anatomy, substernal extension, and restrictions imposed by the bony confines of the thoracic inlet can make identification and preservation of the recurrent laryngeal nerve (RLN) and parathyroid glands challenging. A definition and classification of goiter and substernal goiter has been presented (see Table 16.1 for classification of substernal goiter).

HISTORY

The history of untreated sporadic nontoxic goiter is characterized by slow and inexorable growth. Occasionally hemorrhage into a preexisting nodule in the goiter can result in the development of acute airway symptoms. During initial evaluation, regional symptoms should be assessed including the pattern of respiration, phonation, swallowing, and the presence of a globus sensation. Symptoms may occur first when the patient is in the supine position or in extreme neck extension, in extreme neck flexion, or raising the arms over the head. Similarly, respiratory symptoms may occur nocturnally and be recognized by family members who should be questioned on this point. During the initial surgical evaluation, symptoms and laboratory evidence of hypo- and hyperthyroidism should also be reviewed. CT scanning with contrast can be very helpful, but if a patient is subclinically hyperthyroid and is given iodine-containing contrast, the Jod-Basedow phenomenon may occur with the initiation of frank hyperthyroidism for several months. A preimaging thyroid-stimulating hormone (TSH) is therefore essential as subclinical hyperthyroidism with suppressed TSH is not uncommon in elderly patients with multinodular goiter.

PHYSICAL EXAMINATION

During the physical examination, the size of the goiter must be documented as well as its consistency and the possible fixation of the mass to the laryngotracheal complex. Laryngeal landmarks including the thyroid notch, anterior cricoid arch, and trachea should be examined for deviation from the midline. Distention of the jugular veins should be noted as this implies significant jugular compression. All patients being evaluated for goiter should have an examination of the larynx given the potential for vocal cord paralysis, which may be asymptomatic. The finding of vocal cord paralysis is of extreme importance in terms of surgical planning. If during examination the caudal-most portion of the goiter cannot be identified on the physical examination, substernal extension should be considered. An axial CT scan should be strongly considered in patients who have significant regional symptoms, massive goiter, bilateral circumferential goiter, substernal extension, vocal cord paralysis, or lymphadenopathy. Thyroid function tests must be performed in all patients as subclinical

	Type	Location	Anatomy	Prevalence	Approach, Comment
I		Anterior mediastinum	Anterior to great vessels, trachea, RLN	85%	Transcervical (sternotomy, only if intrathoracic goiter diameter > thoracic inlet diameter)
II		Posterior mediastinum	Posterior to great vessels, trachea, RLN	15%	As above. Also consider sternotomy or right posterolateral thoracotomy if type IIB
	IIA	Ipsilateral extension			
	IIB	Contralateral extension			
	B1	Extension posterior to both trachea and esophagus			
	B2	Extension between trachea and esophagus			
III		Isolated mediastinal goiter	No connection to orthotopic gland; may have mediastinal blood supply	<1%	Transcervical or sternotomy

RLN, recurrent laryngeal nerve.

hypothyroidism is not uncommon in patients with multinodular goiter. Fine needle aspiration should be considered in all patients with a nodular goiter. However, in patients with CT and ultrasonographic findings consistent with benign goiter with a smooth margin and without lymphadenopathy who will be undergoing surgery, histologic diagnosis may be deferred to final pathology.

INDICATIONS

Surgical indications for multinodular goiter include the following:

- Clear-cut, significant regional aerodigestive tract symptoms without other apparent cause
- CT scan demonstrating tracheal compression
- Thyroid masses >5 cm or with interval growth on CT scan
- Patients with subclinical or frank hyperthyroidism (after being medically controlled)
- Patients with suspected or proven malignancy
- All patients with substernal goiter

CONTRAINDICATIONS

Patients who are elderly or are poor operative candidates after complete and thorough medical evaluation may be considered for observation or nonsurgical treatment including radioactive iodine. One must be aware of the potential occurrence of radiation thyroiditis acutely with radioactive iodine treatment for goiter and the potential for the induction of Graves disease.

PREOPERATIVE PLANNING

I strongly favor axial CT scanning with contrast (if the TSH is normal) in all patients with goiter. CT scan can help to define the benign nature of the goiter by demonstrating smooth margins of the thyroid gland and lack of lymphadenopathy. It also gives an exact detailed impression of the extent of the impact of the goiter on surrounding cervical viscera and the extent of substernal extension. In fact in many cases, CT scan provides clear-cut information that helps to define the surgical indication(s) including tracheal compression or substernal extension, which may not be evident until CT scan is performed. CT scan provides the roadmap for subsequent surgery. Clefts in the goiter can be identified preoperatively and may be found at surgery to entrap the RLN, especially when these clefts occur on the right side given the more oblique course of the right RLN through the right paratracheal region.

TABLE 16.1 Substernal Goiter Classification

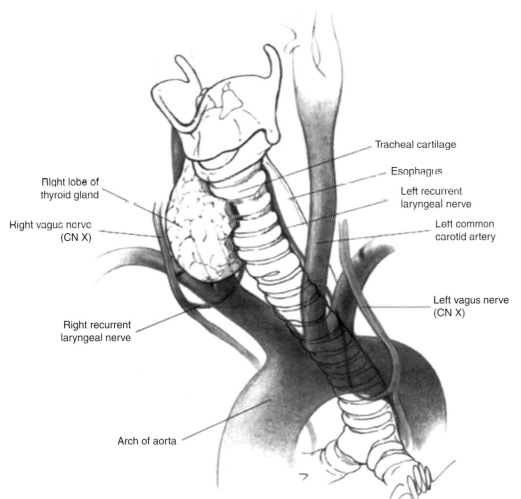

FIGURE 16.1
Neural and vascular anatomy of the base of the neck. Identification of the structures of the carotid sheath and dissection into the mediastinum is essential in early phases of substernal goiter surgery.

Labels on figure:
Tracheal cartilage
Esophagus
Left recurrent laryngeal nerve
Left common carotid artery
Left vagus nerve (CN X)
Right lobe of thyroid gland
Right vagus nerve (CN X)
Right recurrent laryngeal nerve
Arch of aorta

SURGICAL TECHNIQUE

Patient positioning is important, and extension of the head allows cranial movement of the substernal goiter making the mass more accessible. RLN monitoring is used in my unit on all patients undergoing thyroid and parathyroid surgery including patients who have a goiter. The incision should be a generous collar incision incorporated in a normal skin crease at the base of the neck. Strap muscles can frequently be maintained and reflected laterally. If, however, the surgeon feels that the strap muscles represent an encumbrance, they can be sectioned without hesitation. If exposure of the superior pole of the thyroid is limited, the superior portion of the sternothyroid muscle can be sectioned in isolation to provide improved exposure of the superior pole.

It is essential to identify the carotid sheath in the early stages of goiter surgery. The carotid sheath is to the initial steps in goiter surgery what the lateral thyroid region is in surgery of normal size glands. It is extremely helpful to dissect the carotid arteries and jugular veins off of the lateral surface of the goiter and to identify the vagus nerve to allow for testing of the neural monitoring system. The subsequent dissection along the carotid sheath inferiorly into the mediastinum is tremedously helpful in providing key orientation in the initial phases for surgery of substernal goiter (Fig. 16.1).

Preservation of the Recurrent Laryngeal Nerve in Goiter Surgery

Identification of the RLN can be made through inferior, lateral, or superior approaches. Often in large goiters, the nerve can be found through the typical inferior approach used during routine thyroid surgery, identifying the nerve adjacent to the inferior pole after preliminary dissection has cleared the region of the inferior pole. Clips and harmonic scissors can be useful in the management of the middle thyroid veins and inferior pole veins during goiter surgery. In certain cases with large cervical or substernal goiters, the RLN can be identified through a superior approach at the laryngeal entry point at the inferior margin of the cricoid cartilage. This requires an initial dissection and reflection of the superior pole inferiorly. Once the RLN is identified through this superior

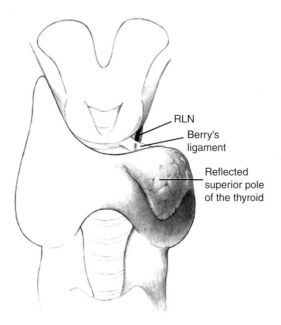

FIGURE 16.2
Superior approach to the RLN can be helpful during goiter surgery.

approach, it can be dissected retrograde off of the undersurface of the goiter and reflected laterally to allow for subsequent safe substernal delivery of the goiter into the neck (Fig. 16.2).

Perhaps the most difficult cases of goiter surgery include those cases of retrotracheal or posterior mediastinal goiter. In these circumstances, posterior elements of the thyroid expand dorsally to the RLN, bringing this nerve ventral to the bulk of thyroid tissue. This places the nerve at extreme risk during surgery. Dorsal excavation of the area deep to the RLN by the goiter can be intuited by careful analysis of the preoperative CT scan, which in these cases documents retrotracheal or posterior mediastinal extension.

It is important in the final phases of surgery to appreciate that the RLN, which early in the dissection is reflected away from the goiter, may be redundant and easily transected in its superior portion during the final phases of goiter surgery if its course is not strictly visualized during all phases of the surgery.

Preservation of the Parathyroid Glands in Goiter Surgery

It is important during goiter surgery to preserve parathyroid tissue. Because of the typical expansion of the inferior pole of the thyroid, it may not be possible in all cases to identify the inferior parathyroid glands. The glands can usually be preserved by observing a strict capsular dissection in this area. The superior gland frequently maintains a more normal position at the cricothyroid junction level of the neck, and the gland can be dissected away from the superior pole of the mobilized thyroid lobe. All adipose tissue must be reflected away prior to resection of the goiter. Before the specimen is sent off the table, it must be examined in all aspects for capsular adipose tissue, which may hide a resected parathyroid. All clefts of the goiter should be meticulously examined, and any parathyroid tissue should be confirmed through frozen section and then autotransplanted.

There are a variety of techniques for the delivery of the substernal goiter. It is essential that the RLN be identified prior to delivery of the substernal goiter. This can be accomplished even with large substernal goiters using the superior approach to the nerve and retrograde dissection of the nerve off the under surface of the goiter as discussed above (Fig. 16.3). In general, after identification of the nerve, delivery of the goiter can be achieved by placing one finger on the lateral capsule surface of the inferior pole and one finger on the

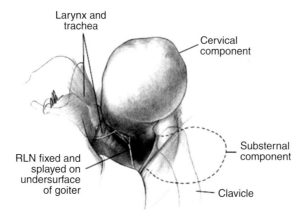

FIGURE 16.3
Adherence of the RLN to the under surface of the large substernal goiter.

corresponding aspect of the capsule of the inferior pole adjacent to the trachea medially. Slow incremental delivery of the substernal goiter into the neck through progressive "drawing up" of the goiter with these two fingers at the medial and lateral edge of the inferior pole is generally successful. A careful analysis of preoperative CT scanning with thoracic surgical colleagues is essential in all patients with significant substernal goiter.

Sternotomy, although rarely needed for typical goiter surgery, can be considered in the following cases:

- Known or suspected malignancy extending to the mediastinum
- Cases with true superior vena cava syndrome identified preoperatively, which suggests mediastinal malignancy
- Large posterior mediastinal goiter especially if associated with contralateral thoracic extension
- Cases in which the blood supply to the goiter is mediastinal
- Large, recurrent substernal goiters
- Cases in which the delivery reveals an immobile substernal component or adherence of the goiter to the surrounding mediastinal vessels or pleura
- Cases in which substernal delivery of the goiter is associated with substantial mediastinal hemorrhage
- Cases in which the mediastinal diameter of the intrathoracic component to the goiter is significantly greater than the diameter of the thoracic inlet
- Cases in which a long thin stalk from the cervical component of the substernal component exists; such stalks may fragment with significant retraction especially if the mediastinal component is wide and bulbous.

POSTOPERATIVE MANAGEMENT

Postoperative management of the airway, recognition and management of RLN paralysis, and recognition and management of the calcium profile postoperatively are essential with surgery for goiter as it is with any thyroid surgery. I typically do not use drains in goiter surgery. The dressing is limited to a folded sponge covered with a clear adhesive dressing, which is removed on the first post operative day. Discharge for hemithyroid patients is in the AM of postoperatiave day one and in the PM of postoperative day one for goiter patients requiring total thyroidectomy.

COMPLICATIONS

One essential component in postoperative surgery for goiter is the avoidance and prompt treatment of a hematoma. This may be a life-threatening problem. Meticulous attention to hemostasis must take place during surgery since it is essential for visualization during surgery as well as for the prevention of postoperative hematoma. Valsalva maneuver repetitively applied at the end of surgery with prolonged and meticulous search of all aspects of the surgical bed is helpful. Nurses, residents, and fellows assisting in the management of patients postoperatively must be trained in identification of a hematoma and its early and urgent management. Hematoma results in blood under pressure and subsequent infiltration of laryngeal mucosa and airway obstruction through glottic and supraglottic edema and tracheal compression. This requires early identification and treatment. Intubation can be difficult if not impossible if there is delay in recognition of this complication. Opening the incision and draining the hematoma at the bedside or in the operating room are important but do not typically prevent the need for obtaining the airway through intubation. In extreme circumstances where the oral airway cannot be obtained through intubation, tracheostomy can be performed through the wound. This is one of the main arguments for complete isthmus dissection and resection in all cases of unilateral thyroid surgery since the trachea is then available in the midline for tracheostomy in this circumstance.

Voice and airway changes should be carefully evaluated with examination of the larynx, and parathyroid function must be assessed following bilateral thyroid surgery. We favor serial calcium/albumin/phosphorus measures every 8 hours postoperatively through postoperative day one, with appropriate replacement of calcium and vitamin D as needed prior to discharge to achieve a stable calcium profile.

Tracheomalacia has been reported in goiter surgery though I have seen this very infrequently. The surgeon should be able to evaluate the contour and adequacy of the trachea through the wound during ventilation subsequent to goiter resection.

RESULTS

- Patients generally recover well with minimal pain medicine necessary.
- I recommend no bending/straining/exercise for the first postoperative week. Many patients will take 1 to 2 weeks off of work.
- TSH assessment is necessary in all patients at 6 to 8 weeks postoperatively and generally is normal for patients in whom an entire lobe is preserved.
- Regional symptoms generally are relieved by resection of the dominant side of the goiter.
- Pathology reports must be evaluated as there is a fairly high incidence of small and microscopic papillary thyroid cancers.

PEARLS

- "Don't see, don't cut rule." During thyroidectomy, any tissue that is not transparent is not cut unless the nerve in that segment of the operative field has been identified visually. In addition, running the nerve stimulator along this tissue is important prior to division of the tissue.
- If the nerve and parathyroid compete for your surgical attention, the nerve wins. Parathyroid left on the specimen intentionally, because of difficulty in nerve dissection, can be autotransplanted.
- Vagal stimulation first and last is a must. Vagal stimulation is required at the beginning of surgery to provide a positive electromyography signal so that neural mapping and search for the RLN can be effectively achieved. Vagal stimulation must be performed also at the end of surgery to provide full and complete segmental testing of the vagus and RLN that has been operated on.
- Watch the nerve as you retract. Especially at the final stages of goiter delivery, significant tension can be placed on the RLN at Berry's ligament. Careful attention to subtle nerve displacement implying significant retraction is important.
- The anterior arch of the cricoid cartilage in the midline is a superb landmark during thyroid surgery. The RLN is at risk until it dives underneath the inferior edge of the inferior constrictor muscle at the inferior edge of the cricoid cartilage laterally.
- After completion of surgery, the nerve may be injured with imprudent suction or the use of small rolled peanut sponges aggressively applied with an instrument.
- Bipolar cautery should only be applied in areas near the nerve and for limited periods of time.
- If the distal nerve looks of thin caliber, then go back toward the mediastinum and redissect to exclude extralaryngeal branching.
- Beware of being misled by a large posterior branch of the nerve and then injuring the unidentified anterior branch as you manage Berry's ligament. Neural stimulation is tremendously helpful in this regard as it segregates sensory and motor fibers information, which is not information which is obtainable through visual neural inspection.

PITFALLS

- Preoperative evaluation must be robust and include symptomatic assessment and examination of the larynx.
- For most large goiters, CT scanning is very helpful in determining the extent of the goiter, the extent of substernal growth, and the relationship of the goiter to cervical viscera.
- Clefts in the goiter seen on CT may be an area where the RLN may be found.
- Great caution should be used when operating on a goiter which extends to the posterior mediastinum given the significant anatomic distortion that may be present in such patients including the ventral RLN.
- Sternotomy may be required in a small subset of patients with substernal goiter. One must be prepared through discussion with thoracic colleagues preoperatively for such patients.
- Great caution should be in place to avoid disturbing capsular vessels during goiter surgery—these can cause troublesome bleeding, which can hinder the remainder of the case.
- RLN identification should be performed prior to substernal goiter delivery and may be accomplished through a superior approach identifying the nerve at the laryngeal entry point.

INSTRUMENTS TO HAVE AVAILABLE

- Fine long tonsil-type hemostat
- Fine jeweler tip bipolar cautery
- Harmonic scissors
- Fine- and moderate-sized metal clips
- RLN-monitoring probe
- DeBakey forceps

SUGGESTED READING

Halsted WS. The operative story of goitre. *Johns Hopkins Hosp Rep* 1920;19:71.
Randolph GW, Shin J, Grillo H, et al. Surgical management of goiter: Part II. Surgical treatment and results. *Laryngoscope* 2011;121:68–76.
Shin J, Grillo H, Mathisen D, et al. Surgical management of goiter: Part I. Preoperative assessment. *Laryngoscope* 2011;121:60–67.
Randolph GW, ed. *Surgery of the Thyroid and Parathyroid Glands*. 2nd ed. Philadelphia, PA: Elsevier Saunders, 2012.

17

TECHNIQUE FOR COMPLETION/ REOPERATIVE THYROIDECTOMY

Gary L. Clayman

INTRODUCTION

Most thyroid lobectomies are performed for definitive pathologic diagnosis as well as treatment in cases of cytologically benign neoplasms, small (<1.5 cm) differentiated papillary thyroid carcinomas in young patients, or follicular lesions that cannot otherwise be further classified. Completion thyroid lobectomy is performed based upon a thorough understanding of the patient's disease process and the risk and potential benefits of the completion surgical procedure. The ultimate goal of completion thyroidectomy is to remove all remaining thyroid tissue with or without central compartment lymphatics in order to improve control of the disease process, provide the ability to deliver effective radioactive iodine in patients who have differentiated thyroid cancer, and provide the feasibility to monitor serologic markers of differentiated thyroid cancers through analysis of thyroglobulin or calcitonin in medullary thyroid carcinomas.

Complications of completion thyroidectomy occur with greater frequency than total thyroidectomy although they are not directly comparable. Scarring and surgical changes in the thyroid bed can occur at a significant distance from prior surgical manipulation. The most common potential complications include transient and permanent hypoparathyroidism as well as vocal cord dysfunction although these risks appear to be reduced in the series in which surgeons have significant experience in thyroidectomy and reoperative central compartment surgical procedures.

Preoperative thyroid function testing including analysis of thyroid-stimulating hormone (TSH) levels is needed in all patients to confirm biochemical euthyroid state prior to surgical intervention.

A thorough review of all pathology by a qualified thyroid pathologist is mandatory prior to proceeding with a completion surgical intervention. Comprehensive analysis of the primary tumor, analysis of surgical margins, assessment of soft tissue extension, excised lymph nodes, lymphovascular invasion, and excised parathyroid tissue should be carried out in all specimens.

An interdisciplinary approach to the evaluation and care of the patient with cancer of the thyroid who has had a thyroidectomy is recommended; therefore, a consultation with an endocrinologist should be obtained for preoperative evaluation, treatment planning, and long-term care considerations.

Although thyroid surgery can be performed without the assistance of magnification, magnification of at least 2.5× facilitates safe surgery. This technique facilitates early identification of the superior and recurrent laryngeal nerves, helps to protect their arborized branches from injury, and allows both identification and meticulous surgery of the thyroid bed and preservation of adjacent parathyroid glands.

HISTORY

A thorough history is required in all patients. The patient should be questioned about matters including transient changes in vocal quality, swallowing, and parathyroid dysfunction following the initial surgical procedure. Any history of radiation exposure or a family history of thyroid malignancies should also be documented.

All information about the patient's previous surgery/surgeries is fundamental to understanding the circumstances and should be collected and analyzed. The pathology slides must be collected and reviewed by a pathologist experienced in pathology of the thyroid gland.

PHYSICAL EXAMINATION

A comprehensive examination of the head and neck should be performed on all patients. Preoperative evaluation of vocal cord function and laryngeal positioning (rotation) is required by either indirect or fiberoptic examination. The absence of symptoms should not prevent the evaluating physician from doing a comprehensive preoperative examination of the head and neck. Subtle alterations in laryngeal function are frequently best evaluated with a comprehensive stroboscopic examination.

INDICATIONS

Relative indications for completion thyroidectomy include patients with

- Differentiated thyroid cancers >1.5 cm in size
- Lymph node metastases in the lateral neck
- Desire of the physician or patient to monitor markers of thyroid malignancy including thyroglobulin, calcitonin, or carcinoembryonic antigen
- A physician or patient desire to evaluate or treat with radioactive iodine
- Symptomatic recurrent benign multinodular goiter

CONTRAINDICATIONS

Completion thyroidectomy is most commonly indicated for patients with differentiated thyroid cancers that are >1.5cm; for patients with cancer of the thyroid with lymph node metastases; or when patients are in their fifth or greater decades of life. Occasionally, completion thyroidectomy is performed in patients with benign diseases, such as recurrent/persistent goiter that has become symptomatic or progressed following a more remote earlier surgery. Completion thyroidectomy is not indicated in anaplastic thyroid cancer since previously incomplete excision of an anaplastic thyroid cancer is rarely resectable and multifocality is generally not the clinicopathologic factor of greatest importance to the patient. Total thyroidectomy with concomitant central compartment dissection is the recommended management for medullary thyroid carcinomas, and therefore this disease is not discussed in this chapter.

PREOPERATIVE PLANNING

Imaging Studies

Ultrasound of the central compartment and lateral necks should be performed on all patients undergoing completion thyroidectomy independent of the histologic diagnosis. Any suspicious lymph nodes should be cytologically analyzed independent of the size of the mass of the thyroid or cytologic diagnosis. It is important to evaluate the paratracheal lymph nodes at levels VI and VII with ultrasound because these lymph nodes are not palpable. A paralyzed vocal cord, prior to the initial surgery, invariably indicates invasive thyroid carcinoma, transient or permanent injury to a previously dissected nerve, or, rarely, idiopathic paralysis. Due to the limited utility of ultrasound in the superior mediastinum and inferior aspect of level IV due to shadowing from the clavicle and the apex of the lung, cross-sectional imaging with contrast-enhanced CT scanning should be considered in patients with central compartment metastatic lymph nodes or laryngeal dysfunction due to neoplastic involvement.

Fine Needle Aspiration Biopsy

Fine-needle aspiration (FNA) cytology is considered the gold standard for any residual masses within the retained thyroid gland as well as analysis of the lymph nodes in the central and lateral neck. Transcervical analysis of the superior mediastinum and analysis of the entire thyroid bed and the lateral neck should be performed in all patients. Lymph nodes with microcalcification, loss of fatty hilum, rounded appearance, or increased central vascularity should be cytologically analyzed with ultrasound guidance if their assessment would alter the extent of the planned surgical intervention.

SURGICAL TECHNIQUE

The time counseling the patient preoperatively, regarding the disease process, the goals and approach of surgery, and the potential complications associated with the surgery, is almost always significantly longer than the surgical procedure itself, but is time well spent. If the initial surgical procedure was done very recently (within 5 days), completion thyroidectomy can be performed at that time without significant central compartment morbidity. However, if the initial thyroidectomy was 7 or more days previously, I prefer in almost all circumstances to wait at least 6 months prior to completing the thyroidectomy. The reasons are self-evident for any surgeon who has attempted surgery in a surgical bed 2 to 3 weeks following any initial surgery. The inflammatory changes are nearing their peak and extend far from the areas of surgical dissection. In the thyroid bed, this implies that even the contralateral unoperated lobe, nerve inlets, and parathyroid beds may be extremely difficult to dissect. But even more importantly, ultrasound, although an incredibly useful tool in the management of thyroid disease, is fraught with difficulties in evaluating the postsurgical bed regarding residual thyroid tissue as well as the regional lymph nodes. Thoughtful education of the patient and delay of reoperation is highly recommended for the benefit of both the patient and the surgeon. The delay for completion surgery at 6 months therefore allows the surgeon and ultrasonographer to carefully assess the previously operated thyroid bed for residual thyroid tissue and metastatic lymph nodes, as well as the unoperated/dissected sites.

The surgical approach to completion thyroidectomy performed via an "open approach" is always an open approach. Despite that fact that the importance of what happens in the surgical procedure is what happens deep to the dermis, in the majority of patients without complications from their surgery, their major focus is frequently the design and outcome of the cervical incision. In completion thyroidectomy, the incision is almost always based upon the location of the initial incision. Despite the minimal risk of neoplastic "seeding" of the incision line, in most circumstances, I prefer to narrowly excise the prior incision line in three dimensions (both cephalad and caudal as well as through platysma). Meticulous care of the skin during incision, retraction, and closure, and protecting skin edges from thermal injury, minimizes the risk of hypertrophic scarring.

Although I generally perform thyroid surgery from a superior to inferior approach, it is best to allow the patient's anatomy to ultimately determine the order of the surgical approach. Due to the usual preceding midline dissection to the thyroid gland, the midline raphe of the sternothyroid muscles is usually scarred but avascular. In reoperation, the key to surgery is always to go "where no man (or woman) has gone before." Therefore, elevating the strap musculature slightly off of midline is frequently advantageous. As long as high-resolution ultrasound shows that the prior surgical bed is devoid of thyroid tissue or metastatic lymph nodes, this thyroid bed need not (and should not) be dissected again. If there is residual thyroid tissue, the amount of residual tissue and the benefit or risk for removal of this remnant should be well thought out. The presence of metastatic lymph nodes in the previously operated thyroid bed requires a dissection of level VI/VII, which is covered in Chapter 19.

In my opinion, completion/reoperative thyroidectomy should not be performed by the occasional thyroid surgeon. The potential risks to the patient are significantly increased among occasional surgeons and nearly equivalent to previously unoperated patients in the series of experienced surgeons. Thyroidectomy requires a thorough understanding of the anatomy and variations of the superior and recurrent laryngeal nerves as well as normal and ectopic location of the parathyroid glands and preservation techniques. These nerves should be routinely identified and preserved. Nerve monitoring is not required but provides surgeons the ability to monitor and stimulate motor laryngeal nerves to verify their function and long-term potential to do so. Although for many years I performed thyroid surgery without nerve monitoring, I now use monitoring routinely in all thyroid surgery primarily for the education of the residents and fellows. I have not used nerve monitoring for intraoperative decision making in my career.

Parathyroid glands should be preserved unless immediately adjacent to gross malignancy. It is advantageous to autotransplant a pathologically confirmed portion of a parathyroid gland to preserve lifelong parathyroid function in the event of a further requirement of a central compartment surgery.

General endotracheal anesthesia is induced without paralytic agents. I use recurrent laryngeal nerve monitoring endotracheal tubes and continuous nerve monitoring on all patients undergoing thyroid surgery. The patient is placed in only a slightly hyperextended position, mostly providing a "chin up" approach. The patient is positioned with the back section of the table elevated to reduce venous congestion, and the table placed in Trendelenburg to facilitate visualization of the superior pedicle (a lounge chair position).

The legs are lowered and compression stockings placed on all patients. The patient is slightly hyperextended in the neck. I leave the patient with the head toward the anesthesiologist and simply request space around the head by moving the table about 2 feet away from the anesthesia machine.

Both arms should be tucked in so that the surgeon and the assistant can easily move up and down without interference. The nerve-monitoring tube is visually verified to be in the correct midglottic position and then the nerve monitor system verified to be functioning. The patient is prepped and draped with the chin to midsternal area exposed.

The previous incision is excised (despite its location whether favorable or not) with a narrow 2-mm margin and excised through to platysma and the midline subcutaneous flap to the anterior jugular prevascular fascia. It would be extremely rare to have to create a new incision in completion thyroidectomy.

The incision is made with a scalpel through to the subcutaneous tissues. Attention to detail in incising and handling skin reduces cicatrix hypertrophy. The proper skin incision in thyroid surgery is critical, keeping the knife blade perpendicular to the skin to achieve satisfactory scaring. It is important to avoid any cautery burns to the surrounding skin or skin edges. After making the skin incision with the knife edge, electrocautery should be used to incise the subcutaneous and platysmal tissue. However, once the subcutaneous tissue is incised, a flat electrocautery should be used because the pointed cautery is likely to injure the anterior jugular veins and other important veins anterior to the thyroid gland. Electrocautery is used to incise the subcutaneous tissues deep to the platysma to the fascia enveloping the strap musculature and the communicating anterior jugular veins.

Although elevation of the skin flap is generally immediately subplatysmal in neck dissections, in thyroid surgery, especially in obese individuals (in the midline), elevating at the level of the investing fascia eliminates the potential for lipectomy and facilitates identification of the linea alba. The flaps are elevated to the level immediately above the thyroid notch, superiorly, and the sternal notch, inferiorly. Skin rake tension on the flaps elevated primarily perpendicular allows the plane above the anterior jugular veins and strap musculature to be readily visualized and opened with the electrocautery. The flaps are suspended with the use of 2-0 silk sutures placed at the very base of the elevated flap with a moistened sponge to keep from drying. Although some individuals prefer self-retaining retractors, I have not used them and prefer suture suspension to anchored drapes on the patient.

The linea alba is first identified inferiorly and incised with the use of electrocautery along its entire length. In most patients, the linea alba or median raphe of the strap musculature is easily identified. The linea alba is unquestionably much easier to define first lower in the neck. In completion thyroidectomy, the scarred area is usually an avascular plane. Gentle lateral tension of the sternothyroid muscle with application of the electrocautery on the raphe from the immediate suprasternal area to the thyroid notch is performed to separate these muscles.

Communicating branches of the anterior jugular veins may be encountered and controlled with suture ligatures or a Harmonic or similar type of ultrasonic device.

The sternohyoid and sternothyroid strap muscles are elevated off of the lateral surface of the gland with the use of electrocautery. In completion thyroidectomy, I first elevate the sternothyroid muscle toward this homolateral side of the prior thyroid lobectomy. I elevate it with the use of electrocautery from the sternal notch to the thyroid notch and laterally dissect the muscle along its ventral surface toward the great vessels. As the muscles are retracted laterally with Army Navy or small Richardson retractors, the muscles are separated from the anterior and lateral surfaces of the previously dissected thyroid bed. This then only takes a moment, and then the sternothyroid and sternohyoid muscles on the side of the retained thyroid tissue are similarly elevated with the use of electrocautery off of the anterior and lateral surfaces of the retained lobe of the thyroid. In any circumstance when there is a question of prior invasion of the strap muscles or inability to separate the strap muscles from the prior surgical bed, a margin should be obtained by resecting the muscle in continuity with the completion thyroid lobectomy.

The superior vascular pedicle is visualized by retraction of the sternothyroid and sternohyoid muscles both superiorly and laterally. Although I rely on all patients and their neoplasm to dictate the ultimate progression (order of events) in their procedure, in general, I prefer to address the takedown of the superior thyroid pedicle first. Takedown of a small portion of the sternothyroid muscle can be performed if there is incomplete visualization of the pedicle with retraction only. The experienced surgeon will rapidly recognize the anatomic variations of location of the thyroid and insertion of the strap muscles that suggest that this release is indicated.

Gently lifting the superior-most portion of the gland allows for identification of a fascial plane enveloping the superior vascular pedicle. A mosquito hemostat is used to dissect the plane beneath the superior thyroid artery and vein, and the superior laryngeal nerve is identified deep to these structures. Branches of the superior laryngeal nerve are frequently arborized.

If the superior laryngeal nerve is difficult to visualize, I prefer to take down the individual vessels of the superior aspect of the lobe in a stepwise fashion to spare variants of superior laryngeal nerve anatomy. Even though there are a variety of different ways to expose the superior thyroid pedicle and ligate the vessels individually, it is important to carefully expose this area, avoiding any bleeding from the minor vessels, and ligate the superior thyroid pedicle close to the thyroid gland in an effort to avoid injury to the superior laryngeal nerve. The best approach is to place a small blunt clamp on the superior pole of the thyroid gland and pull the thyroid laterally and inferiorly. This opens up a space called Joll's triangle, which should be exposed medial to the superior thyroid vessels away from the constrictor muscles of the pharynx. A small right-angle clamp allows both vessels to be isolated, clamped, and then sectioned with electrocautery (Fig. 17.1). Recently I have used Harmonic technology to perform thyroidectomy, thus avoiding suture ligatures. I have always avoided the use of surgical clips in thyroidectomy and neck dissections due to their effect on surveillance with both computerized axial tomography as well as ultrasound.

With the superior vascular pedicle transected, the superior lobe is mobilized in the capsular plane of the thyroid along its medial, lateral, and ventral surfaces such that the superior pole should be totally mobile. The dissection continues along the lateral capsular surface of the gland. Small capillaries and neovascularization are frequently encountered and are controlled with bipolar electrocautery or similar means. The middle and inferior thyroid veins are usually dominant and are transected along the capsule of the gland. As the thyroid gland is dissected, it is mobilized more medially, and the middle thyroid vein is transected (Fig. 17.2).

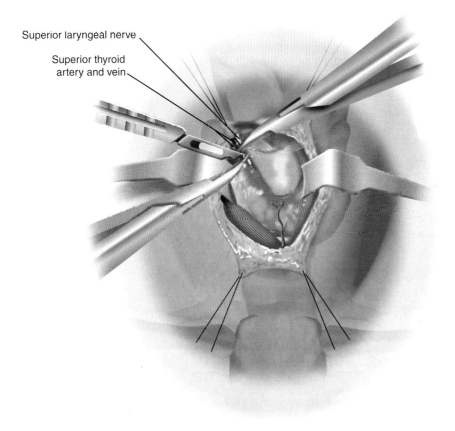

FIGURE 17.1 Joll's triangle (the fascial plane medial to the thyroid gland and lateral to the cricoid and thyroid cartilage) has been opened, and the superior vascular pedicle is ligated once the superior laryngeal nerve has been safely visualized.

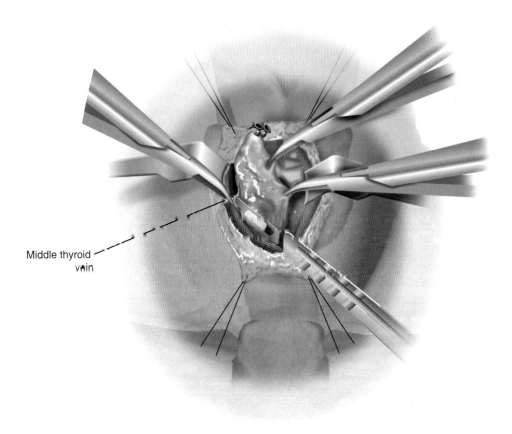

FIGURE 17.2 As the dissection of the thyroid transitions to a more posterior lateral approach, the middle thyroid vein is ligated along the gland capsule.

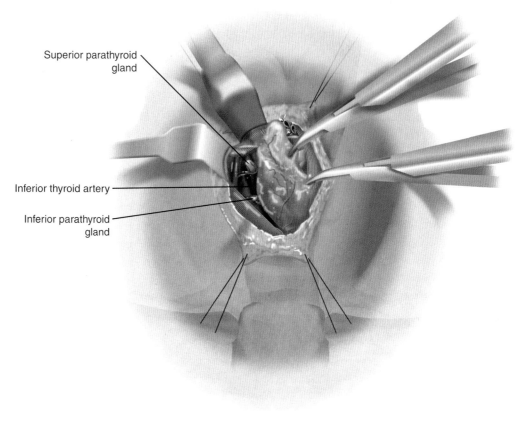

Superior parathyroid gland

Inferior thyroid artery

Inferior parathyroid gland

FIGURE 17.3

This inferior parathyroid gland located along the thyroid capsule is gently dissected from the thyroid gland and laterally displaced.

Karmalt retractors or moistened sponges help to medialize the gland and allow for adequate visualization of the posterolateral component of the dissection. Meticulous dissection and capsular excision technique facilitate maintaining vascularity of the parathyroid glands. With the gland medialized, the inferior thyroid artery and the inferior parathyroid gland can usually be visualized (Fig. 17.3). Bipolar electrocautery and sharp dissection are used to mobilize the parathyroid gland(s) on their vascular pedicle(s). I prefer to use bipolar electrocautery on very small fine vessels at very low settings to minimize compromise of the vasculature of the parathyroid gland.

Identification and Dissection of the Recurrent Laryngeal Nerve

The recurrent laryngeal nerves arise from the vagus nerve, on both sides, and pass deep to the vessels that are derived from the primitive fourth aortic embryologic arch. Therefore, the right recurrent laryngeal nerve passes beneath the right subclavian artery, whereas the left recurs at the ligamentum arteriosum of the aortic arch. Both nerves then ascend toward the larynx in the approximate area of the tracheoesophageal groove. This understanding is critical in safe dissection in that the recurrent laryngeal nerves are never at risk in the superior mediastinum in the dissection of structures lateral to the carotid arteries, aortic arch, innominate, or subclavian arteries.

Due to their sites of redirection, the left recurrent laryngeal nerve assumes a course ascending relatively longitudinally parallel lateral to the border of the trachea, whereas the right recurrent laryngeal nerve tends to be directed more angularly as it ascends medially to the larynx. Depending on the size and location of the lobe, the nerves may pass laterally or primarily beneath the lobes as they approach the cricothyroid membrane. In meticulous microdissection, the recurrent laryngeal nerves, proximally, have a wide range of arborized branches that may originate centimeters from the laryngeal insertion. One or more of the medialized proximal branches usually pass immediately posterior to the lateral suspensory ligament of the thyroid (Berry). Variability is the rule here, and instances of anterior branches' penetration of thyroid tissue in the ligament can be present.

The recurrent laryngeal nerve may be injured in the tracheoesophageal groove, at the crossing of the inferior thyroid artery, or near Berry's ligament. Extensive paratracheal dissection may lead to injury, through either traction or direct irritation of the recurrent laryngeal nerve during dissection in the tracheoesophageal groove. The majority of the time, the recurrent laryngeal nerve is posterior to the inferior thyroid artery; however, approximately 25% of the time, the nerve is anterior to the inferior thyroid artery and anatomically more likely to be injured during dissection. The most common injury to the recurrent laryngeal nerve is near Berry's ligament. This is most likely due to traction or the use of electrocautery very close to the recurrent laryngeal nerve. Most of the time, the injury occurs in an effort to control bleeding from the branches of the inferior thyroid artery near Berry's ligament. These vessels may get retracted behind the recurrent laryngeal nerve, and the nerve may be injured in an effort to control bleeding. Because the dissection is done in the tracheoesophageal groove area, every effort should be made to identify the recurrent laryngeal nerve. If for any reason the recurrent laryngeal nerve is not identifiable in the tracheoesophageal groove, a diligent search should be made for a nonrecurrent recurrent laryngeal nerve, which may occur in <1% of individuals. If the patient had a previous CT scan of the chest, this should be evaluated to rule out arteria lusoria. If the innominate artery is posterior to the esophagus, invariably the patient will have a nonrecurrent recurrent laryngeal nerve. Injury to this nerve is best avoided by using a keen knowledge of the anatomy and careful dissection in the posterior portion of the thyroid gland near Berry's ligament.

The recurrent laryngeal nerve is generally identified within the area of the inferior thyroid artery. Its location, whether deep or superficial to the inferior thyroid artery, is not constant or totally predictable. For practical purposes, the nerve may be identified caudal to the inferior parathyroid gland, but this may lead to a higher risk of compromise to the vascular supply of the parathyroid gland. I generally identify the nerve and its arborized branches immediately in the vicinity of the inferior parathyroid gland once it has been lateralized. Although great attention has been placed on the relationship of the inferior thyroid artery to the recurrent laryngeal nerve, basically the artery may present superficial, posterior, or branch in both locations surrounding the recurrent laryngeal nerve. Independent of the anatomic configuration, the recurrent laryngeal nerve should be identified prior to transection of these vascular structures.

The nonrecurrent laryngeal nerve can only be found on the right side of the neck and is present in about 1% of the population. This occurs due to an anomalous right subclavian artery that is retroesophageal. In such circumstances, the right subclavian artery arises as the final branch of the aortic arch, originating behind the esophagus and terminating into the supraclavicular and axillary regions. The right common carotid artery arises directly from the aortic arch in these circumstances, and therefore the nerve follows a direct course from the vagus, traversing posterior to the common carotid artery and assuming a variable horizontally angulated course beneath the thyroid lobe into the laryngeal inlet.

The philosophy of protecting the nerve by solely dissecting on the thyroid capsule does not necessarily ensure protection of the nerve from injury. In some circumstances, small anterior branches of the recurrent laryngeal nerves may penetrate the capsule especially in the vicinity of Berry's ligament.

The parathyroid glands frequently are situated along the course of the recurrent laryngeal nerves, and preservation of their function is requisite by maintaining their adequate lateral blood supply. The clear identification of the recurrent laryngeal nerves and distal dissection of these nerves allow safe division of the longitudinally and medially directed vascular supply to these glands, which is mandated for their normal function.

From a lateral to medial approach, the branches of the recurrent nerve are identified, small vessels are controlled with bipolar electrocautery, and larger vessels are managed by ligatures. Gentle tracing of the nerve using a cottonoid allows for atraumatic dissection along the nerve sheath.

Thyroid tissue frequently invests into the area of the cricothyroid membrane laterally in the area of Berry's ligament, thus making complete removal of all thyroid tissue unreasonable in some patients due to the interdigitated nature of their recurrent laryngeal nerve branches. In other instances, the ligament may be cauterized or suture ligated with minimal to no thyroid tissue recognized in this area.

The thyroid gland is usually retracted medially, both to identify the recurrent laryngeal nerve and to expose the area of Berry's ligament. Overretraction of the thyroid gland may lead to stretch and traction on Berry's ligament, where the nerve may become tented, causing traction injury to the nerve.

One must be constantly vigilant for premature arborization of the recurrent laryngeal nerve, and all branches are preserved (Fig. 17.4). The pretracheal fascia is entered and electrocautery (on a pure cutting setting) can be used to mobilize the thyroid to the contralateral side of the isthmus. Once the medial-most branch of the recurrent (or nonrecurrent nerve) is identified, the pretracheal fascia can be safely used as a dissection plane. The recurrent laryngeal nerve and its arborized motor branches, if monitored, can be stimulated with a minimal setting of 0.5 to up to 0.9 mA. Although I have not routinely used nerve monitoring, I have begun to use monitoring in resident and fellow education. It has not, however, altered my surgical technique or discontinued completion of thyroid surgery based on nerve stimulation criteria.

The pyramidal lobe and delphian lymph node are mobilized with the thyroid isthmus. The fascia and the thyroglossal remnant area are freed with the use of electrocautery starting superiorly at the inferior level of the hyoid bone and connecting inferiorly to the isthmus and pyramidal lobe dissection. In some instances, the tract and pyramidal remnants may be prominent, and in other instances, they may be vestigial. The dissected thyroid lobe, isthmus, and pyramidal lobe are elevated off of the pretracheal fascia toward the previously excised thyroid until all thyroid tissue has been removed.

The dissected recurrent laryngeal nerve is inspected from the immediate medial carotid area, from level VII until the laryngeal nerve inlet. The paratracheal area is inspected both with cottonoid displacement as well as digital palpation for undiagnosed paratracheal pathology. Recall that a preoperative ultrasound had inspected the previously dissected thyroid bed for the presence of abnormal lymph nodes. As long as no paratracheal pathology was identified at that time, dissection of levels VI and VII is not indicated unless metastatic lymph nodes are pathologically confirmed at the time of completion thyroidectomy.

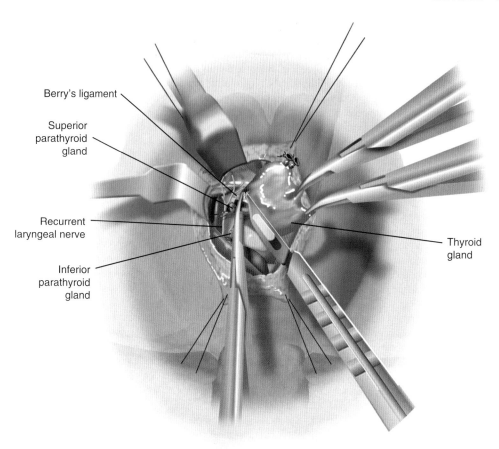

Berry's ligament

Superior
parathyroid
gland

Recurrent
laryngeal nerve

Inferior
parathyroid
gland

Thyroid
gland

FIGURE 17.4

With the most anterior branch
of the recurrent laryngeal
nerve identified and dissected
laterally, a mosquito hemostat
is placed on the vasculature
emanating from Berry's
ligament and then sharply
sectioned to prevent injury
to the immediately adjacent
nerve.

Preservation and Management of the Parathyroid Glands

Identification and preservation of the parathyroid glands are extremely important in patients undergoing completion thyroidectomy. This is most critical in these patients because the complication of permanent hypoparathyroidism may be difficult to manage over a long period and is extremely distressing to the patient. Every effort should be made to preserve the parathyroid glands with their own blood supply, avoiding any devascularization. The incidence of hypoparathyroidism is directly proportional to the extent of thyroidectomy and inversely proportional to the surgeon's experience. The majority of parathyroid glands receive their blood supply from the inferior thyroid artery; however, the superior parathyroid gland may get its own blood supply through the superior thyroid vessels. Careful dissection should be done at the superior pole, both to identify the superior parathyroid gland and to carefully preserve it with its blood supply. Avoid electrocautery injury to the parathyroid glands and excessive irrigation. Suction may damage the glands by causing a surface hematoma, including excessive retraction of the soft tissue of the neck and parathyroid glands. If for any reason the parathyroid gland appears to be devascularized or changes color considerably, every effort should be made to autotransplant the parathyroid gland. However, prior to autotransplantation, it is very important to send a small piece of tissue to confirm that the tissue is actually the parathyroid gland and not metastatic thyroid cancer or a lymph node.

The specimen is removed, and the wound is thoroughly irrigated with sterile water and obtained for meticulous homeostasis. Bipolar electrocautery is used as required. The wounds are not usually drained. The strap muscles are reapproximated in the midline with one interrupted absorbable sutures. Meticulous closure of subcutaneous tissues and skin is performed with fine attention to detail. I use absorbable suture in a subcuticular fashion and further apply adhesive and Steri-strips.

POSTOPERATIVE CARE

Completion thyroidectomy is generally performed as a 23-hour observation hospitalization. However, postoperative verification of normalized parathyroid hormone levels contributes to a safe outpatient surgery as well. The patients are discharged on anti-inflammatory pain medication, with narcotics only for breakthrough discomfort. The patient's first outpatient follow-up is at 1 week for inspection of the wound, further instruction on wound care, and review of the pathology.

Hormone replacement with Cytomel 25 ∝g twice daily is recommended if radioactive iodine is anticipated in the patient's postoperative care. In some situations, recently, Synthroid (T4) may be started immediately since recombinant TSH is widely available and avoids withdrawal of thyroid hormone. An endocrinologist is reconsulted postoperatively for continued follow-up and monitoring.

COMPLICATIONS

The most common complication of completion thyroidectomy is transient hypoparathyroidism. Meticulous preservation of visualized glands and autotransplantation of any vascular compromise limit the long-term risk. Ultimately, the risk of permanent hypoparathyroidism should be <1%. Autotransplantation of approximately one half of a gland in completion thyroidectomy should reduce the ultimate rate of permanent hypoparathyroidism to this acceptable rate. Temporary or permanent injury to the superior or recurrent laryngeal nerve may occur in any case where nerve identification and dissection may occur. Temporary paralysis can occur even in the most minimal dissections with the most meticulous technique, although nerve preservation and gentle care are the best approaches to preserve the integrity and long-term function of these critical nerves.

RESULTS

There is little to no evidence that completion thyroidectomy provides benefit to individuals <45 years of age with tumors <1.5 cm in greatest dimension. Significant debate persists, internationally, on the indications for radioactive iodine in patients with differentiated thyroid carcinomas. Nevertheless, patients with soft tissue extension of differentiated thyroid malignancies or evidence of lymph node or distant metastatic disease are those with the greatest suggestion of clinical benefit of radioactive iodine therapy and thus indication for completion thyroidectomy.

PEARLS

- Prior to surgical management, interdisciplinary evaluation and treatment planning with both the thyroid surgeon and endocrinologist are essential.
- Completion thyroidectomy should be performed within the first 5 days following initial surgery or otherwise delayed for 6 months in order to minimize the difficulty associated with inflammatory and wound healing issues within the surgical field.
- Preoperative evaluation of the central compartment and lateral neck with a high-resolution ultrasound and FNA cytology of abnormal lymph nodes should be performed in all patients.
- In patients with lymph node metastases, I recommend high-resolution CT scanning with contrast to identify sites of disease that cannot be appreciated with ultrasound, as well as the ability to provide a surgical roadmap. When in doubt, cross-sectional imaging should be used to facilitate surgical planning.
- Elevate the skin flaps in the immediate anterior jugular prevascular plane.
- Examination of the larynx should be performed on all patients independent of vocal quality or symptomatology.
- Treat each parathyroid gland as it were the only functioning remaining tissue. Transplant a portion of a gland whenever feasible.

PITFALLS

- Surgery in the 2- to 12-week time period is complicated by difficulty in differentiating normal fascial planes.
- The previously operated side should not be dissected unless there is obvious persistent disease. Rushing into a subsequent surgery to assess postsurgical changes from persistent disease is not warranted over watchful waiting.

INSTRUMENTS TO HAVE AVAILABLE

- Harmonic instrumentation or similar sealant device baby right-angle clamps
- Parotid dissector or similar fine dissection tool
- Insulated bipolar electrocautery
- Cottonoid pledgets
- 4-0 silk stick ties on a tf needle (small vascular pop-off needle)

SUGGESTED READING

Cohn KH, Bäckdahl M, Forsslund G, et al. Biologic considerations and operative strategy in papillary thyroid carcinoma: arguments against the routine performance of total thyroidectomy. *Surgery* 1984;96(6):957–971.

Shaha AR, Shah JP, Loree TR. Patterns of failure in differentiated carcinoma of the thyroid based on risk groups. *Head Neck* 1998;20(1):26–30.

Rafferty MA, Goldstein DP, Rotstein L, et al. Completion thyroidectomy versus total thyroidectomy: is there a difference in complication rates? An analysis of 350 patients. *J Am Coll Surg* 2007;205(4):602–607.

Vaiman M, Nagibin A, Olevson J. Complications in primary and completed thyroidectomy. *Surg Today* 2010;40(2):114–118.

Cohen J, Clayman GL. Subtotal and total thyroidectomy. In: *Atlas of Head and Neck Surgery*. Philadelphia, PA: Elsevier, 2011a.

Cohen J, Clayman GL. Thyroid lobectomy. In: *Atlas of Head and Neck Surgery*. Philadelphia, PA: Elsevier, 2011b.

18 SURGICAL MANAGEMENT OF LOCALLY INVASIVE THYROID CANCER

Ashok R. Shaha

INTRODUCTION

The incidence of thyroid cancer is increasing rapidly worldwide. Approximately 56,000 new patients with thyroid cancer will be seen in the United States in the year 2012. Although the major rise in incidence of thyroid cancer is seen in patients with small cancers, below 2 cm, there also appears to be a slight rise in the incidence of advanced thyroid cancer. There is an increased detection of incidental thyroid nodules seen on imaging studies done for other purposes such as ultrasound (US), carotid Doppler, computed tomography (CT), magnetic resonance imaging (MRI), and positron emission tomography (PET) scans, which may account for this apparent increase in thyroid cancer.

Despite increased detection rates, the mortality from thyroid cancer has remained essentially unchanged over the past two decades. Approximately 1,400 patients die of thyroid cancer every year in the United States, a majority of whom have aggressive well-differentiated, anaplastic, or medullary thyroid cancer. Although death from well-differentiated thyroid cancer is quite rare, these cancers may invade the surrounding structures in the neck, such as trachea, recurrent laryngeal nerve (RLN), esophagus, and larynx. Patients with locally invasive thyroid cancer usually have a long history of the presence of thyroid cancer. However, certain forms of biologically aggressive thyroid cancer such as poorly differentiated tall cell variant or insular thyroid cancer may grow rapidly and be locally invasive.

Thyroid cancer is characterized by slow growth. The prognostic features in thyroid cancer are well recognized through reports from the Mayo Clinic, Lahey Clinic, Memorial Sloan-Kettering Cancer Center which include age, gender, grade of the cancer, size of the cancer, extrathyroidal extension, and distant metastases. Thyroid cancer is generally considered to be more aggressive in patients above the age of 45. In patients above the age of 60 to 65, thyroid cancer is much more aggressive and the incidence of the poorly differentiated form is much higher.

The prognostic factors are crucial in the evaluation, management, and prognosis of patients with thyroid cancer. Based on the prognostic factors, the risk group stratifications such as low and high-risk groups are well described by Blake Cady from the Lahey Clinic and by Ian Hay from the Mayo Clinic. The low risk thyroid cancer group includes younger patients with smaller cancers, while high-risk groups include patients above the age of 45 with more aggressive and advanced form of thyroid cancer.

The data from Memorial Sloan-Kettering Cancer Center were further analyzed leading to the stratification of low-, intermediate-, and high-risk groups. Our patients were divided into low risk (younger patients with small cancers) or high risk (older patients with larger tumors or a more aggressive form of thyroid cancer). An intermediate-risk group was described, which includes younger patients with more aggressive forms of thyroid cancer or older patients with smaller (non aggressive) cancers. There clearly is a survival difference in these three risk categories, and the treatment decisions should be individualized based on risk group analysis. Generally, patients in the low-risk group of thyroid cancer require appropriate and satisfactory surgical excision only, while the high-risk group requires aggressive surgery and additional treatment including radioactive iodine ablation and external beam radiation therapy in a selected group of patients. While the treatment of patients in the intermediate-risk group should be individualized based on the aggressiveness of the primary cancer, this would generally include younger patients having more aggressive forms of thyroid cancer requiring adjuvant treatment such as radioactive iodine ablation, while older patients with small cancers would require surgical excision only.

HISTORY

The history and physical examination are very important in the evaluation of the patient with locally invasive thyroid cancer. The presence and duration of symptoms such as dysphagia, weight loss, shortness of breath, and hoarseness are crucial in appreciating the locally aggressive nature of the disease. Subtle symptoms such as sore throat and mild dysphagia will require further detailed investigation. Occasionally, the patient may give a history of a thyroid nodule being present for a long time with previous benign or indeterminate needle biopsies. The presence of a mass in the neck arouses suspicion of metastasis to the cervical lymph nodes. These patients will require further evaluation to make the diagnosis and determine the extent of the cancer.

PHYSICAL EXAMINATION

A detailed physical examination of the entire neck remains a critically important aspect in the evaluation of the patient suspected of having locally invasive thyroid cancer. The central compartment must be examined to determine the size and configuration of a mass when present. The degree of fixation of the mass to the skin and/or the trachea must be noted. The entire neck should be palpated to determine the presence of metastasis to the lymph nodes. Mirror or fiberoptic laryngoscopy must be carried out to determine whether mobility of the vocal cord/s is impaired. The finding of a mass fixed to the central compartment in the presence of a paralyzed vocal cord suggests locally invasive thyroid cancer.

INDICATIONS

- Locally aggressive thyroid cancer invading the surrounding structures in the central compartment of the neck
- Recurrent thyroid cancer with local invasion
- Patients presenting with vocal cord paralysis or a fixed mass in the central compartment
- Cancer adherent to or invading the trachea, larynx, or esophagus
- Bulky primary cancer with invasion of the strap muscles

CONTRANDICATIONS

- Massive cancer involving the central compartment and encasing the carotid artery/s
- Extensive cancer involving the mediastinum and occasionally the sternum
- Massive cancer causing bilateral vocal cord paralysis and airway obstruction
- Cancer invading the prevertebral fascia and paravertebral musculature
- Massive distant metastases with major loss of pulmonary reserve
- Massive tracheal invasion in close proximity to the carina

PREOPERATIVE PLANNING

Thyroid function tests will confirm the patient to be euthyroid before the surgery. However, thyroglobulin may be of help as a baseline tumor marker. Calcitonin and carcinoembryonic antigen (CEA) are important tumor markers if medullary thyroid cancer is suspected.

Imaging Studies

US is a useful technique in the evaluation of the extent of the cancer, and features suggestive of malignancy such as irregular margin, microcalcification, and hypervascularity are extremely valuable.

Cross-sectional imaging in suspected locally aggressive thyroid cancer is a critical aspect in the evaluation of the extent of the cancer and its invasion into or adherence to the surrounding structures in the central compartment. CT scan with contrast is the best imaging study for the evaluation of the extent of the cancer. While the use of contrast will delay radioactive iodine ablation by 2 to 3 months, if the operating surgeon feels that the information obtained from CT with contrast is crucial in selecting the best surgical procedure for the invasive thyroid cancer, the CT should be performed with no hesitation.

MRI is generally not necessary; however, if the cancer is inseparable from the trachea, MRI is quite helpful to evaluate the relation of the cancer to the trachea. If there is any involvement of the tracheal wall or tracheal lumen, US should be performed for more detailed evaluation of the primary cancer and cervical lymph nodes.

Other imaging studies such as PET scan and bone scans are individualized. For consistency in poorly differentiated cancer, the PET scan may be of value to evaluate the distant organs such as mediastinum, lung, or liver. Routine chest radiography or CT scan may not be helpful in determining the presence of pulmonary metastasis, which is best evaluated in well-differentiated thyroid cancer with a radioactive iodine scan.

Pathology

If the patient has been biopsied elsewhere or has had previous surgery for cancer of the thyroid, the slides should be obtained and reviewed by a head and neck pathologist. If a tissue diagnosis has not been obtained, appropriate biopsies should be done to establish the correct diagnosis. Any suspicious lymph nodes in the neck may require preoperative fine needle aspiration biopsy with cytology or thyroglobulin wash from the aspirant.

SURGICAL TECHNIQUE

In long-standing or biologically aggressive cancer of the thyroid, the wall of the trachea may be directly invaded with extension of the cancer into the lumen. The recurrent laryngeal nerve (RLN) is directly related to the posterior capsule of the thyroid gland, and even though direct invasion of the RLN is rare, the nerve may be embedded in the cancer and it may be extremely difficult or impossible to separate from the cancer requiring sacrifice of the portion of nerve for tumor clearance (Fig. 18.1). Occasionally, cancer in the lymph nodes in the paratracheal area may directly invade the RLN leading to preoperative palsy and the need to resect a portion of the RLN.

The growth of the primary cancer or cancer in the lymph nodes in the tracheoesophageal sulcus may invade vital structures such as the RLN, trachea, or esophagus. The surgeon must be prepared to undertake appropriate surgical resection if these surrounding structures are involved by the primary cancer or metastatic lymph nodes. Involvement of the esophagus is quite rare, and most of the time, the cancer is adherent to the esophageal musculature leading to the need for resection of the esophageal muscles rather than the mucosa itself. However, if the cancer involves the esophageal mucosa, a much more radical resection is required and reconstruction may require a microvascular free flap or a gastric pull up. Cancer involving the region of the cricoid cartilage or cricopharyngeal muscles may be difficult to evaluate even intraoperatively on gross evaluation. The management of recurrent cancer involving this region of the cricothyroid area makes for extremely complex surgical decision making as laryngectomy may be necessary for surgical resection with cancer-free margins. Involvement of other vital structures such as the carotid artery, vagus, and phrenic nerves and sympathetic trunk is quite rare.

The majority of these patients will require a multidisciplinary approach with active involvement of specialists in endocrinology, nuclear medicine, and medical oncology with special expertise in the management of thyroid cancer with targeted therapies. The laryngologist and speech language pathologist play an important

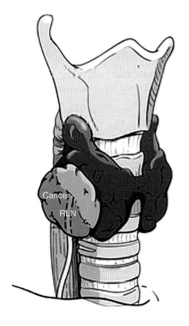
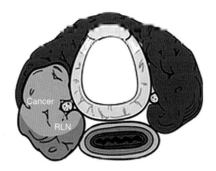

FIGURE 18.1
Involvement of RLN by thyroid cancer.

role in the management of voice problems. The RLN may be directly in contact with cancer, and resection of the RLN or any tedious separation may jeopardize the function of the RLN either temporary or permanently. The superior laryngeal nerve (SLN) is rarely directly involved by the cancer, but surgical intervention may lead to iatrogenic trauma to the SLN, leading to a change in voice and inability to raise the voice, pitch, and tone. The parathyroid glands are adherent to the posterior portion of the thyroid capsule. In locally aggressive thyroid cancer, these glands may be inseparable from the cancer or may be involved in the thyroid capsule leading to unintentional loss of one or more parathyroid glands, resulting in temporary or permanent hypoparathyroidism. Consideration should be given to parathyroid autotransplantation.

Anesthesia Considerations

The anesthesia decisions are also intricate in these complex surgical procedures. Any attempt at awake intubation should be best avoided for the fear of laryngospasm and intralaryngeal trauma. Induction should be smooth with a nontraumatic intubation with a size 6 tube. Larger tubes such as 8 and 9 are not necessary in thyroid surgery. The cuff of the endotracheal tube should be well below the vocal cords. If there is a major concern about a difficult intubation, a fiberoptic nasotracheal intubation may be considered.

Principles of Surgical Management of Locally Invasive Cancer of the Thyroid

The oncologic principles in the management of locally aggressive thyroid cancer dictate that all gross cancer should be removed and clear surgical margins obtained. Pathologists should be readily available for appropriate frozen sections of the lymph node, esophageal musculature, or tracheal wall as necessary. The surgeon should avoid resection of important structures such as the RLN unless it is directly involved by the cancer. One must develop a balance between the best control of the cancer and quality of life.

It is important to review the final pathology report to analyze whether this is a well-differentiated papillary carcinoma or other varieties of papillary carcinoma such as tall cell, insular, or poorly differentiated. The majority of older patients have a pathologically more aggressive form of papillary carcinoma of the thyroid. Occasionally, aggressive follicular Hurthle cell or medullary carcinoma may invade surrounding structures. Understanding the biology of the cancer, its initial extent, and appropriate surgical intervention will offer the best chance of controlling the cancer in the central compartment.

Management of the Central Compartment Lymph Nodes

Generally, the incidence of metastases to cervical lymph nodes is much higher in patients with locally aggressive cancer of the thyroid, gross extrathyroidal extension, older age group, or a large cancer. If there are any suspicious lymph nodes in the paratracheal area, they should be removed, frozen section obtained, and appropriate central compartment clearance should be performed. The lymph nodes may extend to levels VI and VII, and a thorough dissection of this area should be undertaken should there be any suspicious lymph nodes; however, it is important to recognize that Hashimoto's thyroiditis may occasionally present with lymph nodes. These are, however, generally globular in shape, and frozen section can readily confirm this benign nature. Because of the high incidence of central compartment lymph node involvement in larger cancers. The American Thyroid Association guidelines in 2009 were revised to include prophylactic central compartment dissection in patients with larger cancers, gross extrathyroidal extension, or aggressive histology.

Every effort must be made during central compartment dissection to identify and, if possible, preserve the RLN and the parathyroid glands along with their blood supply. If any of the parathyroid glands especially the inferior one is devascularized, it should be autotransplanted in the sternomastoid muscle.

Recurrent Laryngeal Nerve

The preoperative evaluation of the extent of the cancer must include evaluation of the vocal cords either by mirror or fiberoptic examination and is crucial in facilitating the management of RLN during locally invasive thyroid surgery. The cancer can usually be shaved off of the RLN and every attempt should be made to preserve the functioning RLN at the conclusion of the surgical procedure. However, the nerve may need to be sacrificed especially if the cancer is involving it directly or the vocal cord is paralyzed preoperatively. Prior to sacrifice of a functioning RLN on one side, every attempt should be made to evaluate the opposite side and preserve the opposite RLN by careful dissection. A functioning nerve rarely needs to be sacrificed; however, occasionally the cancer may directly encase the RLN either from the primary cancer or from the lymph node metastases in the tracheoesophageal groove. If the nerve is sacrificed and the two ends can be easily visualized, a nerve graft may be entertained such as ansa, greater auricular, or sural nerve. An interposition graft may be performed with the ansa, or one end of the ansa may be used to anastomose with the distal end of the transected RLN. Even though the nerve function is unlikely to recover with vocal cord mobility, most of the time the vocal cord function will improve with nerve grafting. In young patients with well differentiated cancer of the thyroid, every attempt should be made to dissect the cancer and the lymph nodes off the RLN as any microscopic disease that is left behind can be treated with radioactive iodine ablation with satisfactory long-term control of the cancer and best quality of life.

Trachea

Grillo et al. defined various stages of cancer involvement of the trachea:

- Type I includes cancer adherent to the tracheal cartilage, which, however, can be easily separated from the tracheal cartilage.
- Type II includes cancer minimally invading the tracheal cartilage, which can usually be excised with portions of the tracheal ring.
- Type III includes submucosal involvement of the trachea.
- Type IV includes intraluminal extension of the cancer. Types III and IV are challenging problems and generally will require segmental resection of the trachea (Fig. 18.2). A sleeve resection of the trachea up to five rings with end-to-end anastomosis can be performed easily. However, any extended tracheal resection will require appropriate mobilization of the trachea in the mediastinum usually with the assistance of a thoracic surgeon.

Occasionally, the cancer may invade a small segment of the tracheal ring, and a tracheal window can be performed easily, which can be repaired with surrounding soft tissue or periosteal graft from the clavicle. The majority of the time, such small tracheal defects can be converted into a tracheostomy, which can be removed in approximately 10 to 14 days with satisfactory function. Appropriate preoperative endoscopy in the operating room is quite helpful to localize and evaluate the extent of intraluminal invasion and the distance between the subglottic area and the proximal end of the cancer. The evaluation of the distal end is important in relation to the distance from the carina.

Surgical Approaches to Tracheal Resection

Appropriate imaging studies are crucial in the proper evaluation of the extent of the cancer involving the trachea. It would be important to have a definitive evaluation of the extent of the invasion of the trachea and larynx by fiberoptic laryngoscopy. Tracheal resection is much more complex if the cancer involves the subglottic larynx or the cricoid cartilage. If the cancer is very close to the carina, generally it is considered to be unresectable. At the time of surgery, it is important to perform esophagoscopy either fiberoptic or rigid, to determine whether intraluminal invasion has occurred.

Total thyroidectomy should be performed in a standard fashion with preservation of the parathyroid glands. It is important to preserve at least one parathyroid gland with its blood supply. The jugular area should be evaluated as there is a high incidence of paratracheal and lateral jugular nodes.

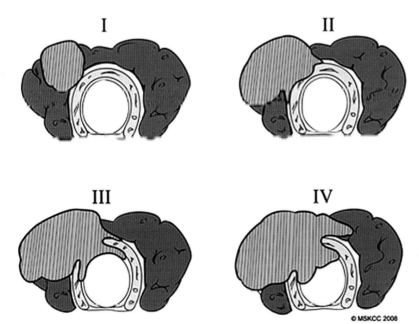

© MSKCC 2008

FIGURE 18.2
Four stages of tumor extension to the trachea.

Preoperative evaluation of the lateral neck nodes with US or CT scan is also crucial since the lymph nodes at levels II, III, and IV may be involved with metastatic cancer, and a neck dissection should be included. Paratracheal lymph nodes should be evaluated. Utmost care must be taken to avoid any traction injury to the RLN on the side of the node dissection.

After completing the total thyroidectomy, the trachea should be opened based on the clinical and radiologic evaluation of the extent of the disease. At least one to two rings inferior to the cancer margin should be resected. After opening the trachea, the endotracheal area can be evaluated. It is important to avoid injury to the cuff of the endotracheal tube to avoid air leak. At this time, the extent of the cancer inside the trachea is evaluated, and the circumferential resection of the trachea is performed carefully avoiding injury to the esophagus.

If the cancer is adherent to the esophagus, the involved esophageal musculature should be resected. The dissection should now be continued in the tracheoesophageal groove posteriorly preserving both of the RLNs or at least the functioning RLN. As the dissection is continued superiorly, the superior portion of the trachea is opened just inferior to the cricoid cartilage unless the cancer is directly invading the cricoid area where the inferior portion of the subglottic area and the cricoid cartilage should be resected. After resecting the trachea circumferentially, the endotracheal tube is partially withdrawn. The cancer and the tracheal sleeve are resected, and the endotracheal tube is repositioned. An experienced anesthesiologist is quite helpful for these technical maneuvers.

After repositioning the endotracheal tube and securing the airway, the primary end-to-end anastomosis of the trachea is undertaken. Flexion of the head on the chest is quite helpful in these circumstances. Extensive lateral tracheal dissection in the mediastinum should be avoided, as it can lead to devascularization of the trachea. A primary anastomosis is undertaken with nonabsorbable sutures such as Prolene, or Monocryl and Vicryl; however, Monocryl is more acceptable as it causes less reaction in the lumen of the trachea. If Prolene sutures are going to be used, they should be passed submucosally avoiding an intramucosal suture line with nonabsorbable sutures, which can lead to granuloma formation and fibrosis. The posterior anastomosis is performed initially followed by the anterior anastomosis with slight rotation of the trachea on either side. At the conclusion of the anastomosis, the wound is filled with saline and hyperventilation performed through the endotracheal tube to make sure there is no air leak. In spite of that, a minor air leak may be expected and generally a drain is placed in this region. A Penrose drain is better than suction drainage, which may cause more air leak. The neck should be kept flexed with a large Prolene suture from the chin to the chest. This is generally retained for a period of 8 to 10 days, and most of the time the patient is discharged with a large suture, which is removed during the first office visit approximately 8 to 10 days after the surgical procedure (Figs. 18.3 to 18.6).

I prefer to extubate the patient in the operating room and observe the airway; however, if the surgical procedure is performed late in the evening or there is considerable manipulation of the RLN, then it would be most appropriate to leave the patient intubated and extubate the next day under close observation. If there is a considerable airway distress or severe stridor, the patient should be reintubated, and further evaluation should be undertaken as to the best way to secure the airway. I try to avoid a tracheostomy in these patients, as tracheostomy will interfere with healing of the tracheal anastomosis.

Larynx

The involvement of the larynx by the primary thyroid cancer is quite rare; however, the cancer may be adherent to the thyroid cartilage, which can be easily peeled off the thyroid cartilage with the perichondrium, or partial framework resection can be performed. Partial laryngeal surgery such as hemilaryngectomy may be considered in select cases of unilateral laryngeal involvement by thyroid tumor. Primary total laryngectomy is rarely necessary unless the cancer is directly invading the larynx, obstructing the airway or destroying the larynx. However, recurrent cancer in the central compartment invading the cricoid cartilage or obstructing the lumen of the larynx requires a total laryngectomy. The difficult area in the laryngeal complex is the cricothyroid complex where the cancer may be difficult to resect if adherent to the cricothyroid region. Rarely, recurrent cancer may invade the entire central compartment of the neck with involvement of the esophagus and larynx, which will require total laryngopharyngectomy with cervical esophagectomy at which time appropriate reconstruction may require a gastric pull-up or microvascular free flap reconstruction with either jejunum or a radial forearm flap. The risks of complications in such an aggressive procedure are quite high and may lead to considerable morbidity and occasional mortality.

Esophagus

Local invasion into the esophagus usually involves the muscular portion of the esophagus rather than the mucosa. In such cases, the cancer can be resected with a portion of the muscular wall without entering the mucosa. Utmost care needs to be taken to avoid tearing the mucosa. If there is a rent in the mucosa, appropriate closure should be undertaken with muscular coverage to avoid esophageal leak and mediastinal infection. Rarely the cancer may invade the entire wall of the esophagus with extension of the cancer into the lumen,

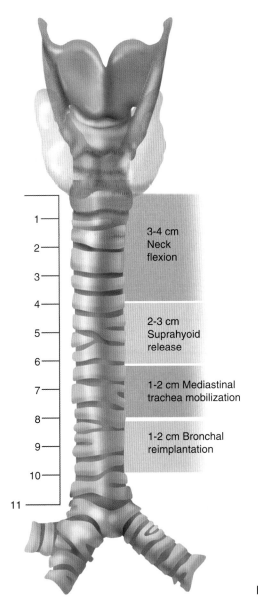

3-4 cm
Neck
flexion

2-3 cm
Suprahyoid
release

1-2 cm Mediastinal
trachea mobilization

1-2 cm Bronchal
reimplantation

FIGURE 18.3 Extent of tracheal resection and reconstruction.

which obviously will require resection of the esophagus usually along with laryngopharyngeal resection and appropriate reconstruction.

Related Structures

The resection of the carotid artery is rarely performed for cancer of the thyroid. However, it may be necessary to obtain the help of a vascular surgeon for appropriate reconstruction of the carotid artery. Occasionally, the tumor may extend into the superior mediastinum requiring appropriate surgical resection with sternal split. The involvement of neural structures such as brachial plexus is quite rare. Occasionally, the recurrent cancer may involve the paravertebral muscles such as the scalene or levator scapulae, the resection of which may be quite difficult. Recurrence rates are quite high in this group of patients. Such patients will benefit with adjuvant therapies.

POSTOPERATIVE MANAGEMENT

The patient's serum calcium levels should be monitored carefully in the postoperative period and hypocalcemia treated appropriately. Thyroid hormone replacement should begin the next day, and patients are generally discharged soon after the removal of the drain. The patient is ambulatory the next day with a regular diet as tolerated. The final pathology report should be carefully reviewed both in terms of the margins of resection

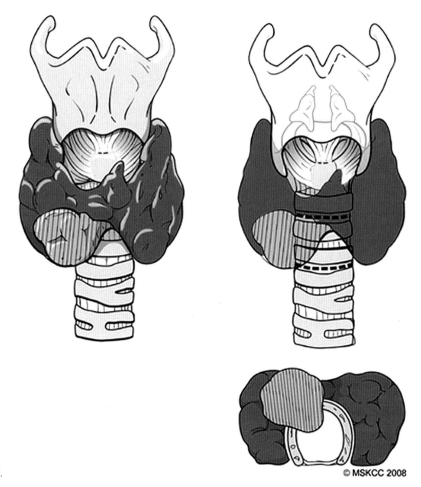

FIGURE 18.4
Sleeve resection of the trachea.

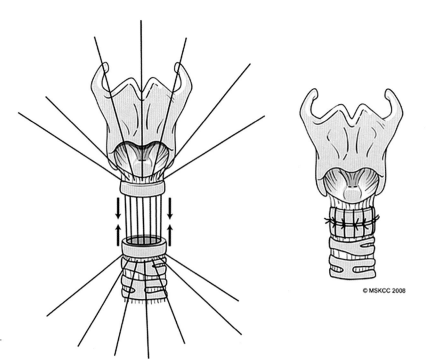

FIGURE 18.5
Primary end-to-end anastomosis of the trachea.

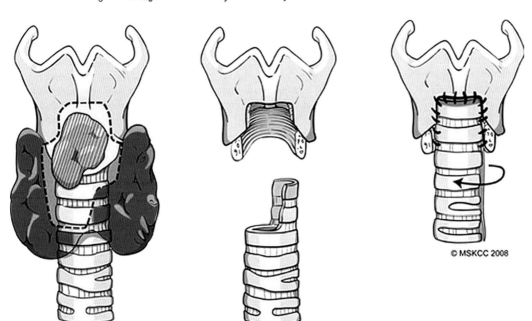

© MSKCC 2008

FIGURE 18.6
Complex resection of the upper trachea and subglottic region.

and the aggressiveness of the thyroid cancer. If the cancer is reported to be poorly differentiated or high grade, postoperative external beam radiation therapy may be considered depending upon the primary extent of the disease and the surgical resection.

Adjuvant Therapy

The majority of these patients will require adjuvant therapy in the form of radioactive iodine. Patients with well-differentiated cancer of the thyroid usually respond quite well to treatment with radioactive iodine; however, patients with poorly differentiated cancers do not respond as well. Radioactive iodine ablation is also helpful to evaluate if there is any suspicious lesion in the lungs. If there is activity in the lungs suggestive of metastatic disease, which can be quite high in this group of patients, larger doses of radioactive iodine may be required.

Radioactive scanning is carried out annually. More recently, the patients are prepared with Thyrogen (recombinant thyroid stimulating hormone) rather than making them hypothyroid for 6 weeks. If there is suspicion of recurrent cancer in the central or lateral neck nodes, appropriate follow-up is important with serial USs. Serum thyroglobulin, stimulated thyroglobulin, and thyroglobulin doubling time are important markers in the follow-up. Calcitonin and CEA are also important in patients with medullary thyroid cancer, especially calcitonin doubling time.

COMPLICATIONS

The major complication of tracheal resection includes bilateral RLN injury leading to airway problems in the postoperative period and securing the airway immediately after the extubation is critical. The patient should be monitored very closely preferably in the recovery room or in the Intensive care unit. The majority of the patients with minor airway problems will improve over 24 to 48 hours. Short-term steroids are routinely used during this period. The patient's neck should be kept flexed at all times. If there is a severe airway issue, the patient should be intubated and observed for a period of time subsequent to which appropriate decisions will have to be made, based on the fiberoptic laryngoscopic evaluation for maintenance of the airway. Occasionally, a tracheostomy may be necessary if the patient has considerable stridor. Tracheostomy is best performed away from the suture line either in the distal portion of the trachea, or a cricothyrotomy may be considered with a small tracheostomy tube. Patients with these airway-related problems can have a complex postoperative course and severe morbidity after tracheal resection.

Postoperative calcium levels should be carefully monitored, and hypocalcemia should be treated appropriately. The incidence of hematoma is between 2% and 3%, and the neck should be closely monitored. Appropriate intervention should be undertaken should they have expanding hematoma. Other complications may be related to neck dissection such as a chyle leak. The majority of the patients with chyle leak have minor problems, which will be corrected in a few days.

RESULTS

The results in patients undergoing treatment for locally aggressive thyroid cancer depend mainly on the age of the patient, satisfactory gross resection of the cancer, histologic variations, and effectiveness of adjuvant therapy such as radioactive iodine or external beam radiation therapy in selected patients. The results are excellent in patients below the age of 45 if all gross cancer has been removed. The long-term survival is equivalent to the patients who do not present with extrathyroidal extension. The 5-year survival in this group is about 80%; however, the survival drops to approximately 50% in individuals above the age of 45 where all gross cancer could not be removed or the histology shows tall cell insular or poorly differentiated thyroid cancer.

The recent results from Sloan-Kettering show the disease-specific survival when stratified by R0/R1/R2 resection to be 96%, 60%, and 63%, while the recurrence-free survival was 83%, 60%, and 65%. Even in patients with M1 disease, R0 resection had excellent locoregional control and better quality of life with over 50% of patients alive at 5 years.

PEARLS

- A true multidisciplinary approach is necessary in the management of patients with locally invasive cancer.
- Preoperative evaluation of vocal cord function is critical.
- Endoscopy should be performed at the time of surgery to evaluate the extent of the cancer involving the trachea or esophagus.
- Surgery should be designed to include removal of all gross cancer and sacrifice vital organs only if they are directly involved by the cancer, such as RLN, trachea, esophagus, or larynx.
- In locally aggressive recurrent cancer of the thyroid, total laryngectomy may be indicated especially if the larynx is directly involved by the cancer. Partial laryngectomy may be considered in select patients.
- If the cancer is adherent to the wall of the trachea and all gross cancer can be removed, a shave procedure should be undertaken.
- If there is intraluminal involvement of the trachea by cancer, appropriate resection should be undertaken using sleeve resection and primary end-to-end anastomosis.
- Most of the patients with locally aggressive cancer of the thyroid will require adjuvant therapy including radioactive iodine ablation and, in selected cases, external radiation therapy.
- If there is a gross extrathyroidal extension or aggressive histology, postoperative radiation therapy in the form of IMRT should be undertaken.
- Patients should be best followed with cross-sectional imaging and a PET scan of the central compartment of the neck, neck nodes, and distal regions.
- Thyroglobulin is commonly used as follow-up marker for cancer recurrence especially the thyroglobulin doubling time.

PITFALLS

- The recurrence rate is quite high in these patients especially if the surgical margins are positive.
- Evaluation of the extent of the cancer in the trachea may be quite difficult.
- Thorough understanding of the extent of the cancer and surgical expertise will result in appropriate intraoperative decision making regarding tracheal shave, window, or sleeve resection.
- Evaluation of the presence of submucosal cancer may be quite difficult.
- Reconstruction of small defects in the trachea may be difficult because of continuous air leak.
- Bilateral RLN injury may lead to life-threatening airway obstruction.

INSTRUMENTS TO HAVE AVAILABLE

- Standard thyroidectomy tray
- Harmonic scalpel
- LigaSure
- Surgical loops
- Bipolar cautery
- Intratracheal nerve monitor

SUGGESTED READING

Grillo HC, Suen HC, Mathisen DJ, et al. Resectional management of thyroid carcinoma invading the airway. *Ann Thorac Surg* 1992;54(1):3–9: discussion 9–10.

Shah JP, Loree TR, Dharker D, et al. Prognostic factors in differentiated carcinoma of the thyroid gland. *Am J Surg* 1992;164(6):658–661.

Patel KN, Shaha AR. Locally advanced thyroid cancer. *Curr Opin Otolaryngol Head Neck Surg* 2005;13(2):112–116.

Shaha A. Treatment of thyroid cancer based on risk groups. *J Surg Oncol* 2006;4(8):683–691.

Price DL, Wong RJ, Randolph GW. Invasive thyroid cancer: management of the trachea and esophagus. *Otolaryngol Clin North Am* 2008;41(6):1155–1168,ix–x.

Cooper DS, Doherty GM, Haugen BR, et al. American Thyroid Association (ATA) Guidelines Taskforce on Thyroid Nodules and Differentiated Thyroid Cancer. Revised American Thyroid Association management guidelines for patients with thyroid nodules and differentiated thyroid cancer. [Erratum in *Thyroid* 2010;20(8):942. (Hauger, Bryan R corrected to Haugen, Bryan R). *Thyroid* 2010;20(6):674–675]. *Thyroid* 2009;19(11):1167–1214.

19 CENTRAL COMPARTMENT NECK DISSECTION

Ralph P. Tufano

INTRODUCTION

Indications for the performance of a central neck dissection (CND) for cancer of the thyroid can be confusing. The reason for this is the lack of good evidence-based data on its utility when performed routinely in the management of differentiated cancer of the thyroid. When reading the pertinent literature, it becomes obvious that one of the limitations is that there is no standardization of the operation. Boundaries and compartments are not well defined, and the reports often fail to report whether these procedures were being performed in the presence or absence of gross lymph node metastasis. These shortcomings prompted the convergence of a subgroup of experts on cancer of the thyroid to come together under the auspices of the American Thyroid Association (ATA) to formulate a consensus statement on the anatomy and terminology pertinent to CND. The group concluded that the CND should consist of level VI and level VII lymph node basins and must contain the prelaryngeal (delphian), pretracheal, and at least one paratracheal nodal basin. The surgery should be designated as elective or therapeutic. Obvious lymph node metastasis in the central neck should be treated with therapeutic intent accomplished by a compartmental dissection. While elective CND for medullary thyroid cancer is advocated, controversy exists in differentiated thyroid cancer. This chapter describes the technical performance of a CND and considerations for when it should be performed.

HISTORY

A patient usually will present to the surgeon with a mass in the thyroid that has been detected by palpation or detected incidentally on radiographic imaging for evaluation of other disease processes (e.g., carotid ultrasound [US], magnetic resonance imaging [MRI] of the spine). A diagnosis is usually established by ultrasound guided fine needle aspiration biopsy (FNAB). Most patients with a diagnosis of thyroid malignancy with or without central neck lymphadenopathy are usually asymptomatic. Patients with larger or more aggressive tumors can present with one or all of the following: hoarseness, dysphagia, and dyspnea.

PHYSICAL EXAMINATION

A patient is nearly always diagnosed with a primary cancer of the thyroid prior to making a determination of whether a CND needs to be performed. The entire neck should be palpated. A firm, fixed thyroid cancer with suspected extrathyroidal spread warrants a CND. Flexible fiberoptic laryngoscopic examination of the vocal folds should be conducted in all patients undergoing thyroid surgery. Vocal fold paralysis, lateral neck lymphadenopathy confirmed as cancer by fine needle aspiration (FNA), central neck lymphadenopathy confirmed on physical examination, radiographic imaging or intraoperative inspection, medullary cancer of the thyroid, and suspicion of more aggressive variants of thyroid cancer are all accepted indications for CND. This is in accordance with the ATA guidelines. A patient who has previously undergone a total thyroidectomy with or without radioactive iodine (RAI) may have an increasing serum thyroglobulin level determined as part of follow-up surveillance. Radiographic imaging (US, computed tomography [CT], MRI, positron emission tomography [PET]) is usually instituted. If a central mass in the neck is found during the surveillance period, a determination as to whether an FNAB should be carried out is made as a multidisciplinary team and usually only if surgery is considered beneficial.

INDICATIONS

- Thyroid cancer with gross lymph node metastasis present in the central or lateral neck compartments
- Medullary cancer of the thyroid
- Select T3 and T4 differentiated thyroid cancer

CONTRAINDICATIONS

- Elective dissection on the side of only one functioning recurrent laryngeal nerve (RLN)

PREOPERATIVE PLANNING

The issues of CND should be discussed with the patient when the procedure is being considered. The CND may be performed electively or therapeutically at the time of thyroidectomy or therapeutically in a reoperative setting. The literature suggests the patient may be at an increased risk of complications compared to total thyroidectomy alone. US evaluation of the central neck is helpful to appreciate the extent of lymph node metastasis as it relates to important structures in the central compartment and is also helpful to confirm recurrent/persistent thyroid cancer by US- or CT-guided FNA. Axial imaging (CT, MRI, and PET–CT) may be helpful in determining the degree of involvement of associated central structures in the neck such as the laryngotracheal complex, esophagus, and carotid artery. Administration of iodinated contrast with CT may preclude early postoperative RAI administration. This usually is not a problem in the setting of recurrent cancer of the thyroid where the tumors are typically non-RAI avid.

SURGICAL TECHNIQUE

The borders of the central compartment for central neck dissection are: superior-horizontal line at the inferior border of the cricoid and the RLN insertion point, inferior plane on level with innominate artery, lateral-common carotid artery, posterior-prevertebral fascia, anterior: sternothyroid muscle, medial border for unilateral central compartment dissection-medial edge of contralateral strap muscles (Figure 19.1).

I will divide the central neck dissection into two categories: Primary or reoperative to emphasize some differences in the techniques.

Primary Central Neck Dissection

Primary CND is usually performed at the time of total thyroidectomy and may be performed en bloc with the thyroid or separately. There are some nuances to the right and left paratracheal dissections that will be discussed. If not already dissected, the prelaryngeal or delphian nodes are excised. The fibroadipose tissue overlying the cricothyroid membrane is incised and dissected off of the cricothyroid membrane. It is important to avoid injury to the cricothyroid muscle or damage the cricothyroid membrane when performing this maneuver.

Adequate exposure of the central neck must be obtained to permit a comprehensive compartmental dissection. The strap muscles must be elevated over the carotid sheath laterally and to the sternum inferiorly. The right paratracheal dissection begins with a skeletonization of the common carotid artery that proceeds inferiorly to the innominate artery and superiorly to the thyroid cartilage. The dissection should not proceed deep to the common carotid artery to avoid injury to the RLN. The vagus nerve in the carotid sheath may be stimulated at 1 mA to determine the neurophysiologic integrity of the RLN. The RLN is then appreciated again in the area of where it was dissected for the thyroidectomy. On the right side, it travels more ventrally and obliquely than the left RLN. It is followed inferiorly until it can no longer be traced under the common carotid artery. Because of its more ventral and oblique location, the RLN divides the right paratracheal compartment into an anterior and posterior compartment as well as a lateral and medial compartment. The RLN must be dissected from its laryngeal point of insertion to its most inferior extent in the neck to be able to safely remove all of the lymph nodes in the right paratracheal compartment. A fine-tip dissector and no. 15 blade are used without a nerve hook. Minimizing tension is important in preserving RLN function and avoiding neuropraxia.

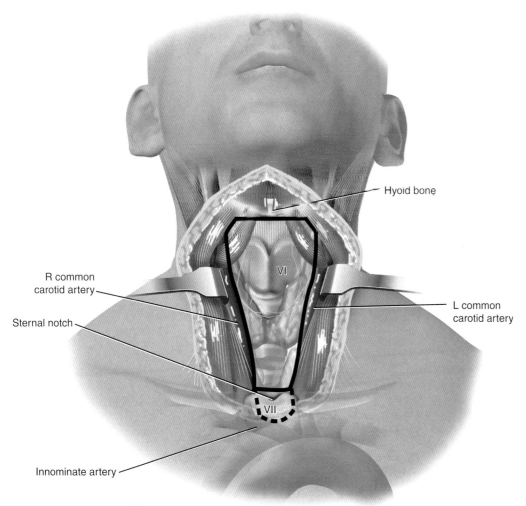

Hyoid bone

R common
carotid artery

L common
carotid artery

Sternal notch

Innominate artery

FIGURE 19.1
The CND borders are outlined
and should include both levels
6 and 7 lymph node stations.

Prudent use of fine-tip bipolar cautery away from the RLN to cauterize small vessels is recommended. Once the nerve is completely transposed, the lymph node–bearing tissue posterior and medial to the carotid artery and posterior and lateral to the RLN can be delivered anteriorly (Fig. 19.2A). The RLN entry point is usually used as the superior border of the dissection. It is essential to preserve the main trunk of the inferior thyroid artery and all of its superior branches to maintain a blood supply to the superior parathyroid gland. The inferior parathyroid gland may need to be dissected away from the adjacent lymph nodes to save its blood supply, but this is often not possible if trying to achieve a complete clearance of all nodal tissue. If the viability of the parathyroid gland appears compromised, it should be harvested and kept in cooled saline. Approximately 10% of it should be sent for frozen section to confirm parathyroid tissue and avoid inadvertent autotransplantation of metastatic cancer in a lymph node. The dissection then proceeds over muscularis of the esophagus with gentle anterior retraction (Fig. 19.2B). The tissue is dissected over the trachea and the pretracheal lymph nodes are elevated and ligated approximate to the medial edge of the left strap muscles. The inferior dissection is completed by carefully ligating all tissue anterior and superior to the innominate artery. This is important because there are usually thymic veins that drain into the brachiocephalic vein and on occasion a thyroid ima from the innominate artery. Level VI does extend to the hyoid bone, but it is uncommon to see lymph node metastasis superior to the level of the RLN insertion site. Routine preoperative US evaluation of the thyroid and lymph nodes of the neck for any patient with FNA-confirmed PTC is recommended by the ATA guidelines, published in 2009. While there may be some limitations of US in the central compartment when the thyroid gland is present, the upper level VI is not subject to those same limitations. If preoperative imaging doesn't suggest metastatic cancer in the upper level VI region, it has been our experience that this area just be kept under observation rather than operated.

The left paratracheal dissection starts with identifying the common carotid artery. Unlike the right, the left common carotid artery has its own takeoff from the aorta and is dissected inferiorly to the level of the clavicle and superiorly to the thyroid cartilage. The RLN is traced from where it was identified during the thyroidectomy inferiorly. Unlike the right RLN, the left runs in a more craniocaudal course and in the tracheo-esophageal groove (Fig. 19.3). It does not need to be circumferentially dissected and transposed. It is followed inferiorly to the level of the clavicle. The lymph node tissue medial to the carotid is brought over the muscularis

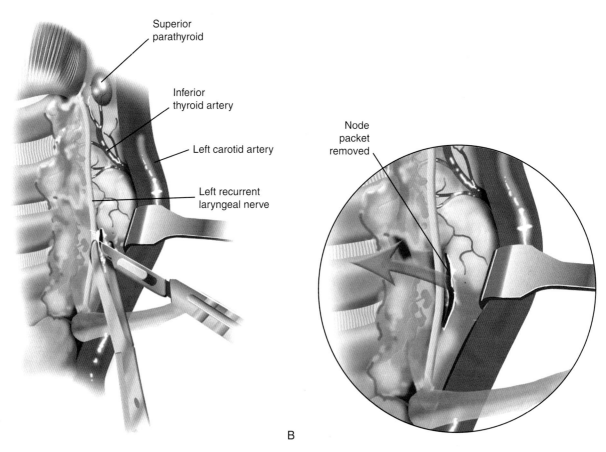

FIGURE 19.2

Right paratracheal dissection: **A:** The right RLN courses ventrally and obliquely in the right paratracheal region. Because of this, the right paratracheal dissection should include lymph nodes deep and lateral as well as superficial and medial to the RLN. The RLN should be carefully dissected and mobilized to allow for this. **B:** Once the RLN has been mobilized, the lymph nodes are dissected free from RLN.

Superior parathyroid

Inferior thyroid artery

Right carotid artery

Recurrent laryngeal nerve

Node packet removed

A

B

of the esophagus and the RLN. The anterior border of the RLN must be freed from the specimen, and this is accomplished with a fine-tip dissector and no. 15 blade without the aid of a nerve hook (Fig. 19.3). One must be careful when dissecting the RLN inferiorly. The RLN is usually tented up with the lymph node–bearing tissue from the superior mediastinal paratracheal region and thymus. An arbitrary ligation of the tissue is then made at the level of the superior border of the innominate artery taking care to meticulously ligate all tissue in this

Superior parathyroid

Inferior thyroid artery

Left carotid artery

Left recurrent laryngeal nerve

Node packet removed

A

B

FIGURE 19.3 Left paratracheal dissection: **A:** The left paratracheal dissection can proceed from lateral to medial once defining the RLN along its course in the tracheoesophageal groove. **B:** Lymph nodes removed after being dissected free from RLN.

area and avoid injury to the RLN. The superior border again is the RLN insertion laryngeal insertion point, and the parathyroid glands are managed similar to the right side. Similarly, the pretracheal lymph nodes are elevated and ligated at the medial border of the right strap muscles.

The operative bed is then inspected. An assessment of parathyroid gland viability is made. The liberal use of autotransplantation is advocated if the viability of the parathyroid gland is questionable. Two percent lidocaine may be used to relieve vasospasm and may help in the decision making to autotransplant. Again, it must be emphasized that if autotransplantation is employed, a frozen section of a small portion of the suspected parathyroid gland must be sent for frozen section confirmation of parathyroid tissue. The integrity of the RLNs is inspected and nerve monitoring, if used, may provide information on the neurophysiologic integrity of the nerve that may help with decision making regarding the usefulness of an elective bilateral paratracheal dissection. A Valsalva maneuver is given and hemostasis is achieved with the judicious use of bipolar cautery or sutures. Hemostatic agents may also be used. The strap muscles are closed with a running absorbable suture. The use of a drain is left to the discretion of the surgeon. The closure proceeds similar to thyroidectomy, and medical-grade skin adhesive glue may be used.

Reoperative Central Neck Dissection

There are some differences between primary and reoperative CND that must be described. Reoperative CND may be considered when there is FNA-confirmed evidence of disease or growth of a mass not amenable to biopsy. It is generally accepted that reoperative CND is fraught with a higher complication rate than primary surgery. Some authors have refuted this belief and have even stated that reoperative CND may be at least as safe, if not safer, than primary CND. Nonetheless, the recommendation for surgery versus observation should be made in a multidisciplinary fashion and tailored to the patient's needs.

All patients undergoing reoperative CND should undergo a fiberoptic laryngoscopy to assess vocal fold mobility. Often, the localization and confirmation of metastatic cancer are made with US and FNAB. It is important to have a clear understanding of the location of the cancer and its relationship to surrounding structures. The cancer may be in lymph nodes or at the primary site. This is important to distinguish because reoperation for metastatic cancer versus recurrence at the primary site has a strikingly different risk profile. In our experience, when the recurrent disease is at the primary site, there is a much higher risk of vocal fold (VF) paralysis (33%) versus metastases to the lymph nodes (<1%). If US can't resolve this issue, then axial imaging such as CT or MRI with contrast may be helpful, especially if there is also concern for local invasion. US is also very helpful in defining whether a unilateral or bilateral paratracheal lymph node dissection will be useful. In our experience, elective reoperative paratracheal lymph node dissection of an US designated clear paratracheal compartment is not indicated as the risk of metastasis ultimately manifesting in the US negative paratracheal nodal basin is low (0%). This may be due to the improved sensitivity of US to detect subcentimeter lymph node metastasis in the central neck when the thyroid is not present.

Reoperative CND can be performed through the existing thyroidectomy incision. The original incision may be excised if necessary and is generally recommended to achieve the best cosmetic result. The approach may be either through the midline raphe of the strap muscles with elevation of the strap muscles over the thyroid bed or from a lateral approach. The lateral approach may be warranted when extensive scarring is present. In this circumstance, the carotid sheath is identified and the strap muscles are elevated over the thyroid bed from lateral to medial. It may be advantageous to divide the sternothyroid muscle to achieve better access to the cervical paratracheal nodal compartment. The strap muscles are then elevated over the thyroid bed superiorly and inferiorly taking great care to avoid excessive cautery as you proceed superiorly to avoid injury to the RLN.

The main difference in technique compared to primary CND is in the method used to identify the ILNs. The region where the RLN is typically found during thyroidectomy may be scarred, and familiar landmarks for identification of the RLN are not present. RLN monitoring may be useful during reoperative CND. I recommend that the vagus nerve be stimulated at 1 mA prior to beginning the dissection to get the baseline amplitude on the waveform. Once the carotid artery is identified in the same fashion as in primary surgery, the right RLN may be searched for medial and deep to the common carotid artery above the innominate and subclavian artery junction and the left RLN medial to the common carotid artery inferior in the neck and in the tracheoesophageal groove. The remainder of the operation proceeds in the same fashion as described for primary CND (Fig. 19.4).

POSTOPERATIVE MANAGEMENT

Patients undergoing CND are typically admitted overnight for observation. Postoperative considerations are similar to total thyroidectomy. I recommend monitoring the serum calcium trend developed by assessing 6- and 12-hour post op levels. Alternatively, one could elect to administer oral calcium and vitamin D supplementation per routine and taper accordingly. Observation for bleeding and hematoma formation is also important.

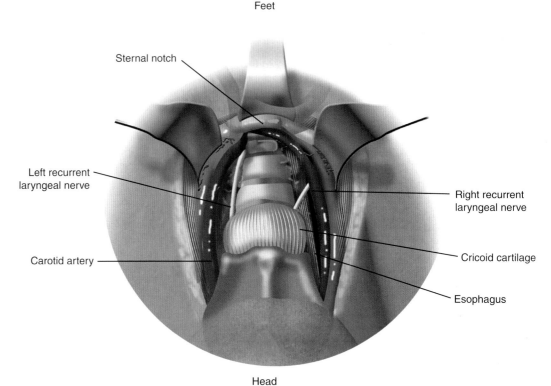

Feet

Sternal notch

Left recurrent
laryngeal nerve

Right recurrent
laryngeal nerve

Carotid artery

Cricoid cartilage

Esophagus

Head

FIGURE 19.4
A completed reoperative CND
with removal of prelaryngeal,
pretracheal, and bilateral
paratracheal nodal basins.

COMPLICATIONS

The complication profile is similar to that of total thyroidectomy. The risk of ILN paralysis has generally been documented by many authors to be the same as with thyroidectomy for primary surgery but may be higher for reoperative surgery. Nonetheless, the true incidence of vocal fold paralysis with these operations is difficult to discern because of the variability in techniques used to assess vocal fold paralysis. Most studies demonstrate an increased incidence of hypoparathyroidism, especially when the CND includes both paratracheal nodal basins. The hematoma rate is similar to conventional thyroidectomy.

RESULTS

The functional results of a primary or reoperative CND are reviewable shortly after surgery. Hoarseness should be evaluated with flexible fiberoptic laryngoscopy. Patients with hypocalcemia from hypoparathyroidism should be repleted accordingly. Oncologic long-term results will be determined by serial follow-up. US is typically used for surveillance of the central neck after thyroid surgery with or without CND. Any suspicious lymphadenopathy in the previously operated central neck should be monitored if it is <5 to 8 mm and biopsied if it is larger than 8 mm.

PEARLS

- Skeletonizing the RLN in its entire cervical course is necessary to achieve a complete compartmental dissection.
- The right paratracheal compartment is divided into an anterior and posterior compartment as well as a lateral and medial compartment by the RLN.
- Liberal autotransplantation of frozen section proven parathyroid glands will help to minimize long-term hypocalcemia.
- Preservation of the main trunk of the inferior thyroid artery and superior terminal branches helps to minimize hypoparathyroidism.
- Reoperative CND poses unique challenges for RLN, and parathyroid preservation and its risk–benefit profile must be carefully weighed in a multidisciplinary fashion.

PITFALLS

- Excessive but unintended traction may result in injury to the RLN.
- If the main trunk of the inferior thyroid artery and its superior branches to the superior parathyroid glands are not preserved, hypoparathyroidism may occur.
- Incomplete clearance of lymph nodes may be the result of attempts at preserving the inferior parathyroid glands pedicled to their blood supply.
- "Berry picking" can lead to the need for additional surgery.

INSTRUMENTS TO HAVE AVAILABLE

- Fine tip dissectors for RLN.
- Fine-tip bipolar cautery
- Nerve monitoring system

SUGGESTED READING

Farrag TY, et al. The utility of evaluating true vocal fold motion prior to thyroid surgery. *Laryngoscope* 2006;116(2):235–238.

Roh JL, et al. Total thyroidectomy plus neck dissection in differentiated papillary thyroid cancer patients: patterns of nodal metastasis, morbidity, recurrence and postoperative levels of serum PTH. *Ann Surg* 2007;245(4):604–610.

Carty SE, et al. Consensus statement on the terminology and classification of central neck dissection for thyroid cancer. *Thyroid* 2009;19(11):153–158.

Shen WT, Ogawa L, Ruan D, et al. Central neck lymph node dissection for papillary thyroid cancer: comparison of complication and recurrence rates in 295 initial dissections and reoperations. *Arch Surg* 2010;145:272–275.

Tufano RP, et al. Reoperative central compartment dissection for patients with recurrent/persistent papillary thyroid cancer: efficacy, safety and the association of the BRAF mutation. *Laryngoscope* 2012;122(7):1634–1640.

20 MANAGEMENT OF THE SUPERIOR LARYNGEAL NERVE DURING THYROIDECTOMY

Claudio R. Cernea

INTRODUCTION

During the years 1930s, Amelita Galli-Curci was probably the most famous soprano in the world. Unfortunately, a fairly large goiter was diagnosed, and she underwent a thyroidectomy under local anesthesia, with careful identification and preservation of both recurrent laryngeal nerves. However, her voice became permanently hoarse due to damage to the superior laryngeal nerve, and she could sing no more. Since that time, the external branch of the superior laryngeal nerve (EBSLN) has been known as "the nerve of Amelita Galli-Curci."

The EBSLN is the only motor supply to the cricothyroid muscle (CTM). This muscle causes an elevation of the cricoid cartilage, shortening the distance with the thyroid cartilage, thus increasing the length and tension of the vocal fold. This increased tension is crucial for the emission of high-frequency sounds, especially among females and professional voice users.

The injury of the EBSLN causes a complete paralysis of the CTM, evidenced by a so-called electrical silence at electromyography (EMG). Functionally, the fundamental frequency of the voice is lowered and voice performance is markedly worsened, especially when producing high-frequency sounds. The impact of this paralysis can be devastating.

The EBSLN may be injured during a thyroidectomy, due to its close anatomic relationship with the superior pole and thyroid vessels. Generally, the nerve crosses the superior thyroid artery and vein well superior to the superior border of the superior pole. However, sometimes it is dangerously close to the superior pole or, in some instances, is even caudal to it.

In 1992, I proposed the following surgical anatomical classification of the EBSLN, based on the relationships between the nerve, the superior thyroid vessels, and the superior border of the superior pole of the thyroid (Fig. 20.1).

* Type 1. Nerve crossing the superior thyroid vessels one or more centimeters superior to a horizontal plane passing through the superior border of the superior pole of the thyroid
* Type 2a. Nerve crossing the vessels <1 cm above the aforementioned horizontal plane
* Type 2b. Nerve inferior to the plane

Clearly, type 2b has the highest risk of damage during thyroidectomy. Using cadaver dissection studies, I found that 20% of the EBSLN were of this type. In the clinical setting, I have observed 14% type 2b nerves in a series of normally sized or slightly enlarged thyroid glands. Conversely, type 1 nerves were the most common anatomic presentation (60% in cadaver anatomical series and 68% in our clinical series).

The anatomic classification proposed by me in several recent papers has been widely accepted. Some authors have reported similar proportions of the high-risk type 2b EBSLN as in my original results.

Some individual biometric features can be related to an increased incidence of type 2b EBSLN. Furlan et al. conducted an anatomic study on 36 fresh cadavers. Type 2b nerves were statistically more prevalent among individuals with shorter stature ($P = 0.0006$) and with increased volume of the gland ($P = 0.0007$).

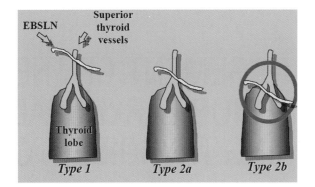

FIGURE 20.1

Surgical classification of the EBSLN. Please refer to suggested reading no. 1.

SURGICAL TECHNIQUE

The surgical management of the superior pole of the thyroid is necessary in most operations involving the thyroid gland. In fact, after opening the midline raphe between the strap muscles, I always prefer to start the thyroidectomy with dissection of the superior pole. The exposure of the superior pole usually starts with initial mobilization of the entire lobe. If present, the middle thyroid vein is ligated, to facilitate this initial mobilization. Presently, I favor the use of the harmonic scalpel, which in my opinion provides much safer hemostasis and reduces the operative time. In most instances, when the thyroid lobe is of normal size or only slightly enlarged, there is no need for complete section of the strap muscles. However, in many situations, a partial incision of the sternothyroid muscle with cautery or with the harmonic scalpel may improve access to the superior thyroid pedicle.

The superior thyroid vessels usually divide into three branches that embrace the superior thyroid pole; two are located anteriorly, and one runs dorsally. I strongly recommend that the surgeon dissect and ligate these branches individually, placing sutures as caudally as possible. In most instances, the EBSLN will be located cranial to the superior border of the thyroid lobe and, therefore, will be protected against injury. However, as previously mentioned, in 15% to 20% of cases, the nerve may be type 2b (Fig. 20.2). Thus, in all cases, ligature of the superior pole vessels and dissection in the sternothyroid–laryngeal triangle and along the medial surface of the superior pole of the thyroid lobe must be performed meticulously, with wide exposure. I have been using a 3.5 wide-angled loupe for the last 25 years, and I find it very important to ensure proper visualization of the EBSLN, which can be quite delicate and difficult to identify without magnification. Moreover, I have always used a simple nerve stimulator, set for an intensity of 1 or 2 mA. When the nerve is electrically stimulated, a quick but powerful contraction of the CTM is observed within the operative field, proving unequivocally that I have identified the nerve. After the positive identification, the EBSLN must be kept under direct vision constantly during the entire dissection of the superior pole. After completion of this dissection, the integrity of the nerve may be documented once again through electrical stimulation.

In recent years, intraoperative nerve monitoring systems have been developed and have become an important tool in the identification of the inferior laryngeal nerve and to graphically document its integrity at the end of a thyroid lobectomy. The most popular system is produced by Medtronic (NIM). When available, I use this system during a thyroidectomy. I believe it is very useful for the identification of a type 2b EBSLN at the beginning of the dissection of the superior pole. Even when the nerve is not visible at this point, that is, is a type 1 nerve, I try to look for it at the end of the operation. After the thyroid lobectomy is completed, I always check for any residual bleeding under pulmonary hyperpressure (Valsalva). At this moment, using the headlight

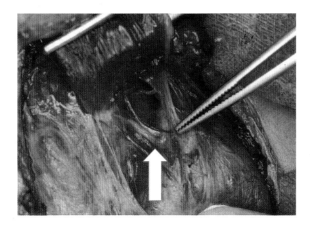

FIGURE 20.2

Type 2b external branch of the superior laryngeal nerve (arrow).

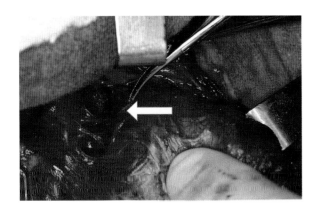

FIGURE 20.3 Type 2b EBSLN in a patient with a very large goiter (arrow).

attached to my loupes, I carefully search for the EBSLN in the superior aspect of the operative field, where the superior pole was originally situated. In many cases, the nerve can then be identified and stimulated, producing a response that is recorded for documentation of its integrity. It should be noted that the magnitude of this complex is much smaller than the one obtained after the electrical stimulation of an intact inferior laryngeal nerve. Some authors have based their identification and preservation of the EBSLN only on surgical anatomical findings. Nevertheless, I always favor positive electrical identification of the nerve.

The dissection of the superior pole is much more difficult when the patient has a large goiter. In this situation, the superior border of the pole is elevated markedly, increasing the contact with the EBSLN (Fig. 20.3). The superior thyroid vessels are also larger, and extra care must be taken during their dissection and ligation. In this situation, I usually divide the strap muscles to ensure better and safer exposure of this area. In addition, it is very important to keep in mind that the chance of finding a high-risk type 2b nerve in these patients may be as high as 54%, according to a study I published in 1995. Hence, it is essential to obtain a positive identification of the EBSLN in such large goiters before ligating the superior vessels.

Recently, some authors have employed minimally invasive techniques to approach the thyroid gland, including video-assisted thyroidectomy. It is important to emphasize that the anatomic classification that I have proposed in 1992 was developed using nonpreserved cadavers after *rigor mortis*, in order to enable the neck to be hyperextended, exactly in the same position as in a conventional thyroidectomy. However, no neck hyperextension is applied during a video-assisted thyroidectomy, thus approximating the EBSLN more closely to the superior pole of the thyroid. In a series of 12 cases, Dedivitis and Guimarães were able to clearly identify the nerve in 83.3% of the cases, noting that it coursed medially to the branches of the superior thyroid vessels in 80% and laterally in 20%. On the other hand, the magnification and illumination offered by the scope probably facilitated the visualization and preservation of the EBSLN. In 2009, Inabnet et al. published a prospective study of ten patients submitted to minimally invasive thyroidectomy under local anesthesia, with nerve monitoring of the EBSLN. Among the 15 nerves at risk, 8 were identified and successfully preserved, with their normal function assessed during the operation by the nerve monitoring and postoperative by video laryngoscopy.

PEARLS

- The EBSLN may be found in the operative field of a thyroidectomy in 15% to 20% of the cases.
- Avoid mass ligatures of the superior pole vessels.
- Use nerve monitoring or, at least, a nerve stimulator, especially when performing a thyroidectomy in a voice professional.

PITFALLS

- Risk of EBSLN injury is much higher in large goiters.
- Excessive cautery with the Bovie near the CTM can cause a negative functional impact on voice performance.

INSTRUMENTS TO HAVE AVAILABLE

- Surgical loupes with at least 2.5× magnification
- NIM system, including endotracheal tube with electrodes
- Stimulation probe
- External unit for intraoperative EMG recording

SUGGESTED READING

Cernea CR, Ferraz AR, Furlani J, et al. Identification of the external branch of the superior laryngeal nerve during thyroid-ectomy. *Am J Surg* 1992;164:634–639.

Cernea CR, Ferraz AR, Nishio S, et al. Surgical anatomy of the external branch of the superior laryngeal nerve. *Head Neck* 1992;14:380–383.

Cernea CR, Nishio S, Hojaij FC. Identification of the external branch of the superior laryngeal nerve (EBSLN) in large goiters. *Am J Otolaryngol* 1995;16:307–311.

Cernea CR, Brandão LG, Hisham AN. Surgical anatomy of the superior laryngeal nerve. In: Randolph GW, ed. *Surgery of the Thyroid and Parathyroid Glands.* 2nd ed. Elsevier Saunders, Philadelphia, 2012:736:300–305. ISBN: 978-1-4377-2227-7.

Cernea CR, Dedivitis RA, Ferraz AF, Brandao LG. How to avoid injury of the external branch of the superior laryngeal nerve. In: Cernea CR, Dias FL, Fliss D, eds. *Pearls and Pitfalls in Head and Neck Surgery.* 2nd ed. Karger AG, Basel, Switzerland, 2012:4–5.

21 SURGERY FOR SECONDARY HYPERPARATHYROIDISM

Brendan C. Stack Jr

INTRODUCTION

Secondary hyperparathyroidism (sHPT) is not often a surgical disease. sHPT is in fact more prevalent than primary hyperthyroidism and is often not diagnosed or even considered by the surgeon evaluating the patient with hyperparathormonemia. Because of the high prevalence of sHPT, many patients presenting with primary hyperparathyroidism from either single- or multiple-gland disease in fact will have coexisting sHPT.

sHPT is most commonly a result of vitamin D deficiency. Vitamin D deficiency is now appreciated to be extremely prevalent but is not a surgical disease. If surgery is not urgent/emergent, it is advisable to hold off on surgery until the vitamin D level has been repleted to at least 30 ng/mL. This will remove confounding circumstances that might interfere with the proper treatment of the primary hyperparathyroidism, when postoperative parathyroid hormone (PTH) is elevated after a normal measurement(s) in the operating room.

sHPT has been recognized clinically for many decades. Classic sHPT is the second most common cause of sHPT and typically is seen in patients on chronic renal dialysis as a result of chronic renal insufficiency. Twenty-six million Americans have chronic kidney disease, and virtually all dialysis-dependent patients develop sHPT.

HISTORY

The classic history for sHPT is that of chronic renal failure requiring hemodialysis. These patients suffer from bone demineralization and chronic hypocalcemia, which serves to stimulate all parathyroid glands. This chronic parathyroid gland stimulation results in multigland hyperplasia. Usually years of dialysis are required before patients are referred for evaluation of sHPT, often with PTH values >500 ng/dL. These patients are evaluated for parathyroidectomy for a variety of reasons at this point but principally for an anticipated receipt of a donor kidney or to assist in the management of severe biochemical derangements that accompany chronic dialysis.

PHYSICAL EXAMINATION

Patients who have the suspicion of sHPT should undergo a comprehensive otolaryngologic and head and neck examination. Specific attention should be paid to the central and the inferior portions of the neck. There is a significant coexistence of thyroid lesions, and any thyroid lesions should be evaluated and managed based on their merits independent of the underlying diagnosis of sHPT. If surgery is contemplated, examination of the larynx should be undertaken to insure normal vocal cord function preoperatively. If a parathyroid is present as a palpable mass in the neck, concern is raised for parathyroid carcinoma.

INDICATIONS

The indication for surgery for sHPT is to correct hyperparathormonemia. This is desirable in patients being considered for renal transplant and patients in whom it is anticipated will be dialyzed for the rest of their life. Patients in the latter category may proceed to surgery for reasons of intractable bone disease, calciphylaxis, or other biochemical disorders refractory to medical treatment.

CONTRAINDICATIONS

The main contraindication to surgical treatment for sHPT is the poor medical condition of many of these patients on presentation for surgical consultation. These patients require inpatient observation, and their course can be complicated with profound postoperative hypocalcemia requiring intensive replacement therapy due to their significantly demineralized bones.

PREOPERATIVE PLANNING

Imaging Studies

Ultrasound (US) has become the most popular form of imaging of thyroid and parathyroid disease. Most US examinations can be performed in the outpatient setting, preferably by the thyroid/parathyroid surgeon. Dedicated thyroid ultrasonographers have a higher level of expertise in imaging in the central and inferior regions of the neck than the average radiologist who would customarily supervise a US technician in the radiology department and review only static images. The US imaging will not be able to see parathyroids that are not pathophysiologically enlarged. While US has more than 90% sensitivity in detecting single-gland parathyroid disease, in multigland sHPT the sensitivity is only 40% to 60%. The superior glands can be more challenging to image by US due to their posterior location and the overlying thyroid tissue. Inferior glands have a more variable location and higher likelihood of being ectopic. sHPT from vitamin D deficiency is a milder form, in which it would be uncommon to image any enlarged parathyroid glands by US in this patient population.

Sestamibi imaging is also frequently used for parathyroid localization, particularly if radio-guided surgical excision is planned. In patients in whom surgery is not indicated, this modality would not typically be required for the diagnosis or medical treatment of sHPT. Radio-guided surgery is a helpful adjunct in cases of renal-induced sHPT where the PTH is elevated above 1,000 pg/mL. Hyperplastic glands take up the radiotracer, assisting in the identification and confirmation of the identity of a hyperplastic gland.

Laboratory

A clear biochemical diagnosis of hyperparathyroidism should be the goal of the preoperative evaluation. For sHPT serum calcium and intact parathormone (PTH) should be measured. Typically the calcium is low normal or low, and the PTH is very elevated. Overall, low calcium reflects chronic depletion of the body's calcium stores. Vitamin D testing is also very important in the sHPT patient population. If a patient is operated on for parathyroid disease with preexisting vitamin D deficiency, this could confound the results of any intraoperative parathyroid testing that might be used as part of the operative procedure, returning inappropriately elevated. Additionally, postoperative parathormonemia could result from vitamin D deficiency and not simply be viewed as a surgical failure.

SURGICAL TECHNIQUE

In the event of severe parathormonemia (>1,000 pg/mL) in patients with chronic renal insufficiency in which renal transplant is being contemplated, subtotal parathyroidectomy is indicated for sHPT. It is anticipated that with these patients, renal transplant will be successful, the kidney function will return to normal, and the chronic stimulation causing the parathyroid tissue to be hyperplastic will resolve. Therefore, a normal functioning parathyroid gland would be left in the neck with a small chance of needing additional revision surgery. If renal transplant is not contemplated or previously failed, total parathyroidectomy should be considered. This can be done in conjunction with primary or delayed autotransplantation in the forearm. I prefer primary autotransplantation. Cryopreservation is a critical resource to have when managing sHPT patients.

The Minimally Invasive Radio-Guided Parathyroidectomy

Once the diagnosis has been made and US imaging has been obtained, preoperative injection of sestamibi may facilitate the radio-guided approach to the parathyroidectomy. A 2-cm incision is made halfway between the

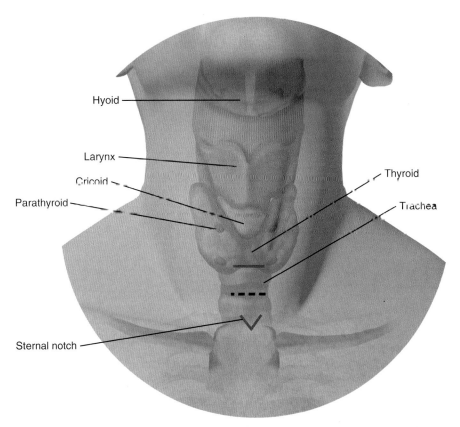

FIGURE 21.1 External neck anatomy with shadowed relevant internal structures indicating ideal incision placement for parathyroidectomy.

cricoid cartilage and the sternal notch as has been described by Norman. Once the incision is open, subcutaneous adipose tissue is removed down to the level of the strap muscles in the midline. This provides exposure and working space through this minimal access incision. Blunt dissection is then used in this pocket, and the incision is then kept open with a retractor. The midline is opened with a Bovie cautery. Both the superficial and deep levels of strap muscles are separated in the midline vertically. Both the unilateral and bilateral exploration can then be performed through this approach (Figs. 21.1 to 21.3).

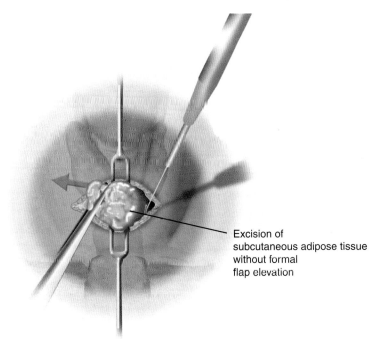

Excision of
subcutaneous adipose tissue
without formal
flap elevation

FIGURE   21.2 Excision   of subcutaneous adipose tissue creates skin flaps and a subcutaneous working space for the procedure.

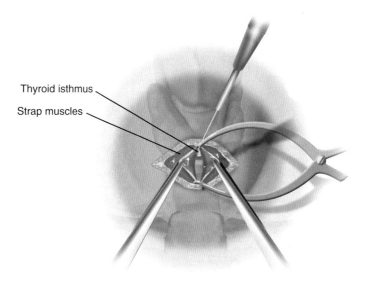

FIGURE 21.3

Strap muscles are divided vertically along the midline raphe.

A unilateral exploration will now be described, which is repeated on the contralateral side in the event a bilateral exploration is indicated. Typically when a parathyroidectomy is being performed for renally derived sHPT, 3 or 3½ glands are removed, which would require a bilateral procedure. The straps are undermined with great care using blunt Kittner dissectors in order not to disturb the thyroid capsule or blood vessels on the surface of the thyroid. A retractor is then placed in the wound, elevating and lateralizing the strap muscles. Blunt dissection of the tracheoesophageal groove is then performed. Generally, the thyroid is retracted medially, and the contents of the carotid sheath are retracted laterally with bimanual Kittner dissectors to expose the tracheoesophageal groove. As a patient safety maneuver, I identify both recurrent laryngeal nerves (RLNs) during bilateral dissections. Using a safe blunt technique and minimal focused hemostasis with bipolar cautery makes this "nerve friendly" and may obviate the need for a formal nerve dissection (Figs. 21.4 and 21.5).

Identification of both the superior and inferior parathyroid glands with their vascular pedicle is the next step. Once those glands are identified, all four glands can be examined prior to excision. The healthiest and smallest appearing gland can be the one left in situ as a remnant. The other half of that gland should be biopsied and cryopreserved. This point is moot if the objective is total parathyroidectomy with autotransplantation and/or cryopreservation. But, similar to the above, the most normal-appearing gland should be biopsied, autotransplanted, and/or cryopreserved.

Once this assessment has been made, blunt dissection around the gland allows for further mobilization of the gland, and the vascular pedicle can be then be divided with a hemoclip or bipolar cautery and divided with the scissors. Care is taken not to rupture the capsule of the glands. This could result in diffuse implantation of gland contents (parathyromatosis), which is a difficult problem to subsequently localize and treat. The glands are removed and kept in their proper orientation, that is, superior and inferior and right and left. The glands can then be examined with the radio-guided examination as described by Norman. The PTH should be measured

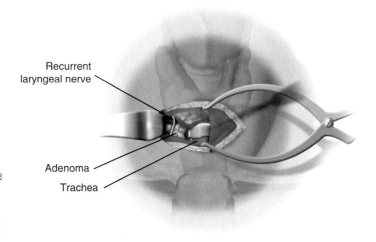

FIGURE 21.4

The key to the approach to the tracheoesophageal grove is to "hug" the underside of the strap muscle while dissecting and simultaneously retracting it laterally.

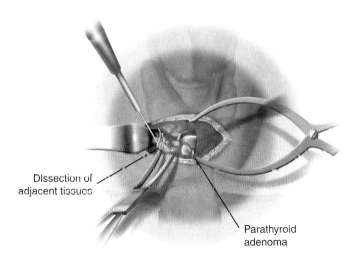

Dissection of adjacent tissues

Parathyroid adenoma

FIGURE 21.5 Once the tracheoesophageal groove is exposed, the adenoma(s) can be identified through careful blunt dissection. When required, tissue is divided with bipolar cautery once, assuring the RLN is not contained within it.

at the beginning of the surgery, and at any time during the surgery, additional PTH levels can be drawn. My preference is to measure the PTH 10 and 20 minutes following an exploration of each side or removal of all planned parathyroid material in a particular case.

Radio-guided examination of the parathyroid tissue when used is done in the following manner. A baseline or background in counts per second is obtained from the right shoulder or right lateral neck and serves as a reference point. A secondary reference point, which is a negative control, is the adipose tissue that was excised as part of the approach for the operation. The parathyroid gland is then placed on top of the tip of the inverted gamma probe to eliminate detection of background radiation, and counts per second are recorded. Typically hyperplastic parathyroid glands in cases of sHPT will have 10% to 15% of the background activity. If the glands are higher than 20%, one or more of the glands may have undergone a transformation to an adenoma because of chronic stimulation from chronic renal insufficiency. This is often the case in tertiary hyperparathyroidism (tHPT). The counts per second are charted in the operative record.

Once the surgeon is satisfied that the targeted parathyroids have been removed, with a concomitant decrease in the PTH, the procedure is concluded. Hemostasis is obtained; the wound is irrigated and is closed in layers. The skin is closed with a subcuticular suture and reinforced with surgical tape. A drain is not usually required.

Intraoperative PTH Assay

Decrease in intraoperative parathyroid hormone (IOPTH) is often not as brisk in patients with sHPT because of chronic renal insufficiency and the dependency of the PTH half-life on adequate renal function. In these cases it is prudent to send both a 10-minute postexcision and 20-minute postexcision values, and if there is an adequate correction with the first value, it is not necessary to maintain the patient under general anesthesia while waiting for the second value to return. Recent data have demonstrated that IOPTH testing is effective in surgery for sHPT and perhaps can guide the specific number of glands resected in tHPT.

Cryopreservation

I cryopreserve parathyroids in all cases of sHPT. Cryopreservation is absolutely required in cases of delayed autotransplantation or if a repeat autotransplant is required. Parathyroid tissue is prepared in like manner for autografting. Given current regulations on implants and biologic/donor material, it can be a daunting task to establish a local parathyroid bank. Using other tissue banks may be limited by regulatory requirements. Parathyroid tissue cannot be stored in an operating room or laboratory freezer. Several large institutions offer parathyroid banking as a fee for service option.

Autotransplantation

I am an advocate of primary autotransplantation. There is recent literature to support total parathyroidectomy with autotransplantation being left as a secondary option. If a patient will remain on dialysis for life, hypocalcemia can be managed with oral calcium and dialysis techniques.

The technique for autotransplantation can be varied. I prefer to mince the most normal-appearing parathyroid tissue into 1-mm pieces and to implant four to six of these into a pocket in the nondominant brachioradialis muscle in the forearm. The pocket is closed and marked with permanent suture or a hemoclip. The remaining fragments are placed in cell culture fluid and placed on ice for shipment to the tissue banking facility.

Autotransplants can have a measurable PTH production and reduction of serum calcium within 8 to 12 weeks following implantation.

Calciphylaxis

The population with chronic renal failure is at risk of developing calciphylaxis. Calciphylaxis is the spontaneous calcification of the intima of small and medium blood vessels, in the soft tissue and in the dermis. It can result in soft tissue necrosis and organ damage, and usually this infarction process is complicated by a superinfection that then results in sepsis and carries a significant mortality. When the total serum calcium is multiplied by the total serum phosphorus and the product of these two numbers exceeds 60, the risk for the development of calciphylaxis is significant. Approximately 1% of patients with chronic renal failure and 4.1% of patients on dialysis have been shown to develop this disorder. The age of onset varies widely, ranging from 6 months to 83 years; the mean is reported to be between 48 and 57 years. A higher incidence has been noted in women; reports of the female:male ratio range from 3:1 to 12:1. The cause for the higher female distribution is not known. Most studies indicate a higher incidence of calciphylaxis among whites, although this finding is not consistent and may reflect a disproportionate availability of dialysis among industrialized societies.

Parathyroid Carcinoma

Large, firm, and adherent parathyroids are characteristic of parathyroid carcinoma. Ultimately this is a diagnosis that can only be made on pathologic examination of the tissues. Several reports have stressed the importance of an en bloc resection including thyroid lobectomy with the isthmus and paratracheal and central neck lymph node dissection. This procedure, when performed as the initial therapeutic step, offers the patient the best chance for cure. Unfortunately, the diagnosis of parathyroid carcinoma is frequently made following permanent pathologic review. Controversy exists as to whether the patient without obvious extension of the cancer should be taken back to the operating room for ipsilateral thyroidectomy, isthmusectomy, and excision of paratracheal and central neck lymph nodes after the diagnosis is obtained from the pathology report. Some advocate close observation of calcium levels for evidence of recurrence, holding en bloc excision in reserve in the event of recurrence. Most agree that recurrent cancers that can be identified and are amenable to resection should be excised, even multiple times if necessary, for palliative relief from hypercalcemia. Because patients with parathyroid carcinoma are at a relatively high risk of multiple relapses over prolonged time periods, they should be monitored for life using serum calcium and intact parathyroid hormone (iPTH) levels. Carcinoembryonic antigen (CEA) is also an alternative tumor marker for this disease. If elevations of these disease markers are noted, signs of recurrence should be evaluated with localizing imaging studies such as ultrasonography, computed tomography, magnetic resonance imaging, sestamibi scanning, or positron emission tomography scanning.

POSTOPERATIVE MANAGEMENT

The chief concern postoperatively, assuming there are no RLN complications, is postoperative hypoparathyroidism/hypocalcemia. This is often inevitable if total parathyroidectomy is performed. Even if there is primary autotransplantation, this graft will take 8 to 12 weeks before it contributes a physiologically meaningful amount of parathormone to maintain normal calcium levels. Hypoparathormonemia is aggravated by the fact that most of these patients have demineralized skeletons. A "hungry bone syndrome" may develop when chronic hyperparathormonemia is relieved, allowing for osteoblasts to acutely remineralize the skeleton.

Therefore, it is important to preempt a hypocalcemic crisis postoperatively, and this can be done with oral calcium supplementation with or without 1,25 dihydroxycholecalciferol. This is started on post-op day 0, and the patient should be monitored every 6 hours. IV calcium can be administered but should be used to treat symptoms, not just a low number. Once calcium levels have trended upward, discharge may be possible. Often the above demands need to be balanced with scheduled dialysis for patients who have not yet had a kidney transplant (renal sHPT).

COMPLICATIONS

The complications associated with surgery for sHPT are the same as surgery for primary hyperparathyroidism or thyroid surgery. There is a 1% to 3% risk of permanent injury to the RLN, thus mandating a preoperative evaluation and laryngoscopy. There is an 8% to 10% incidence of transient, mild hoarseness following surgery, which is self-limited.

Two potential complications are related to the patient's parathyroid status. The surgery can be a failure, that is, the PTH is not reduced adequately. This usually is a result of residual parathyroid tissue producing excess PTH. Alternatively, there could be an undiscovered supernumerary or ectopic parathyroid gland that was not located. Conversely, the patient can be made hypoparathyroid, which is actually a more challenging clinical condition than hyperparathyroidism.

To avoid postoperative hypoparathyroidism, prudent handling of parathyroid tissue during surgery is recommended. If there is any question with regard to the viability the parathyroid or parathyroid fragment that was left in situ after the operation, there should be a low threshold for autotransplantation. As an additional maneuver, in the event of postoperative hypoparathyroidism, it is prudent to cryopreserve parathyroid tissue for a subsequent parathyroid implantation. It is important to note that in the event of primary or metachronous autotransplantation of parathyroid tissue, 8 to 12 weeks may be required for the parathyroid autograft to function and correct the hypoparathyroidism. In the interim it will be important to support the patient with calcium supplementation and calcitriol (1,25 hydroxy vitamin D) supplementation. Occasionally intravenous calcium may be required. In the case of delayed or metachronous parathyroid autotransplantation, it is also important to note that up to 30% of autografts are unsuccessful. Management of postoperative hypoparathyroidism is easier when the patient is on dialysis since calcium can be added to the dialysate.

RESULTS

Successful surgery for sHPT for chronic renal insufficiency results in a dramatic lowering of parathormonemia. Ideally the PTH will be reduced to a 100 ng/dL or less. This is an ideal situation for a patient who is suffering from significant hyperparathormonemia and helps prepare them biochemically for receipt of a renal transplant. This will help insure a lower risk of graft-related failure or complications. This may also improve symptoms related to HPT such as bone pain. This will help in cases of osteopenia or osteoporosis.

PEARLS

- Prior to contemplation of surgery, it is important to do a complete biochemical profile on a patient with sHPT and be in close consultation with the treating nephrologist and renal transplant surgeon as necessary (total calcium, ionized calcium, intact PTH, magnesium, phosphorus, creatinine, 250H Vitamin D, and chloride).
- Understanding the stage of renal disease and the appropriate timing and indications for parathyroid surgery for renal sHPT
- Use good surgical practice in exploring and excising parathyroid tissue, similar to other endocrine surgical procedures.
- Increase vigilance with these patients is necessary, as they are more medically challenged and more susceptible to electrolyte abnormalities and, in the case of sHPT from chronic renal insufficiency, may still require dialysis perioperatively.
- Complication rates can be higher in this patient population due to extensive bilateral tracheoesophageal grove dissection (5% to 10% for nerve injuries) and extensive parathyroid resection (20% to 75% hypocalcemia).

PITFALLS

- Bilateral recurrent nerve injury requiring tracheostomy, due to bilateral exploration
- Severe hypoparathyroidism. "The only thing worse than HYPERparathyroidsim is HYPOparathyroidism."
- Inadequate reduction in parathormone levels

INSTRUMENTS TO HAVE AVAILABLE

- Standard head and neck surgical instruments
- Technetium-99 sestamibi, preferable with ST-SPECT
- Intraoperative, rapid, iPTH assay
- Operative gamma counter
- Frozen section pathology
- Approved cryopreservation facilities
- Endotracheal nerve monitoring (optional)

SUGGESTED READING

Costello D, Norman J. Minimally invasive radioguided parathyroidectomy. *Surg Oncol Clin N Am* 1999;8(3):555–564.
Ruda J, Hollenbeak CS, Stack BC Jr. A systematic review of the diagnosis and treatment of primary hyperparathyroidism from 1995 to 2003. *Otolaryngol Head Neck Surg* 2005;132(3):359–372.
Stack BC Jr. Minimally invasive radioguided parathyroidectomy (MIRP). *Oper Tech Otolaryngol Head Neck Surg* 2009;20(1):54–59.
Stack BC Jr. Secondary Hyperparathyroidism. British Medical Journal (BMJ) Point of Care: www.pointofcare.bmj.com. Online beginning September 2009, updated annually. https://online.epocrates.com/u/29111107/Secondary+hyperparathyroidism

22 VIDEO-ASSISTED PARATHYROIDECTOMY

David J. Terris

INTRODUCTION

The management of the patient with primary hyperparathyroidism (PHPT) has changed dramatically in the last 10 years with the introduction of robust preoperative imaging and the availability of rapid intraoperative parathyroid hormone (PTH) assays. Single-gland surgery (described variously as targeted, directed, focused, or minimally invasive) is now preferred for the vast majority of patients with uncomplicated PHPT. With the high success rates and low morbidity of a modern parathyroidectomy, attention can now be shifted to patient-centered issues such as convenience of surgery and cosmesis. These considerations have spawned outpatient management and video-assisted techniques, among other novel approaches. The application of high-resolution endoscopy has permeated most areas of surgery, and the endocrine field is now no exception. The intense illumination and high-fidelity magnification may help improve visualization of critical structures during surgery and have allowed surgeons to use quite small incisions in order to retrieve parathyroid adenomas. Many patients can now enjoy a sutureless, drainless, outpatient procedure that leaves a scar of ½ to ¾ of an inch.

HISTORY

The proper indications for surgery should be met prior to contemplating a video-assisted or any other type of parathyroidectomy. The history is therefore focused on soliciting the classic symptoms associated with PHPT ("moans, bones, groans, and stones") as well as the less discrete but sometimes disabling symptoms such as depression, fatigue, memory loss, anorexia, constipation, nausea, poor sleep, and irritability.

PHYSICAL EXAMINATION

It is so unusual to be able to palpate a parathyroid adenoma that when this is possible, one should anticipate the presence of a parathyroid carcinoma. Assessment for lymphadenopathy should be undertaken for the same reason. Preoperative examination of the larynx is encouraged as patients with an unsuspected vocal cord paralysis can maintain a normal voice. Assessment of body habitus is important for the video-assisted technique and may include calculation of a body mass index.

INDICATIONS

All patients with symptomatic PHPT should undergo surgery if possible. National Institutes of Health panels have been convened several times (most recently in 2008) to issue guidelines for surgical intervention in patients with asymptomatic PHPT that are somewhat strict but serve as a starting point in defining surgical eligibility. These indications include creatinine clearance <60 mL/minute, age <50, calcium levels more than

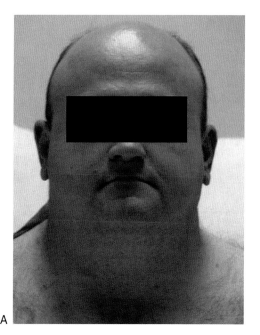
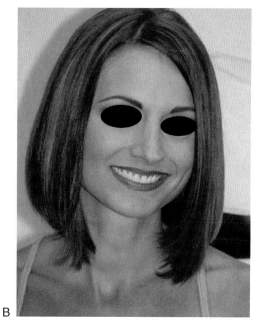

FIGURE 22.1 Our philosophy has been to customize surgery to patients and their disease characteristics. This patient with a 26-inch neck will not be eligible for minimally invasive procedure **(A)**. By contrast, this television commentator from North Carolina is an ideal candidate for an endoscopic minimally invasive procedure **(B)**.

1 mg/dL above normal, and reduced bone mineral density (T score on a dual-energy x-ray absorptiometry scan of <2.5 at any site). Despite these commonly recognized guidelines, there are many who believe that confirmation of the diagnosis of hyperparathyroidism is sufficient to recommend surgery, particularly with the availability of modern techniques. Therefore, most surgeons extend beyond the published indications for surgery on a regular basis after careful consultation with both the patient and the referring endocrinologist.

Once a decision for surgery has been reached, the eligibility criteria for a video-assisted parathyroidectomy technique include the presence of localizing studies (usually either an ultrasound or a sestamibi scan), nonobese neck (Fig. 22.1), and no suspicion of cancer. While some European authors have reported on four-gland exploration using an endoscopic approach, I prefer an open exploration when all glands will be examined. Obese necks demand sufficient additional depth of dissection for exposure that a minimally invasive nonendoscopic technique is preferred. Patients with cancer should have open surgery.

CONTRAINDICATIONS

A patient who has had prior neck surgery or in whom a cancer is anticipated should not undergo video-assisted surgery. Most patients with nonlocalizing studies or those whose imaging suggests an ectopic location such as the mediastinum or submandibular triangle should undergo conventional surgery (Fig. 22.2). Patients who are infirm or have substantial medical comorbidities are probably best served by conventional techniques (although as a targeted, single-gland exploration).

PREOPERATIVE PLANNING

Planning falls into one of three principal areas: confirmation of the diagnosis, imaging of the affected gland(s), and the acquisition of informed consent. While most patients are referred with a diagnosis of PHPT, confirmation by laboratory assessment of ionized and total calcium, PTH level, vitamin D level, and in some cases a 24-hour urine calcium level may be helpful.

My preferred imaging modalities consist of both surgeon-performed office ultrasound and a high-quality Tc-sestamibi scan with fused CT images. The CT may be particularly helpful for defining the depth of the adenoma and to help to prevent the commonly missed overly descended superior gland that masquerades as an inferior adenoma. If neither of these imaging studies are localizing, a four-gland exploration is anticipated and video-assisted techniques are not utilized.

Patients are made aware of the usual risks and complications of thyroid compartment surgery, and in this case, including a small risk of persistent hyperparathyroidism and a remote risk of transient or permanent hypoparathyroidism.

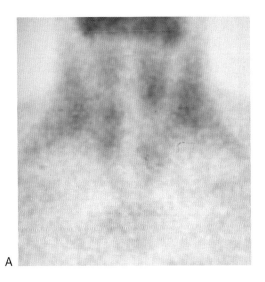

A

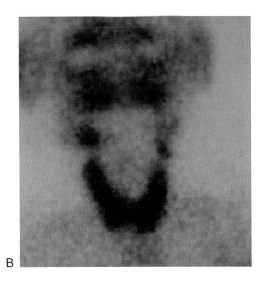

B

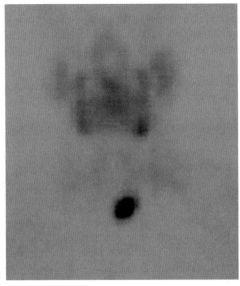

C

FIGURE 22.2 Decisions regarding procedural approach depend to some extent on localizing studies; a nonlocalizing sestamibi **(A)** or one that suggests an ectopic gland **(B)** would favor a conventional open surgery. Localizing scans, such as this so-called "lightbulb" sestamibi **(C)**, facilitate performance of video-assisted surgery.

SURGICAL TECHNIQUE

The patient is marked for the surgical incision while seated upright in the holding area to facilitate identification of the optimal location in the neck (Fig. 22.3), which is typically just above the sternal notch in a natural skin crease. Once in the operating room, the patient is positioned supine on the table, and the arms are tucked in papoose fashion. The patient is intubated with a conventional endotracheal tube as laryngeal nerve monitoring is not needed for these cases. (Alternatively, these operations can easily be accomplished under local anesthesia

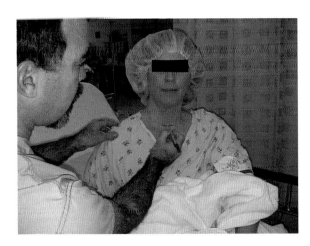

FIGURE 22.3 Cosmetic considerations have become increasingly important for patients undergoing thyroid and parathyroid surgery. To optimize the location of the scar, I recommend marking the patient's incision while the patient is seated upright in the holding area. (Reprinted from Terris DJ. Novel surgical maneuvers in modern thyroid surgery. *Op Techn Otolaryngol Head Neck Surg* 2009;20(1):23–28, with permission.)

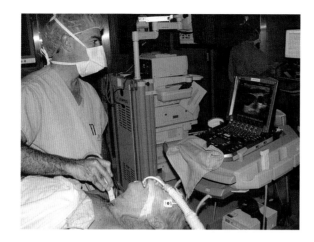

FIGURE 22.4
I find it helpful to perform an immediate, preincision ultrasound to confirm the location of the anticipated adenoma.

in motivated patients who are properly selected.) I prefer to rotate the operating table 180 degrees from the anesthesiologist, and blood samples are drawn from a peripheral vein in the foot.

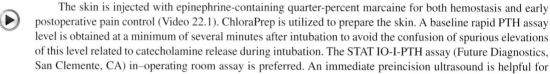

The skin is injected with epinephrine-containing quarter-percent marcaine for both hemostasis and early postoperative pain control (Video 22.1). ChloraPrep is utilized to prepare the skin. A baseline rapid PTH assay level is obtained at a minimum of several minutes after intubation to avoid the confusion of spurious elevations of this level related to catecholamine release during intubation. The STAT IO-I-PTH assay (Future Diagnostics, San Clemente, CA) in–operating room assay is preferred. An immediate preincision ultrasound is helpful for confirming the precise location of the adenoma and is done just prior to sterilizing the skin (Fig. 22.4).

A 15- to 20-mm incision is made corresponding to the previous marking, and electrocautery is used to dissect down to the strap muscles. These are vertically separated without raising subplatysmal flaps. Terris retractors (Medtronic Inc., Jacksonville, FL) are placed on the strap muscles and directly on the thyroid gland to create and maintain the optical pocket (Fig. 22.5). A 30-degree 5-mm laparoscope (the Endo-Eye from Olympus Corporation, Tokyo, Japan, is preferred) is held by the camera assistant at the opening of the incision and angled downward to provide magnified visualization. The second assistant holds both retractors, thereby allowing the surgeon to use both hands to operate (Fig. 22.6).

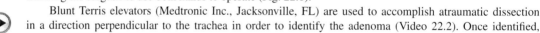

Blunt Terris elevators (Medtronic Inc., Jacksonville, FL) are used to accomplish atraumatic dissection in a direction perpendicular to the trachea in order to identify the adenoma (Video 22.2). Once identified,

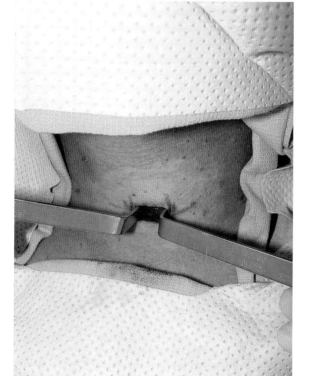

FIGURE 22.5
The proper placement of the retractors is critical; one is placed on the strap muscles and one is placed directly on the thyroid gland, to help deliver it up and out of the tracheoesophageal groove and maintain the optical pocket.

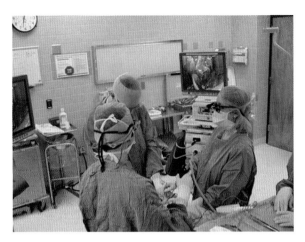

FIGURE 22.6 The proper arrangement of the equipment and the operating staff is essential in order to facilitate the conduct of video-assisted surgery and is depicted in this photograph. The technique requires a surgeon and two assistants; the camera assistant uses both hands to hold the endoscope, and the retractor assistant holds both retractors (one in each hand). This allows the surgeon to use both hands to operate. The addition of a slave monitor improves the ergonomic comfort of the camera assistant who can therefore face the image squarely. (Reprinted from Terris DJ, Seybt MW. Modifications of Miccoli minimally invasive thyroidectomy for the low-volume surgeon. *Am J Otolaryngol* 2011;32(5): 392–397, with permission.)

circumferential blunt dissection is pursued until the adenoma remains attached only by its vascular pedicle (Video 22.3; Fig. 22.7).

The vascular supply to the gland may be divided by one of two techniques: for small vessels, monopolar electrocautery is usually sufficient, but for larger vessels, medium vascular clips are used to control the vessel with one or two clips on the patient side and one clip on the adenoma side. Scissors are used to divide the vessel, and then the adenoma is retrieved (Video 22.4). For inferior adenomas, the recurrent laryngeal nerve need not be sought. For superior adenomas, this nerve is usually identified in order to prevent injury (Fig. 22.8).

Intraoperative rapid PTH levels are obtained 5, 10, and 15 minutes following removal of the adenoma. When a 50% reduction and a postexcision level in the normal range are achieved, the operation is concluded. The wound is irrigated. A sheet of Surgicel is placed into the surgical pocket, and the strap muscles are reapproximated with a single figure-of-eight suture of 3-0 Vicryl. Prior to closure, a sliver of skin edge may be resected to minimize the chances of a hypertrophic scar (Fig. 22.9). One, or at most two, interrupted subcutaneous sutures of 4-0 Vicryl are placed. A skin adhesive is used to seal the skin edges. A small ¼-inch Steri-Strip is placed horizontally directly on top of the glue to facilitate removal of the glue 2 to 3 weeks after surgery (Fig. 22.10).

Importantly, the patient is extubated deep to minimize coughing and bucking on emergence. The patient is transferred to the gurney and taken to the recovery room where postoperative laryngoscopy is performed to confirm vocal fold function. The patient is discharged to home 60 to 90 minutes after surgery with a 3-week tapering course of calcium supplementation.

POSTOPERATIVE MANAGEMENT

This surgery is almost always performed on an outpatient basis, and therefore the patient moves from the recovery room to the same day surgery area. When the patient is awake and alert, is able to take liquids and void, and is emotionally prepared, he or she is discharged to home with an accompanying individual. Patients who come from more than 2 hours' drive away are encouraged to spend the night in a local hotel.

The postoperative calcium supplemental regimen is completed (1 g of Oscal-D three times daily for 1 week, then twice daily for the 2nd week, and then daily for the final week), and no wound care is necessary.

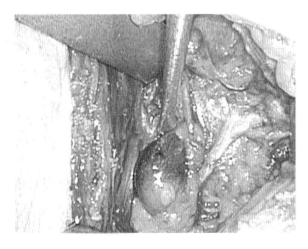

FIGURE 22.7 A typical adenoma is depicted and in experienced hands is distinguishable from a lymph node, thymus, adipose tissue, thyroid nodule, or normal parathyroid tissue.

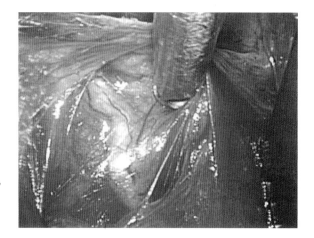

FIGURE 22.8
The recurrent laryngeal nerve need not always be visualized, but if it is thought to be at risk should be sought and protected.

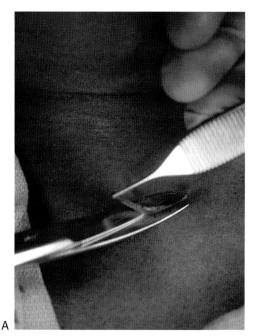

A

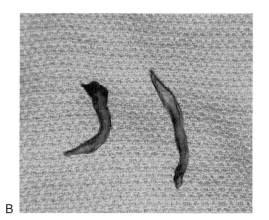

B

FIGURE 22.9
When substantial retraction has been required, the skin edges may manifest ischemic changes. Resection of a sliver of the skin edge **(A,B)** is recommended to minimize the risk of hypertrophic scarring **(C)**. (Reprinted from Terris DJ, Seybt MW, Chin E. Cosmetic thyroid surgery: defining the essential principles. *Laryngoscope* 2007;117(7):1168–1172, with permission.)

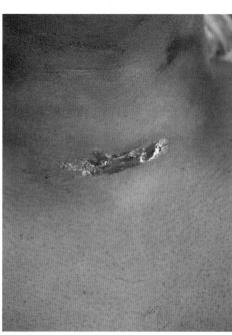

C

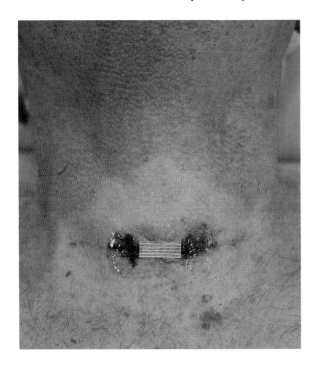

FIGURE 22.10 The incision is closed and sealed with Dermaflex skin adhesive (allowing the patient to shower the evening of surgery), and a single horizontal Steri-Strip is placed on top of the glue to facilitate removal 2 or 3 weeks after surgery.

Showering is permitted as early as the evening of surgery. Two or three weeks after the surgery, the patient may remove the Steri-Strip, and most of the glue comes with it.

Only a single postoperative visit is arranged, for 1 month after the surgery. This way, the calcium and PTH levels can be checked while the patient is no longer on postoperative calcium supplementation. Assuming normal levels, the patient is referred back to the primary care physician or endocrinologist. A repeat calcium level should be obtained at 6 or 12 months after surgery by the primary care physician.

COMPLICATIONS

The potential complications of video-assisted parathyroidectomy are identical to those associated with conventional parathyroid surgery, including temporary or permanent recurrent injury to the laryngeal nerve, temporary or permanent hypoparathyroidism, and persistent hyperparathyroidism. There are also the risks associated with any surgical procedure including pain, bleeding, infection, and the risks associated with anesthesia.

It is worth mentioning that in the event that a patient requires subsequent surgery, either for a missed adenoma or for recurrent hyperparathyroidism, one can anticipate an easier reoperative surgery when only a single quadrant of the thyroid compartment is violated.

RESULTS

The safety and efficacy of this procedure has been established by a number of European investigators and confirmed after widespread application elsewhere in the world. A 96% to 98% success rate can be anticipated when accomplished in experienced hands. The cosmetic results are superb (Fig. 22.11).

PEARLS

- This is a three-person surgery, requiring an individual dedicated for retraction, a second assistant whose exclusive role is handling the camera, and the third person who is the primary surgeon.
- For optimal cosmesis, incision should be marked prior to anesthesia with the patient in an upright position (as is typical of plastic surgery procedures).
- An immediate preincision ultrasound done just prior to sterilizing the skin is helpful for confirming the precise location of the adenoma.
- Proper retraction is essential, with the thyroid retractor placed in such a fashion that the thyroid is delivered up and out of the tracheoesophageal groove, and the second retractor on the strap muscles to maintain an adequate operative space. Narrow but deep retractors with a lip on the end are required in order to adequately maintain the optical pocket.

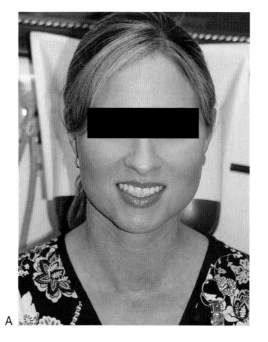 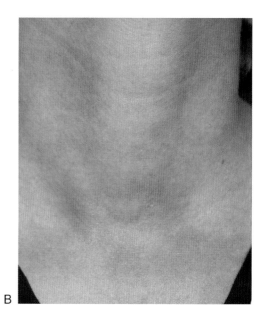

FIGURE 22.11
Excellent cosmetic outcomes may be anticipated **(A)**, and well-placed incisions heal with a virtually unnoticeable scar **(B)**.

- The use of a slave monitor allows both the camera assistant and the surgeon to enjoy favorable ergonomics during the procedure.
- The camera is generally angled downward, although for superior adenomas, it may be angled upward.
- Atraumatic dissection with blunt elevators is key to exploiting avascular planes and minimizing bleeding, which might make endoscopic visualization challenging.

PITFALLS

- Fracture of the capsule of the adenoma should be avoided to minimize the chances of parathyromatosis.
- Closure is very rapid, particularly with the skin adhesives, and may be completed while waiting for the postexcision IOPTH levels to return.
- Careful counseling of both the patient and the family members regarding the signs and symptoms of hypocalcemia is essential to undertaking safe outpatient surgery.

INSTRUMENTS TO HAVE AVAILABLE

- A 5-mm, 30-degree laparoscope with a high-definition monitor and tower is needed.
- A thyroid instrument set (such as the Terris set from Medtronic or the Miccoli set from Storz) vastly facilitates the performance of the procedure.
- A pediatric right-angle clamp can be helpful if dissection of the recurrent laryngeal nerve is necessary.
- Automatic clip appliers may be helpful for controlling the vascular pedicle.
- Skin adhesives allow rapid closure and prevent the need to return for suture removal at a proscribed time after surgery.

SUGGESTED READING

Miccoli P, Berti P, Materazzi G, et al. Results of video-assisted parathyroidectomy: single institution's six-year experience. *World J Surg* 2004;28(12):1216–1218.

Steward DL, Danielson GP, Afman CE, et al. Parathyroid adenoma localization: surgeon-performed ultrasound versus sestamibi. *Laryngoscope* 2006;116(8):1380–1384.

Terris DJ, Stack BC Jr, Gourin CG. Contemporary parathyroidectomy: exploiting technology. *Am J Otolaryngol* 2007;28(6):408–414.

Lombardi CP, Raffaelli M, Traini E, et al. Advantages of a video-assisted approach to parathyroidectomy. *ORL J Otorhinolaryngol Relat Spec* 2008;70(5):313–318.

Seybt MW, Loftus KA, Mulloy AL, et al. Optimal use of intraoperative PTH levels in parathyroidectomy. *Laryngoscope* 2009;119(7):1331–1333.

23 REOPERATIVE PARATHYROID SURGERY FOR PRIMARY HYPERPARATHYROIDISM

Alfred A. Simental

INTRODUCTION

Primary hyperparathyroidism is a disorder involving oversecretion of parathyroid hormone (PTH) from the parathyroid glands resulting in elevated serum calcium, increased calcium extraction from the bone, increased calcium reabsorption in the kidneys, and altered phosphorus metabolism. The majority of cases are caused by a single overactive gland (adenoma), which can be localized by sestamibi nuclear scanning in approximately 80% of adenoma cases. In patients with a single adenoma, 20% or more will result in no abnormal uptake of the sestamibi/technetium study and thus will be classified as "nonlocalizing." Approximately 15% to 18% of patients with hyperparathyroidism are a result of multiple or all glands being involved in overproduction (hyperplasia) of PTH. While some patients with hyperplasia may erroneously localize on sestamibi, the majority will also result in a nonlocalizing study. Initial exploration may result in successful resolution of the hyperparathyroid state in 70% to 80% of patients in the hands of surgeons who do perform a low volume of parathyroid surgery and up to 95% to 97% of patients in the hands of experienced surgeons using current localizing and intraoperative monitoring techniques. Some patients, however, may require reoperation to control ongoing complications or conditions associated with hyperparathyroidism. Reoperation presents an additional challenge as the scar tissue may hide the abnormal parathyroid tissue and make it more difficult to avoid surgical complications.

HISTORY

The symptoms of hyperparathyroidism include fatigue, listlessness, memory loss, depression, renal stones, renal failure, osteopenia, diffuse bone pain, peptic ulcer disease, and increase in cardiovascular risk. Currently, the majority of patients who are diagnosed with hyperparathyroidism will be asymptomatic and will report having routine blood chemistry tests identify them as being hypercalcemic. Patients who have already undergone thyroid surgery or unsuccessful parathyroidectomy should be carefully questioned and their symptoms carefully documented to ensure that the increased risk of reoperation is warranted.

PHYSICAL EXAMINATION

Evaluation of the central and lateral compartments of the neck is of paramount importance in the evaluation of patients with hyperparathyroidism. Markedly enlarged thyroid glands and nodules may be a great surgical hindrance at time of parathyroid surgery. All known thyroid nodules 1 to 3 cm should be evaluated with fine needle aspiration biopsy prior to exploration of the parathyroids. Patients with markedly enlarged glands or a substernal goiter should be considered for concomitant thyroidectomy. Vocal fold function should be evaluated and documented in all cases of parathyroid surgery, especially in the setting of reoperative treatment. Paralysis of the vocal fold and palpable parathyroid nodules suggests the presence of parathyroid carcinoma, especially in the setting of significantly elevated calcium and the absence of a previous history of surgery on the paralyzed side. Approximately 5% of the normal population may exhibit a Chvostek sign despite having normal calcium levels, which would compromise the utility of the test in the postoperative evaluation of calcium levels.

INDICATIONS

The diagnosis of primary hyperparathyroidism is generally established with a concomitant elevation of serum calcium and intact PTH level. Some patients with significant osteoporosis may only demonstrate a high normal serum calcium in the presence of elevated PTH. Serum and 24-hour urine creatinine and calcium levels can be used to rule out the presence of benign familial hypocalciuric hypercalcemia. All patients with sequelae of hyperparathyroidism (kidney stones, overt bone disease, proximal myopathy, and arrhythmia) who are healthy enough for parathyroid surgery should be considered for reexploration and removal of hyperfunctioning glands. When carefully questioned and evaluated, the majority of patients will exhibit some signs or symptoms of hyperparathyroidism. The current consensus guidelines established in 2008 for surgical indications for asymptomatic patients are listed below:

- Age <50
- Elevation of serum calcium 1.0 mg/dL above normal
- Glomerular filtration rate <60 mL/min
- Bone mineral density T-score <−2.5 at any site

Patients who do not undergo surgical exploration should be monitored closely for the development of symptoms or presence of qualifying criteria.

CONTRAINDICATIONS

Patients with a history of Roux-en-Y gastric bypass surgery or patients with malabsorption syndromes should be carefully screened for their ability to absorb calcium from the gastrointestinal tract. This may result in an instance of secondary hyperparathyroidism, in which surgery may be detrimental to the patient. Patients failing an oral calcium challenge study should be considered for observation as postoperatively they may require intravenous (IV) calcium as their sole source of calcium.

While initial parathyroid explorations can be done under local anesthesia, the presence of scarring makes this much more difficult in the reoperative setting. Patients who are not fit for general anesthesia should be strongly considered for medical therapy and observation rather than surgery.

PREOPERATIVE PLANNING

The medical records should be obtained from previous thyroid or parathyroid surgery. The pathology and surgical records should be carefully reviewed to determine areas of previous exploration and documentation of previously removed glands. Tissues removed at previous parathyroid surgery should be analyzed by the head and neck pathologist. Preoperative imaging for patients confirmed with the diagnosis of hyperparathyroidism should include a thyroid ultrasound to determine the size of the thyroid lobes and the presence of intra- or extrathyroidal masses, which may represent an enlarged parathyroid gland. Empiric thyroidectomy in the absence of intrathyroidal masses rarely results in resolution of the hyperparathyroid state and can make reexploration more dangerous for recurrent nerve injury. A sestamibi nuclear scan should be obtained to attempt to localize the site of the hyperactive gland. Patients who have previously undergone bilateral exploration should be explored in situations in which the abnormal parathyroid gland can be localized. Hyperactive parathyroid glands that fail to localize on imaging studies and require surgical exploration due to complications of persistent hyperparathyroidism should be explored in a facility with the capability to perform rapid PTH assay (Table 23.1).

SURGICAL TECHNIQUE

After induction of local or general anesthesia and prior to creating an incision, a baseline intact PTH level should be drawn. An arterial line or reliable peripheral IV should be established to allow for intraoperative sampling throughout the surgical procedure. Successful removal of overactive parathyroid tissue will result in a 50% drop in intact PTH 10 minutes postexcision and an additional 20% to 25% drop at 15 minutes postexcision. PTH levels at the 15-minute level that fail to continue to drop from the 10-minute level draw

TABLE 23.1	Location of Aberrant Parathyroid Glands

Carotid sheath
Intrathyroidal
Paratracheal
Retroesophageal
Superior mediastinal/thymus

are worrisome for residual hyperfunctioning parathyroid tissue. Placement of a transoral esophageal probe will allow for proper identification by intraoperative finger palpation of pharyngeal and esophageal boundaries thus decreasing the risk of inadvertent injury. The existing collar incision should be used if possible. Subplatysmal flaps are raised to the level of the laryngeal cartilage and inferiorly over the sternoclavicular joints. Minimally invasive approaches are difficult and often impossible in the setting of reoperative parathyroid surgery. Directed exploration is undertaken in patients with localizing studies and radio-guided parathyroidectomy may be of most benefit in sestamibi-positive patients. In cases where the parathyroid gland does not localize by sestamibi or ultrasound, the internal jugular veins (IJVs) are exposed low in the neck by retracting the sternocleidomastoid muscles laterally and the strap muscles medially. Using a 22-gauge needle and Luer Lock syringe, 3 to 5 mL of venous blood is drawn out of both IJVs and labeled separately. These samples are then sent for rapid PTH assay and the side with the higher level is explored first. The strap muscles are then split in the midline and retracted laterally over the thyroid gland. Lateral retraction of the strap muscles and medial retraction of the thyroid gland should result in early identification of the carotid artery, thus marking the lateral extent of standard dissection. Dissection should then expose the entire lateral aspect of the thyroid gland and extend to the carotid sheath, being cautious to avoid injury to the recurrent laryngeal nerve (RLN) when dissecting below the level of the cricoid cartilage. Once the entire thyroid has been mobilized up to the level of the superior pole, the search for enlarged glands is performed, realizing that the majority of parathyroids will be in close proximity to the thyroid gland especially in the region near the intersection of the RLN and inferior thyroid artery. The RLN should be identified if initial exploration behind and next to the thyroid gland is unsuccessful. At this time, the area between the carotid artery and RLN should be explored thoroughly up to the inferior thyroid artery and up to the level of the thyroid cartilage and superior thyroid artery. Great care must be taken to avoid injury to the hypopharynx and esophagus when searching the paratracheal and retroesophageal regions. In cases where previous thyroidectomy has been carried out, dissection lateral to the strap muscles may be employed to identify and expose the carotid sheath. In reoperative cases, the region around the trachea and thyroid are usually encased in scar (Fig. 23.1). In these cases, a lateral to medial approach may be helpful as the undiscovered abnormal parathyroid is often located just outside the field of previous dissection where the scarring is less (Fig. 23.2). A limited search medial to the RLN and over the trachea is undertaken. The thymus and pretracheal lymph nodes and adipose tissue on the ipsilateral side should be explored down to the great vessels in the superior mediastinum. If parathyroid tissue is not identified and associated with a drop in intraoperative PTH level, dissection is then carried into the contralateral neck in a similar fashion to the side initially explored by exposing the carotid, mobilizing the thyroid, identifying and tracing the RLN down to mediastinal carotid, and inspecting the retroesophageal and paratracheal regions lateral to RLN up to level of the superior thyroid artery and thyroid cartilage. If the exploration persists and is unsuccessful, the remaining thymus and pretracheal mediastinal adipose tissue and lymph nodes are then removed down to the innominate artery. In the absence of significant thyroid nodules, the thyroid gland is not removed as this will greatly increase reexploration risks as the strap muscles will become adherent to the trachea and RLN. For thyroid nodules >1 cm, especially when on the ipsilateral side to the higher IJV PTH level, thyroid lobectomy may be considered if PTH levels remain elevated. Upon removal of abnormal parathyroid tissue, 10 and 15 minutes postexcision PTH levels are drawn. Successful removal is predicted by a decrease of 50% from preincision PTH level at 10 minutes and 70% to 75% at 15 minutes. However, once the PTH level falls into the normal range, the level may not continue to drop appreciably. Thus, in patients with preincision PTH levels <100, intraoperative monitoring may have limited utility. If no abnormal parathyroid tissue is identified and removed after complete bilateral exploration, the surgery is then discontinued and repeat imaging is undertaken to attempt to identify the location of the missing gland. The strap muscles must be reapproximated with absorbable suture in the midline to prevent the skin from adhering to the trachea, which can contribute to dysphagia and be cosmetically unsightly.

A video demonstration of a patient undergoing a third operation for hyperparathyroidism is included. In this instance, the two previous operations have resulted in bilateral paratracheal exploration and total thyroidectomy. The strap muscles are adherent to the trachea and likely RLN. The mass localizes to the right on imaging studies so exploration begins on that side. Dissection lateral to the strap muscles and skeletonizing the carotid allow for safer dissection from lateral to medial, markedly decreasing the risk to the recurrent nerve, which is almost certainly encased in scar around the cricoid and tracheal junction (Video 23.1).

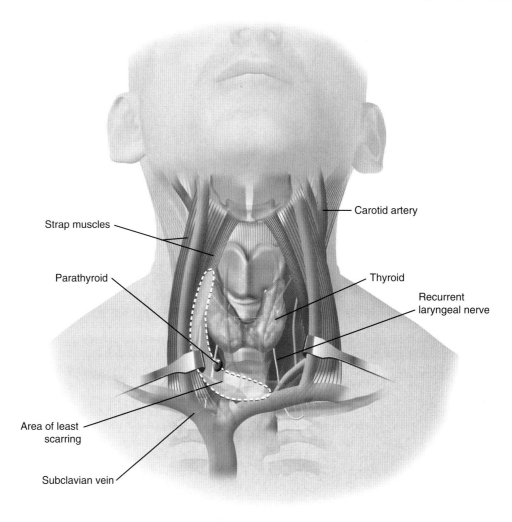

Strap muscles

Parathyroid

Carotid artery

Thyroid

Recurrent
laryngeal nerve

Area of least
scarring

Subclavian vein

FIGURE 23.1
Area of least scarring from
previous surgery.

POSTOPERATIVE MANAGEMENT

In cases where bilateral exploration or reexploration is undertaken, a postoperative PTH level is drawn an hour after the patient arrives in the recovery room to determine the function of the remaining glands. No calcium supplementation is given if persistence of PTH elevation is identified. If the PTH level normalizes, calcium supplementation should be started as the serum calcium levels may dramatically fall due to bone absorption of calcium. Overnight observation may be required for patients with recovery room PTH levels of 15 or less, as IV calcium may be required. Patients using antacid medications such as proton pump inhibitors or histamine (H2) blockers may experience decreased absorption of elemental calcium and may require altered intake of the antacid or use of Citracal for improved calcium absorption. Patients should be restricted to light activity for 1 week postoperatively to minimize the risk of hematoma formation.

COMPLICATIONS

Although uncommon, the earliest complication of parathyroid surgery is vocal fold paralysis. In the cases of bilateral injury, patients often exhibit a normal voice but with subjective dyspnea and inspiratory stridor. This is usually noted upon extubation or in the recovery room. If clinical circumstances allow, fiberoptic laryngeal examination can confirm the diagnosis. In some cases of simple paresis, the patient may be observed without a tracheostomy. However, most patients will require a tracheostomy. Whether this condition is temporary or permanent, only time will tell. Unilateral vocal fold paralysis usually resolves spontaneously and only requires treatment in asymptomatic patients.

While rare, a hematoma from parathyroid surgery usually manifests itself in the first 6 to 12 hours after surgery and often presents as difficulty swallowing, difficulty breathing, or a pressure sensation in the neck. Swelling of the neck may be noted but is not common due to routine closure of the strap muscles trapping the expanding hematoma in the deep neck space. Optimum treatment relies on early recognition of the condition and opening the incision with evacuation of the hematoma with control of any bleeding vessels, ideally in the operating room. This

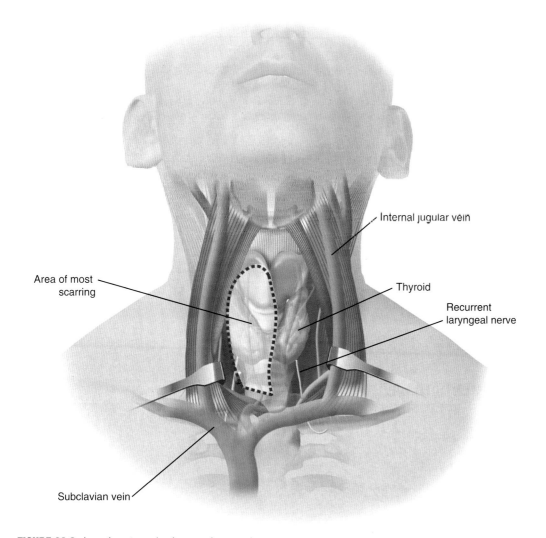

Internal jugular vein

Area of most
scarring

Thyroid

Recurrent
laryngeal nerve

Subclavian vein

FIGURE 23.2   Area of most scarring from previous surgery.

will relieve the pressure on the trachea and relieve the airway obstruction. Postoperative intubation for 1 to 2 days may be required after significant hematoma formation secondary to laryngeal edema from vascular congestion.

Hypocalcemia is also a condition that may occur in the first 6 to 12 hours following parathyroid surgery. Paresthesias such as a tingling sensation in the perioral region, hands, or feet may be the first initial manifestation. Cramping in the larger muscles may occur if persistent hypocalcemia is present. Unfortunately, this may occur in the setting of unilateral exploration and removal of a single gland, or bilateral exploration with removal of no glands. Postoperative PTH assay in the recovery room is likely the best predictor of this occurrence, especially when the PTH level is <20 after parathyroid surgery. This is managed with calcium replacement, IV or PO, and possible vitamin D supplementation.

Wound infection is exceedingly rare in parathyroid surgery in the healthy patient and raises the concern for possible inadvertent injury to the trachea or esophagus. This is usually managed by simply opening the wound with wick type drainage and antibiotics. The injuries are often small and will usually heal with time.

Hypercalcemia can result secondary to recovery of hypofunctioning remaining parathyroid glands in the setting of aggressive calcium and vitamin D replacement. This is seen more commonly in the younger population as a result of early recovery but may also be seen in the elderly as a result of confusion about medication with the addition of calcium when the requirements of several times a day regimen are added to an already crowded medication formulary.

RESULTS

Patients undergoing reoperative surgery can expect a 50% to 80% chance of resolution of their hyperparathyroid state due to postsurgical scarring and ectopic locations of hyperfunctioning glands. Patients who have their calcium levels return to normal levels despite a surgical complication such as vocal fold paralysis are more likely to be satisfied than patients who remain hypercalcemic without complication after reexploration.

PEARLS

- Obtain and read all previous operative and pathologic reports.
- Repeat all localization studies such as sestamibi, ultrasound, and computed tomography /magnetic resonance imaging prior to reexploration.
- Consider the 2002 Consensus Guidelines as indications in reoperative patients who are asymptomatic.
- Counsel patients that reexploration and removal of a single gland may render them permanently hypoparathyroid.
- Avoid removal of parathyroid glands <1 cm (60 mg).
- Bilateral, intraoperative, IJV PTH sampling may direct laterality of exploration.
- Avoid indiscriminant removal of the thyroid gland, especially in the absence of significant (<1 cm) nodules on preoperative ultrasound.
- In cases of extensive scarring after previous surgery, a "lateral to medial approach" may minimize the risk of complication while maximizing the chance of early localization of an abnormal gland.

PITFALLS

- RLN injury on side of previously removed parathyroids
- Inability to monitor intraoperative PTH levels
- Failure to recognize concomitant thyroid pathology preoperatively
- Operating on patients without hyperparathyroidism
- Potential for injury to the pharynx and esophagus

INSTRUMENTS TO HAVE AVAILABLE

- Head light
- McCabe surgical dissector
- Army Navy retractors
- DeBakey and Adson forceps
- Intraoperative PTH Assay
- Radio probe and Gamma monitor

SUGGESTED READING

Shen W, Duren M, Morita E, et al. Reoperation for persistent or recurrent primary hyperparathyroidism. *Arch Surg* 1996;131:861–869.

Morita SY, Somervell H, Umbricht CB, et al. Evaluation for concomitant thyroid nodules and primary hyperparathyroidism in patients undergoing parathyroidectomy or thyroidectomy. *Surgery* 2008;144(6):862–868.

Richards ML, Thompson GB, Farley, et al. Reoperative parathyroidectomy in 228 patients during the era of minimal-access surgery and intraoperative parathyroid hormone monitoring. *Am J Surg* 2008;196(6):937–942.

Pitt SC, Panneerselvan R, Sippel RS, et al. Radioguided parathyroidectomy for hyperparathyroidism in the reoperative neck. *Surgery* 2009;146(4):592–599.

Silberfein EJ, Bao R, Lopez A, et al. Reoperative parathyroidectomy: location of missed glands based on a contemporary nomenclature system. *Arch Surg* 2010;145(11):1065–1068.

Shin JJ, Milas M, Mitchell J, et al. Impact of localization studies and clinical scenario in patients with hyperparathyroidism being evaluated for reoperative neck surgery. *Arch Surg* 2011;146(1):1397–1403.

24 NONLOCALIZING PARATHYROIDECTOMY

Keith S. Heller

INTRODUCTION

For many years, the standard operation for primary hyperparathyroidism (HPT) was a bilateral cervical exploration identifying all four parathyroid glands and removing the one(s) that were abnormal. Abnormal parathyroid glands were recognized by their size and substance when palpated directly. Some surgeons routinely biopsied normal and abnormal parathyroid glands to confirm their identity, but most did not. As imaging techniques were developed and improved, particularly ^{99}Tc sestamibi scanning, high-resolution ultrasonography, and computed tomography (CT) scanning, surgeons used them with increasing frequency to help localize the abnormal parathyroid glands but continued to identify all four parathyroid glands at the time of surgery. These imaging studies, either alone or in combination, can accurately predict the location of solitary parathyroid adenomas in most patients but are much less reliable in identifying the 15% of patients who have more than one hyperfunctioning parathyroid gland. Whether or not preoperative imaging was employed, the success rate for this approach was >95%.

More recently, many surgeons have adopted the practice of focused, single-gland exploration. In this approach, preoperative imaging identifies the parathyroid adenoma. Without performing a complete bilateral exploration, the adenoma is identified and removed. Most surgeons confirm the adequacy of the procedure by measuring parathyroid hormone (PTH) levels intraoperatively (IOPTH). A fall in IOPTH of at least 50% from a baseline value and into the normal range is considered sufficient evidence that the remaining parathyroid glands are normal, so the operation can be terminated without identifying the remaining parathyroid glands. This approach results in cure rates comparable to conventional bilateral exploration.

Although focused, single-gland exploration is performed with increasing frequency, there remain situations in which conventional bilateral exploration is required. In some patients, imaging studies fail to identify any abnormal parathyroid glands. This can occur in the presence of a multinodular goiter that makes the preoperative identification of enlarged parathyroid glands difficult. Small, but abnormal, parathyroid glands can be difficult to image particularly in the presence of four-gland hyperplasia where all four parathyroid glands may be only minimally enlarged. In some clinical situations (secondary and tertiary HPT, familial HPT, multiple endocrine neoplasia syndromes) routine bilateral exploration is recommended regardless of the results of preoperative imaging because of the prevalence of four-gland hyperplasia. A standard, systematic surgical approach is required to identify all abnormal parathyroid glands in these situations.

HISTORY

Most patients with HPT are identified by the finding of an elevated serum calcium level on routine blood tests. The presence of elevated PTH levels and elevated calcium levels is virtually always diagnostic for HPT. In about 15% of patients, however, normocalcemic HPT is discovered during the evaluation of a patient with renal calculi, osteoporosis, or subjective symptoms suggestive of HPT. Once the diagnosis is established and the decision made to proceed with surgery, appropriate imaging studies are ordered.

PHYSICAL EXAMINATION

Enlarged parathyroid glands are almost never palpable. A palpable mass in the midline inferior in the neck in a patient with HPT is usually a thyroid nodule that should be evaluated by ultrasonography and fine needle aspiration (FNA) if appropriate. Rarely, very large parathyroid adenomas or carcinomas can be palpated. The latter are extraordinarily rare and are usually associated with very high serum calcium levels. Lethargy, confusion, and frank coma can occur in the presence of severe hypercalcemia, but many patients with serum calcium as high as 12 or 13 mg/dL have no abnormal physical findings or symptoms. The presence of a scar or scars in the inferior aspect of the neck should alert the examiner to possible previous thyroid or parathyroid surgery. Tracheal deviation is suggestive of a substernal goiter. These findings can make parathyroid exploration more difficult. In addition, a patient with a short, thick neck, frequently associated with the cricoid cartilage at the level of the sternal notch, can be very challenging technically.

INDICATIONS

The number of patients referred for parathyroid surgery continues to increase. Reasons for this trend include the recognition that significant HPT can exist in the presence of normocalcemia (15% of patients undergoing surgery), a greater awareness of the relationship of osteoporosis to chemically mild HPT, and better patient acceptance of parathyroid surgery particularly when focused, single-gland exploration is performed. This operation is frequently done under local anesthesia without overnight hospitalization with minimal postoperative discomfort or disability. Objective indications for parathyroid surgery include the following:

- Serum calcium >1 mg/dL above normal
- Renal calculi
- Osteoporosis
- Age <50 years
- Creatinine clearance <60 mL/minute

Other factors that can be considered in deciding whether or not surgery should be performed include subjective neurocognitive symptoms, bone pain, and fatigue as well as patient preference. The absence of any of the indications listed above is not a contraindication to surgery. Many endocrinologists and surgeons recommend parathyroid surgery for totally asymptomatic patients. Of course, prior to recommending surgery, the diagnosis of primary HPT must be confirmed. In general, imaging studies are used to help in the planning of surgery but are not required to establish the diagnosis of HPT.

CONTRAINDICATIONS

There are virtually no contraindications to parathyroid surgery other than severe coexisting medical conditions. It might be reasonable, however, to avoid difficult reoperative surgery with a higher risk of complications and a lower success rate in a patient in whom observation is a reasonable alternative to surgery.

PREOPERATIVE PLANNING

Imaging

Most patients in whom parathyroidectomy is planned undergo preoperative imaging studies. It is not the intent of this chapter to go into a detailed discussion of the different imaging studies available. Each has its advantages and disadvantages. Ultrasonography is inexpensive and risk free. It can also be performed at the time of initial consultation by the operating surgeon. Ultrasonography is not useful in identifying adenomas that are retrosternal or located deep in the neck (behind the trachea or esophagus). ^{99}Tc sestamibi radionuclide scans (usually performed as single photon emission computed tomography scans sometimes with CT image fusion) can detect adenomas in ectopic locations. CT scanning with contrast is gaining increasing popularity. It is important to remember that the accuracy of each of these techniques is very dependent on the experience of the radiologist interpreting the study. There is also considerable difference of opinion as to whether one imaging study or multiple imaging studies should be performed. Most surgeons use a single study or a combination of ultrasonography with one of the other studies. If the two studies are negative or discordant, it is reasonable to perform a third study in selected cases particularly if a focused, single-gland exploration is planned. A magnetic resonance imaging scan is unlikely to add further information to the other three studies. Angiography and selective venous sampling are not recommended as part of the evaluation of patients who have not had previous, parathyroid surgery. If imaging is negative or discordant or if imaging suggests more than one abnormal parathyroid gland, then a conventional bilateral exploration is planned.

Fine Needle Aspiration

Ultrasound-guided FNA can be used to confirm that a mass detected on imaging is a parathyroid gland rather than a lymph node or a thyroid nodule. In general, this is not necessary and not recommended. Surgery following FNA of a parathyroid adenoma is more difficult because of the disruption of the normal tissue planes. FNA may be helpful in planning a difficult reoperation. If an FNA is performed, the needle should be rinsed with saline after the slides have been prepared and the rinsate sent for PTH measurement. The cytologic appearance of parathyroid adenomas is easily confused with follicular thyroid neoplasms if the cytopathologist is not aware that a parathyroid adenoma is suspected.

Intraoperative PTH Measurement

IOPTH is a tremendously valuable addition to the technology available to the parathyroid surgeon. Because of the short half-life of the intact PTH molecule, PTH values usually fall into the normal range within 10 minutes after the hyperfunctioning parathyroid tissue is removed. Most authors suggest a decrease of at least 50% from a preoperative baseline and that the final IOPTH be within the normal range. While focused single-gland exploration can be performed without IOPTH measurement, a failure rate of about 7% can be anticipated because of the inability of the various imaging studies to detect multigland disease.

Although bilateral exploration can be performed successfully without measuring IOPTH, it nevertheless can be helpful. Ideally, all four glands are identified and the abnormal glands removed. Not infrequently one abnormal and fewer than three normal glands are identified. If IOPTH has fallen adequately, a fruitless, time-consuming search for a normal gland can be avoided. Sometimes, four minimally enlarged parathyroids are identified. Failure of IOPTH to fall following removal of 3½ of these will prompt a search for an adenoma in a supranumerary parathyroid. If an adenoma is fortuitously identified on the side explored initially, exploration of the contralateral side is not necessary if IOPTH falls appropriately.

Frozen Section

Intraoperative frozen sections are used to confirm that removed tissue is indeed parathyroid. Usually it is possible to distinguish hypercellular parathyroid tissue from normal parathyroid tissue but even this can be difficult. The pathologist cannot differentiate parathyroid adenomas from parathyroid hyperplasia by histologic criteria.

SURGICAL TECHNIQUE

In patients undergoing parathyroidectomy without preoperative localization or with imaging studies that are negative or suggest multigland disease, a conventional bilateral exploration is planned. This is usually performed under general endotracheal anesthesia. Surgery under local anesthesia can be performed in carefully selected patients. The patient is placed in the supine position with the neck gently extended. Intermittent leg compression devices on the lower extremities are employed to decrease the risk of a thromboembolic event. If IOPTH measurement is planned, a peripheral venous catheter in the antecubital fossa is usually sufficient for blood sampling during the procedure. Alternatively a radial intraarterial cannula can be inserted. The baseline IOPTH should be drawn in the operating room before the neck is palpated or the patient intubated if possible. A midline transverse incision is planned. The incision should be 1 to 2 cm inferior to the cricoid cartilage but need not be more inferior than 3 cm above the sternal notch. Incisions that are too low make exploration behind the superior pole of the thyroid difficult. Prior to making the incision, local anesthesia is infiltrated to enhance postoperative analgesia. An incision 4 to 5 cm in length is generally sufficient unless the neck is very thick.

The incision is deepened through the platysma muscle. Skin flaps are elevated in the subplatysmal plane. For maximum exposure flaps can be elevated to the superior edge of the thyroid cartilage and to the sternal notch inferiorly. The cervical fascia is incised in the midline and the strap muscles are retracted laterally. It is usually not necessary to divide the strap muscles. If necessary, exposure of the superior pole region can be facilitated by partially dividing the insertion of the sternothyroid muscle. If a middle thyroid vein is present, it should be divided and ligated.

The carotid sheath is then retracted laterally and the thyroid lobe mobilized and retracted medially. It is not necessary to divide any of the arteries to the thyroid gland at this point. Traction on the thyroid lobe is maintained using peanut sponges or by grasping the gland gently with Allis clamps. Care needs to be taken to avoid bleeding from the thyroid lobe. These maneuvers provide adequate exposure to the lateral and under surface of the thyroid lobe and to the retroesophageal and thymic regions in most patients and permit the identification of the parathyroid glands in their most common locations (Fig. 24.1). If the parathyroid glands are easily seen, identification of the recurrent laryngeal nerve is not always mandatory, but it is generally safest to identify the nerve early in the dissection. Both normal and abnormal parathyroids are usually found within small packets of

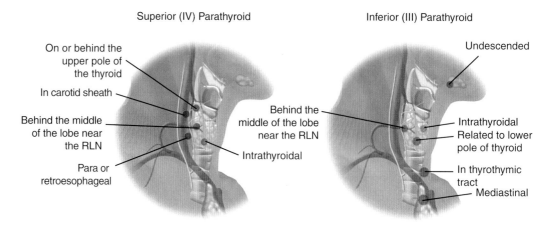

Superior (IV) Parathyroid

On or behind the
upper pole of
the thyroid

In carotid sheath

Behind the middle
of the lobe near
the RLN

Para or
retroesophageal

Behind the
middle of the lobe
near the RLN

Intrathyroidal

Inferior (III) Parathyroid

Undescended

Intrathyroidal
Related to lower
pole of thyroid

In thyrothymic
tract
Mediastinal

FIGURE 24.1

Possible locations of
parathyroid glands.

adipose tissue. They are typically tan or light brown and darken once they are exposed. They have fine blood vessels on their surface that are not seen in the surrounding adipose tissue. Hypercellular parathyroid glands generally have substance to them and can be palpated as firm nodules when exposed even when they are only minimally enlarged. Normal parathyroid glands are flaccid and not palpable when exposed. If an obvious enlarged parathyroid gland is found, it should be removed. There is usually an avascular plane around the gland. By spreading gently in this plane with a fine dissecting clamp, the gland can be mobilized and its feeding artery ligated and divided. The parathyroid gland is then submitted for confirmation by frozen section. While awaiting the results of the frozen section, further exploration is performed on the ipsilateral side to identify the other parathyroid gland. If IOPTII measurement is available, the exploration can be terminated if it decreases appropriately. If IOPTH is not available or if the level does not decrease, exploration of the contralateral side should be performed in a similar fashion. Double parathyroid adenomas do occur. The identification of an adenoma and a normal parathyroid on one side is not a guarantee that the parathyroids on the other side are normal. If multiple abnormal parathyroid glands are identified, a portion of the most normal appearing gland should be left in place with its blood supply intact and the remaining glands removed. As an alternative to this, all four parathyroid glands can be removed and a portion of one cut into small pieces and autotransplanted into either a muscle in the neck or the brachioradialis muscle. If available, cryopreservation of a piece of parathyroid tissue should be considered when a subtotal parathyroidectomy is performed.

If the initial exploration of one side does not reveal an adenoma or if two normal parathyroid glands are identified, exploration of the contralateral side should be performed before further extensive exploration of the initial side is undertaken. It is frequently easier to identify an adenoma than to find the normal parathyroids. If the initial bilateral exploration does not result in identification of an adenoma or if several enlarged parathyroids are identified but all four are not found and IOPTH does not drop or is not available, further exploration is required.

To permit further mobilization of the thyroid lobe, the superior thyroid vessels are divided and the thyroid lobe is mobilized medially. This permits exploration of the area adjacent to or medial to the insertion of the recurrent laryngeal nerve (Fig. 24.2). The area inferior to the thyroid lobe is carefully explored and the thymus gland mobilized and inspected. The substernal thymus gland can be mobilized into the neck by exerting gentle traction on it and using careful blunt dissection around it (Fig. 24.3). By dissecting medial to the carotid sheath, the retroesophageal space can be explored. This is a common site in which ectopic parathyroid glands may be found. It is important to remember that retroesophageal parathyroid glands are superior parathyroids (IV) even when located at or caudal to the level of the lower pole of the thyroid lobe. Their blood supply arises from superiorly and they must be passed under the inferior thyroid artery as they are mobilized in order to safely remove them (Fig. 24.4). Parathyroid glands can similarly be found in the retropharyngeal space. Parathyroid glands can rarely be found in the carotid sheath. This can be opened and explored if necessary. The location and extent of exploration is determined by the surgical findings. If two normal parathyroid glands are found on one side and one on the other, further extensive exploration is performed on the side with one parathyroid gland. If only one parathyroid gland is identified and it can be determined whether it is a superior or inferior parathyroid gland, further exploration based on the expected location of the missing gland is facilitated. Truly intrathyroidal parathyroid glands are rare. Most so-called intrathyroidal parathyroid glands are on the surface of the thyroid immediately under its capsule and can be easily removed without performing a thyroidectomy. If three normal parathyroids are identified and confirmed with biopsy, ipsilateral thyroid lobectomy on the side where only one parathyroid was identified can be considered, but unfortunately is usually not successful. Lateralization of a missing parathyroid can sometimes be performed intraoperatively if IOPTH measurement is available by directly sampling from the jugular vein low on each side of the neck.

If four seemingly normal parathyroid glands are identified, each should be biopsied in order to confirm their identity and help determine if they are hypercellular. If frozen section reveals hypercellularity, subtotal parathyroidectomy preserving a vascularized portion of one gland in situ is recommended. If four biopsy-proven normal parathyroid glands are identified, they should not be removed in the futile hope that this will cure

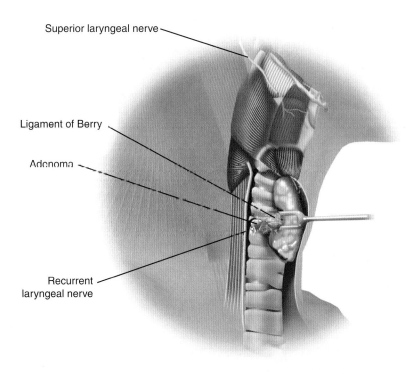

Superior laryngeal nerve

Ligament of Berry

Adenoma

Recurrent
laryngeal nerve

FIGURE 24.2
Identification of the
parathyroid between the
insertion of the nerve and
Berry's ligament.

the disease. This mistake results in hypoparathyroidism when reexploration identifies a parathyroid adenoma in a supranumerary parathyroid gland.

At the completion of the exploration, the wound is irrigated and hemostasis assured. Drains are usually not required. The patient is extubated in the operating room.

POSTOPERATIVE MANAGEMENT

Perioperative antibiotics are not required. Because the patient can usually ambulate immediately after surgery, pharmacologic deep vein thrombosis prophylaxis is not required unless unusual risk factors are present. The patient is rapidly advanced to a regular diet. Patients who undergo bilateral exploration, particularly those in

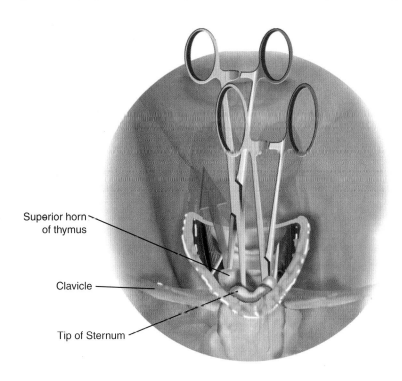

Superior horn
of thymus

Clavicle

Tip of Sternum

FIGURE 24.3
Cervical thymectomy.

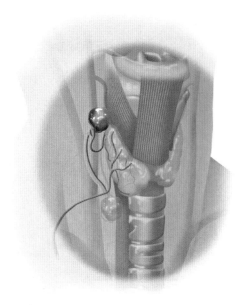

FIGURE 24.4
Mobilization of descended superior parathyroids.

whom multiple parathyroids are removed or manipulated, are observed overnight and discharged the morning following surgery. If only one parathyroid is removed, patients are given 1 g of calcium daily by mouth. If a subtotal parathyroidectomy is performed, the patient is given 3 g of calcium daily as well as 0.5 µg of calcitriol. Serum calcium levels are obtained prior to discharge.

COMPLICATIONS

Complications are rare following parathyroidectomy. Postoperative hematoma requiring reoperation occurs in <1% of cases. Wound infection is very uncommon. Transient vocal cord paralysis is much less common than after thyroidectomy, and permanent recurrent laryngeal nerve injury should virtually never occur.

Symptomatic hypocalcemia is the most common postoperative complication. Some patients are symptomatic after removal of a solitary adenoma although their serum calcium level is rarely low. Significant hypocalcemia is common after subtotal parathyroidectomy. It can be minimized by the calcium and vitamin D regimen suggested above. If it does occur, increasing doses of calcitriol are given. Intravenous calcium is rarely required except in patients with secondary HPT and renal failure who can become profoundly hypocalcemic.

RESULTS

The success rate for parathyroidectomy should be better than 95%. Many authors report cure rates of between 98% and 99%.

PEARLS

- Preoperative imaging should be performed in all patients undergoing surgery for HPT.
- IOPTH measurement is useful even if bilateral exploration is planned.
- Meticulous hemostasis is mandatory during the exploration to avoid tissue staining, which makes parathyroid identification difficult.
- Adequate mobilization of the thyroid gland is needed to identify parathyroid glands in ectopic locations.
- Frozen section confirmation of the adenoma should be obtained particularly if IOPTH is not used.
- Biopsy confirmation of all parathyroids visualized should be performed if an obvious adenoma is not identified.

PITFALLS

- It is easy to convince oneself that pieces of adipose tissue or lymph nodes are actually parathyroid glands.
- Do not remove normal parathyroid glands and "hope for the best."

INSTRUMENTS TO HAVE AVAILABLE

- Dissection is performed with fine clamps and retraction with McBurney or Richardson retractors.
- The decision as to whether vessels should be ligated or controlled with unipolar or bipolar cautery or ultrasonic devices is left to the surgeon's individual preference.
- Many surgeons find that the use of optical magnifying telescopes and headlights provides better visualization of the surgical field.

SUGGESTED READING

Udelsman R. Six hundred fifty-six consecutive explorations for primary hyperparathyroidism. *Ann Surg* 2002;235(5): 665–672.

Irvin GL III, Carneiro DM, Solorzano CC. Progress in the operative management of sporadic primary hyperparathyroidism over 34 years. *Ann Surg* 2004;239(5):704–711.

Bilezikian JP, Khan AA, Potts JT Jr. Guidelines for the management of asymptomatic primary hyperparathyroidism: summary statement from the third international workshop. *J Clin Endocrinol Metab* 2007;94:335–339.

Johnson NA, Tublin ME, Ogilvie JB. Parathyroid imaging: technique and role in the preoperative evaluation of primary hyperparathyroidism. *AJR Am J Roentgenol* 2007;188(6):1706–1715.

Greene AB, Butler RS, McIntyre S, et al. National trends in parathyroid surgery from 1998 to 2008: a decade of change. *J Am Coll Surg* 2009;209(3):332–343.

25 SUPERFICIAL PAROTIDECTOMY

Pavel Dulguerov

INTRODUCTION

Pathologic swellings of the parotid gland are the main indication for parotidectomy. Swellings of the parotid gland may be divided into two broad categories: diffuse and localized. Diffuse swellings usually represent inflammation of the parotid gland and/or infections that are generally treated with medication or sometimes sialendoscopy. Localized swellings represent tumors in the parotid gland or cyst-like conditions (Table 25.1), and their treatment consists of some form of parotidectomy.

Both benign and malignant tumors occur in the parotid gland. The majority (~80%) of parotid tumors are benign, and the most common tumor of the parotid gland is pleomorphic adenoma. This peculiar benign tumor tends to recur if not completely excised and may degenerate with time into its malignant form, carcinoma ex pleomorphic adenoma. Surgery for recurrent pleomorphic adenoma is associated with a higher incidence of complications, in particular, facial paralysis.

The goals of parotid surgery are:

- Prevention of recurrence, which requires a complete removal of the tumor, ideally with a cuff of normal parotid tissue and without tumor seeding by spillage
- Protection and preservation of the facial nerve unless the nerve is directly involved by a neoplasm (almost always malignant)
- Prevention of Frey syndrome
- Prevention of other complications, such as salivary gland fistula, hematoma, wound infection, and anesthesia of the skin
- Optimal cosmetic results

To achieve these goals, the parotid surgeon should have extensive knowledge of parotid pathology, including the exact clinical significance of each parotid tumor (Table 25.1) and intimate knowledge of the anatomy of the facial nerve.

Relevant Anatomy

In addition to the parotid gland, the parotid space contains (a) arteries (the external carotid and its terminal branches, superficial temporal and internal maxillary); (b) veins (the retromandibular or retrofacial, which is generally (in 71%) posterior to the branches of the facial nerve); (c) lymphatic vessels and lymph nodes draining the scalp and face and contained within the gland because these structures develop before the gland is completely surrounded by fascia; and (d) nerves (the facial, the greater auricular, and the auriculotemporal).

Fascias

The fascia in the neck is divided into a superficial and a deep layer. The superficial fascia is usually a thin connective tissue layer under the dermis, and, as a rule, vessels and nerves are located deep to it. The superficial

TABLE 25.1   Etiology of Parotid Masses and a Concise Summary of Treatment

Lesion	Foote	Spiro	Woods	Wang	Treatment
Locations considered	Major Salivary Glands	All Salivary Glands	Parotid Gland	All Salivary Glands	
Number of patients	776	2,751	1,360	1,176	
1. **Adenomas**	66%	53%	84%	75%	Surgery is the main and only universally accepted treatment.
1.1. *Pleomorphic adenoma*	58%	46%	60.5%	53%	Universal agreement about the type of parotidectomy is still lacking; most often, superficial parotidectomy is the minimal operation for superficial "lobe" tumors, while total parotidectomy is used for deep "lobe" adenomas.
1.2. *Monomorphic adenoma*	8%	6.8%	23%	22%	
1.2.1. Adenolymphoma (Warthin tumor)	6.5%	6.6%	22%	17%	Postoperative radiation therapy has been debated in the past for pleomorphic adenoma but has been abandoned in most centers.
1.2.2. Others: Myoepithelioma Basal cell adenoma Oncocytoma Canalicular adenoma Sebaceous adenoma Ductal papilloma Cystadenoma				2.3%	Observation only is recommended for patients who are not good surgical candidates.
2. **Carcinomas**	24%	47%	16%	25%	
2.1. *Acinic cell*	3%	3.0%	2.5%	3%	A: Superficial or total parotidectomy, preservation of facial nerve, no radiation therapy — A
2.2. *Mucoepidermoid carcinoma*	12%	15.9%	4.5%	6%	Low grade: A; High grade: B
2.3. *Adenoid cystic carcinoma*	2%	10.2%	2.1%	4.4%	B
2.4. *Adenocarcinoma* Polymorphous low grade Basal cell Papillary cystadenocarcinoma Mucinous Adenocarcinoma NOS (not otherwise specified)	4%	8.1%	3.9%	2%	B — Treatment A should be changed to B, if tumor size >4 cm (T3).

2.5.	Carcinoma expleomorphic adenoma	6%	5.8%	1.1%	1%	B
2.6.	Squamous cell carcinoma	3%	1.9%	1.6%	0.2%	B
2.7.	Undifferentiated carcinoma	4%	1.3%	0.8%		3
						B: Total parotidectomy, selective supraomohyoid neck dissection (N0) or complete neck dissection (N+), resection of facial branches if grossly involved, postoperative radiation therapy. If extraparotid spread is present, then involved structures should be resected.
3.	**Nonepithelial Tumors** Angiomas, lipomas, neurogenic tumors, mesenchymal tumors, sarcomas					Surgery
4.	**Malignant lymphomas**			1.5%		Radiation therapy ± chemotherapy
5.	**Secondary tumors**			0.3%		Depends on the histology of the primary
6.	**Unclassified tumors**					Depends upon the histology
7.	**Tumor-like lesions** Sialoadenosis, oncocytosis necrotizing sialometaplasia (benign lymphoepithelial lesion, salivary gland cysts (mucocele, salivary duct, lymphoepithelial, dysgenetic, chronic sclerosing sialadenitis, cystic lymphoid hyperplasia in AIDS Sarcoid					Variable indications for parotidectomy

FIGURE 25.1

Anatomical cross section showing the fascial layers lateral to the parotid gland. M, mandible and masseter muscle; P, parotid gland; S, submandibular gland; SCM, sternocleidomastoid; SF, superficial fascia; T, temporalis muscle; Z, zygomatic bone. The discussion is centered about the fascia layers included in the fascia marked by ?. It should contain the SMAS, which is the facial extension of the platysma and its fascia, and the facial extension of the deep cervical fascia. Whether this fascial layer can be divided into two layers, with a separate parotid fascia, is debatable. The superficial fascia below the epidermis is clearly seen.

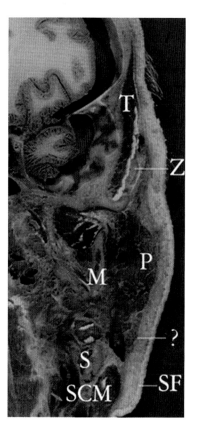

cervical fascia covers the superficial aspect of the platysma muscle and splits to also cover its deep surface. It is attached to overlying skin with thin fibrous septa and continues on the face and scalp to extend all the way to the vertex where it covers the epicranius muscle.

The recognition of the superficial musculoaponeurotic system (SMAS) and its importance in face-lift surgery added to the controversy about the exact composition of the fascia overlying the parotid gland (Fig. 25.1). While it is now accepted that the SMAS layer is a continuation of the superficial fascia–platysma layer in the neck, it is unclear (1) whether there is a distinct superficial fascial layer lateral to the SMAS, (2) whether the parotid fascia is a separate layer deep to the SMAS, and (3) whether the deep cervical fascia participates in the lateral parotid coverage. The SMAS is a thick solid layer below the subcutaneous adipose tissue from which fibrous septa extend laterally to the skin, interpreted by some as a separate fascia; a distinct parotid fascia is present covering the gland, but it is extremely thin. In addition, significant individual variation is present in the thickness of these different layers.

Facial Nerve

The facial nerve, after exiting the stylomastoid foramen, is almost immediately surrounded by the parotid gland. The nerve enters the parotid space between the digastric and stylohyoid muscle. The nerve is lateral (more superficial) to the styloid process and to the most superior extension of the posterior belly of the digastric muscle. The point of entry of the facial nerve into the parotid gland has been described along a line uniting the tip of the tragus to the angle of the jaw. Within the parotid gland, the facial nerve takes an upward and median-ward concave course. It is in close relation to the stylomastoid artery, which arises from the occipital or post-auricular branches of the external carotid artery and is responsible for vascularization of the mastoid segment of the facial nerve. The distance between the main trunk of the facial nerve and the closest point of the digastric muscle was found to be 9 ± 2.7 mm, and the depth of the trunk of the facial nerve from the skin surface was measured in cadavers as 20.1 ± 3.1 mm.

The facial nerve always branches within the parotid gland into two main divisions: the temporofacial and cervicofacial divisions. Several generalizations can be made about the intraparotid anatomy of the facial nerve (Fig. 25.2):

- The buccal ramus can originate from either the temporofacial or the cervicofacial division.
- Branches located at the extremities of the nerve distribution receive fewer anastomosis with other branches.
- The majority of anastomosis occurs between the buccal and zygomatic divisions, forming the so-called plexus.
- The number of anastomosis decreases in caudal branches, with the marginal mandibular branch receiving anastomosis in only 6.3%.
- There is no anastomosis between the cervical and other branches.
- The anastomosis is more extensive when the buccal branch arises from the cervicofacial division.

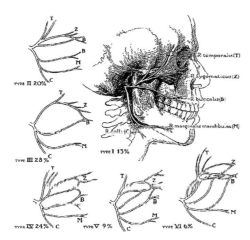

FIGURE 25.2 Branching patterns of the extratemporal facial nerve. The data were obtained from the dissection of 350 cervicofacial halves. The division patterns of the facial nerve are classified in types (I to VI), and the relative frequency of each type is marked. Type I: no anastomosis between facial branches. Type II: numerous anastomosis between zygomatic and buccal branches (parastenon anastomosis, zygomatic loop). Type III: single anastomosis between zygomatic and buccal branch, located distal anterior to the parotid tissue. Type IV: anastomosis between temporal and zygomatic branches and extensive anastomosis between zygomatic and buccal branches. Type V: combination of type II and III with extensive anastomosis between zygomatic and buccal branches. Type VI: plexiform anastomosis between temporal, zygomatic, buccal, and marginal mandibular rami. Type VII: double main facial trunk (3%). (Reprinted from Davis RA, Anson BJ, Budinger JM, et al. Surgical anatomy of the facial nerve and parotid gland based upon a study of 350 cervicofacial halves. *Surg Gynecol Obstet* 1956;102:385–412.)

Anterior to the parotid gland, the facial nerve branches are covered by the SMAS and the masseteric fascia. Further nerve divisions are observed as branches approach the muscle they innervate, always on the deep aspect of the muscle.

Parotid Lobes

The parotid gland was viewed as having two lobes, where "the facial nerve is like the meat of the sandwich," and this concept helped devising partial parotid resections, such as superficial parotidectomy. While this lobe concept was abandoned, the facio-venous plane is an important concept in parotid surgery. It is important to realize that neither is this plane strictly vertical, nor is the same amount of parotid tissue found superficial to the facial nerve: In the superior portion of the gland, the temporal and zygomatic branches of the facial nerve are more superficial than the facial nerve branches in the inferior portion of the parotid. In addition, as the plane of the facial nerve is followed anteriorly, it becomes more superficial, with less parotid tissue covering the nerve.

Parotidectomy Classification

Surgical resection of the parotid gland includes some form of parotidectomy. Because of the great confusion about the various naming in parotid surgery, The European Salivary Gland Society (ESGS) recently organized a classification of parotidectomies: the gland is divided in five levels (Fig. 25.3) and the operation termed according to the level removed. The classical superficial parotidectomy corresponds to the removal of levels I and II; it is thus called parotidectomy I–II.

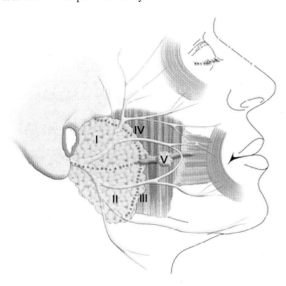

FIGURE 25.3 ESGS division of the parotid gland in five levels. The division in five levels: I (lateral superior), II (lateral inferior), III (deep inferior), IV (deep superior), and V (accessory). The superior level is the area corresponding to the branch of the temporofacial nerve and the inferior level the area of the cervicofacial branch. (Modified from Quer M, Pujol A, Leon X, et al. Parotidectomies in benign parotid tumours: "Sant Pau" surgical extension classification. *Acta Otorrinolaringol Esp* 2010;61:1–5.)

HISTORY

Most patients who are candidates for parotidectomy present with the history of a slow-growing painless mass in the parotid gland and no other associated symptoms. While a complete medical history is necessary prior to ordering further tests, it will most often remain unremarkable.

A patient with such a slow-growing mass in the parotid gland will typically have a pleomorphic adenoma. If a heavy smoking history is present or if bilateral parotid masses are present, Warthins tumor is a likely diagnosis. A malignant tumor will be suggested by a constellation of symptoms including a rapidly growing mass, pain, facial weakness, infiltration of the skin, and cervical lymphadenopathy. The history of treatment for skin cancer should make one suspicious of a metastatic cancer to a peri- or intraparotid lymph node.

Obstruction of the duct with secondary infections usually presents with pain that typically increases during meals and could thus be differentiated from a parotid tumor by history.

PHYSICAL EXAMINATION

A careful examination of the head and neck is necessary, starting with inspection of the parotid region, looking for the location of the mass or skin erosion. Thorough evaluation of the skin of the pinna, preauricular and malar area, forehead, and scalp is mandatory to look for a previously treated or undiagnosed primary cancer of the skin. Otoscopy should be performed, again looking for skin lesions but also for infiltration of the skin of the external auditory meatus from an adjacent parotid tumor. Ipsilateral and contralateral facial nerve function should be evaluated with a standardized grading system. I prefer the regional modification of the House-Brackmann scale because the global scale gives little information about individual branches.

After inspection, palpation of the gland and the mass is carried out assessing its size, consistency, mobility, and location. Intraoral examination should investigate the palate and lateral pharynx for asymmetry suggesting parapharyngeal extension. The neck is then palpated to detect a lymphadenopathy.

INDICATIONS

The treatment of most localized masses in the parotid gland is surgical excision, and only rarely could any form of medical therapy be curative or observation recommended.

CONTRAINDICATIONS

The general teaching is that any mass in the parotid gland should be excised to provide a final diagnosis and usually definitive treatment. There are several exceptions to this attitude:

- Lesions of the parotid gland in infants are hemangiomas until proven otherwise and require radiologic evaluation and initial treatment with β-blockers. The role of surgery in the management of hemangiomas of the parotid gland is evolving.
- Parotidectomy for sialadenitis is associated with high complication rates, and surgery should be avoided if possible. Some types of sialadenitis, such as tuberculosis, present with a mass in a lymph node in the parotid gland and should be diagnosed prior to surgery with fine needle aspiration biopsy (FNAB), core needle biopsy (CNB), or even imaging.
- Patients with limited life expectancy (elderly or high anesthesia risk) could be spared parotidectomy if the diagnosis of a benign tumor or lesion could be made with high certainty. Probably, the accuracy of FNAB is sufficient to diagnose a Warthins tumor. For pleomorphic adenoma, the results of FNAB are not so convincing, and the decision of surgery versus follow-up should be individualized. Further studies are required to determine the diagnostic value of CNB in this setting.
- Patients with cystic lesions should be evaluated for human immunodeficiency virus (HIV), and treatment with sclerosing agents instead of parotidectomy is preferred because the risk of developing similar lesions is high.
- If lymphoma is suspected preoperatively, lymph nodes in other sites, where surgery is associated with less risks, should be searched for and excised for diagnosis and staging.
- Tumors metastatic to the parotid lymph nodes will probably not be cured by parotidectomy, except when the primary neoplasm is located on the skin of the face and scalp.

PREOPERATIVE PLANNING

Extent of surgery correlates with the duration of the procedure and usually with the importance of postoperative complications. As shown in Table 25.1, a vast variety of histologic types can present as a mass in the parotid, and the extent of surgery varies according to the histology. Therefore, it is important to know the diagnosis prior to planning surgery. FNAB and CNB are two techniques helpful in this assessment. Other important preoperative considerations determining the extent of surgery are the location of the tumor and its extension to adjacent structures, and these are best assessed by imaging.

The role of imaging in the evaluation of a mass in the parotid gland is controversial because, despite a few reports for magnetic resonance imaging (MRI), no imaging technique can differentiate between benign and malignant lesions. Imaging is not necessary for the evaluation of a patient with an easily identifiable mass in the parotid gland with benign characteristics on history and physical examination. There are three situations where imaging could be useful: (1) the presence of the mass is uncertain, (2) the location (superficial or deep lobe) is unclear, and (3) an extension outside the parotid gland is suspected.

MRI with gadolinium is the preferred modality because different sequences provide different information. T1-weighted sequences demonstrate protein-rich content often seen in Warthin tumor. On T2-weighted sequences, high-signal lesions tend to be pleomorphic adenoma, while a low-signal lesion favors to other types of parotid neoplasm. Fat saturated T1 sequences differentiate cystic and solid areas/lesions. Diffusion-weighted and perfusion-weighted sequences are supposed to help distinguish between malignant and benign tumors. T2-weighted turbo spin-echo sequences are useful in examining salivary ducts in the so-called MR sialography.

CT is rarely necessary but could be used as a less-expensive modality to locate the lesion and determine whether extraparotid extension is present, especially in the base of the skull. The role of FDG–PET is also limited but could be useful in the evaluation of distant metastasis of an aggressive cancer of the parotid gland prior to extensive surgery or in the evaluation of masses of the parotid gland of uncertain diagnosis.

The exact role of FNAB is controversial because of its variable accuracy, which is dependent on the experience of the cytopathologist. Getting the aspirate under ultrasound guidance and having the pathologist immediately evaluate the specimen seem to improve the accuracy of the procedure. The false-negative rate for diagnosis of malignancy has remained about 20%, and thus, it is not advised to rely solely on FNAB in the diagnosis of a benign tumor and avoidance of surgery. One situation in which FNAB is quite reliable is Warthin tumor, with accuracy around 95%. Finally, FNAB lacks accuracy in the diagnosis of the exact subtype of salivary gland malignancy.

Larger-needle biopsy allows for the examination of a core of tissue instead of individual cells and has been proposed as a new tool with excellent accuracy (100%). In 76 patients, an adequate sample was obtained in 73 (96%) of which two diagnoses were inconclusive (both basal tumor); in the remaining 71 patients, there was no false-positive or false-negative for malignancy! Furthermore, the exact correct histology was found in 78% and in the same histologic subtype in 91%; only in three patients was the diagnosis inexact, although with limited clinical consequences. My preliminary experience with this technique has been excellent.

SURGICAL TECHNIQUE

Most parotid surgery is done under general anesthesia without paralytic anesthetic agents. Curare derivatives are usually used for induction of anesthesia, but their effects wear off within 20 minutes, allowing for stimulation of the facial nerve and monitoring of facial movements and/or facial muscles electromyography (EMG).

The patient is placed in a supine position, with the head and thorax elevated at least 20 degrees, in order to promote venous return from the head and neck and to decrease vascular congestion. The head is rotated to the opposite side and slightly extended. If necessary, the entire operating table can be rotated 10 to 15 degrees toward the opposite side (Fig. 25.4).

I use local infiltration of an adrenaline solution (1:50,000) without local anesthetic. The solution is injected over the planned incision, in the subcutaneous dissection plane, and vertically in the gland, around and away from the tumor. Pledgets soaked in a similar solution can be used during surgery to optimize local vasoconstriction and thus hemostasis around the branches of the facial nerve.

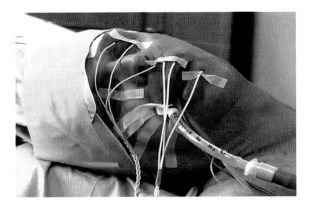

FIGURE 25.4 Positioning of the patient for parotid surgery.

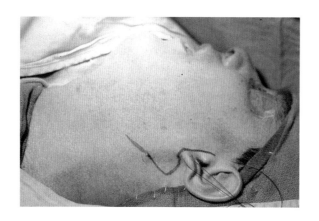

FIGURE 25.5

Typical lazy S parotidectomy incision.

Usually, minimal retroauricular shaving is required. Ocular ointment is placed, and the eyelids are taped shut. Skin disinfecting is accomplished with a solution that does not harm the cornea (e.g., Betadine or chlorhexidine). After disinfecting, sterile electrodes for EMG-based facial nerve monitoring are inserted in the ipsilateral orbicularis oculi and oris muscles with wires directed to the nonoperated side. Reference electrodes are placed near the nasal alae (Fig. 25.4).

The entire half of the face is left exposed in the operative field in order to allow for the visualization of facial movements during surgery. Usually, the drapes are placed close to the midline, and a transparent sheet covers the eye, mouth, and EMG electrodes. The entire neck is left exposed in the operating field for a possible neck dissection. A sterile cotton ball covered with an ointment is placed in the external auditory meatus to prevent the entry of blood during the procedure, since this can result in a postoperative external otitis.

The two most popular incisions are the so-called "lazy S" (Blair) and the rhytidectomy incision. The usual incision has a sigmoid or a "lazy S" shape with a vertical preauricular limb, a curvature under the ear lobule, and a somewhat horizontal limb in a natural skin crease of the neck (Fig. 25.5). The vertical limb follows established rules for scar camouflage by being placed at the junction between two facial esthetic units—the pinna and the lateral face. A variation consists in hiding part of this vertical limb in the concha, behind the tragus. The retroauricular portion of the incision should not be too narrow (>2 cm) to prevent skin flap necrosis. The neck portion of the incision rarely needs to go beyond the level of the anterior border of the sternocleidomastoid (SCM) muscle. The exposure is adequate in most cases, the scar is small and well hidden, and the direction of the incision can be modified, should a neck dissection or extended base of skull resection become necessary.

Recently, the use of a rhytidectomy incision with the same vertical preauricular limb and a horizontal retroauricular limb near the neck hair line (Fig. 25.6) has been promoted as being more cosmetic. Whether this incision is worth the extra time and gives a better cosmetic result remains to be demonstrated in randomized trials with blinded evaluation of the results. Furthermore, the rhytidectomy approach is less versatile with difficulties to extend the incision for neck dissection and limited exposure for anteriorly located lesions.

Obviously, modifications of these incisions are required when skin has to be resected because of invasion by a tumor, malignant or benign. In these cases, the tumor is usually large enough to serve as a natural tissue expander, and rarely are any difficulties encountered with the closure. During reoperation, especially for recurrent pleomorphic adenoma, the scar and any suspicious subcutaneous tissue must be excised at the beginning of the procedure.

Although early parotidectomy techniques did not raise the superficial facial skin flap before beginning dissection of the gland, it is now standard. The dissection of the skin flap is facilitated by prior infiltration. The flap can be raised in the subcutaneous adipose tissue, avoiding injury to the hair follicles. This plane of dissection is superficial to the SMAS and to the superficial cervical fascia. Dissection in this plane is advised if the tumor is very superficial, and this plane of dissection is the safest anteriorly where the distal branches of the

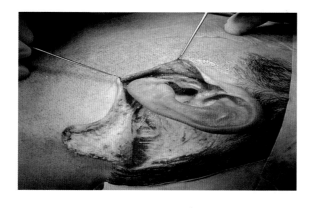

FIGURE 25.6

Rhytidectomy incision for parotidectomy.

facial nerve become more superficial. Usually, dissection in the supra-SMAS adipose tissue is easier, is more expeditious, and results in less bleeding.

The dissection can also be made in a plane deep to the SMAS and is described as providing more esthetic results and as a technique to prevent Frey syndrome. An advantage of sub-SMAS dissection is the better vascularization of the skin flap. In sub-SMAS dissection, progression beyond the anterior extension of the parotid gland should be cautious because here facial nerve branches rapidly become superficial.

I use elements of both; the skin is elevated superficial to the SMAS for a few centimeters after which we search for the level of the parotid lobules and elevate the SMAS/parotid fascia layer to expose the entire gland. Unless some form of "minimalistic" resection is planned, the entire gland must be exposed to allow for better visualization of the lateral aspect of the tumor.

The dissection can be carried out either with a scalpel or with scissors probably with similar results. When using scissors, emphasis has been placed on doing the dissection parallel to facial nerve fibers and placing the scissors shafts at right angles to the underlying parotid gland.

Most of this dissection is "blind," since the skin flaps are put under tension in a posterior direction. The edge of the instrument can be seen as its tip elevates the skin. After elevation of the skin flap, stay sutures can be placed on the flap and the ear lobule to help the retraction.

The next step is to free the posterior aspect of the parotid gland. The gland is easily separated from the SCM muscle, a step requiring sectioning of the superficial layer of the deep cervical fascia. At this point, it often becomes obvious that the anterior branch of the greater auricular nerve has to be transected. Some believe that the nerve should be tied to prevent the occurrence of a postoperative neuroma. The posterior and "lobular" branch of the greater auricular nerve can usually be preserved, although over time anesthesia of the skin seems to recover, even when the entire nerve is transected.

Deep to the SCM muscle, the parotid gland is attached to the posterior belly of the digastric muscle, which is a key landmark in this operation. The parotid gland must be completely freed from the digastric muscle, all the way to its origin on the mastoid; a step that leads to the identification of the main trunk of the facial nerve. The external jugular vein and the retromandibular vein should be preserved during the initial stages of dissection, in order to decrease the intraparotid venous pressure and thus decrease bleeding. While dissecting along the digastric muscle, the subdigastric region should be examined for the presence of suspicious lymph nodes.

The gland is also separated from the anterior aspect of the cartilaginous external auditory meatus, cutting the fascial attachments and exposing the so-called cartilaginous pointer, another landmark helpful in the identification of the facial nerve. It is important to stay against the cartilage during this dissection, to decrease bleeding, to avoid injuring branches of the facial nerve within the parotid gland, and most importantly to use it as a guide during the dissection.

The dissection continues by the identification of the junction between the cartilaginous and bony external auditory meatus. During this dissection, the posterior extension of the parotid fascia is sectioned, as it inserts on the tympanomastoid suture (sometimes referred to as Lore fascia).

The tail of the parotid can be dissected before or after the preauricular dissection. The dissection should not proceed too deep before the nerve trunk is identified. On the other hand, a common error is to start looking for the facial nerve too early; the nerve is a deep structure and is never superficial to the cartilaginous pointer or to the posterior belly of the digastric muscle.

Before trying to identify the facial nerve, good exposure and excellent hemostasis are paramount. Good exposure is achieved by the previously described dissection of the posterior aspect of the parotid gland. The gland is retracted anteriorly by a retractor held by an assistant, and the external ear canal is retracted posteriorly by a suture attached to a weight or to the drapes (Fig. 25.7). Careful hemostasis is important because any blood in the wound will collect in its deepest portion, which is where the facial nerve will be found (Fig. 25.8). Above the level of the cartilaginous pointer, a regular monopolar electrocoagulator can be employed, while deep to this level, a fine bipolar forceps is used.

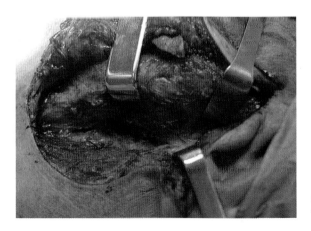

FIGURE 25.7 Dissection of the posterior portion of the parotid gland.

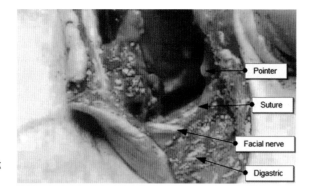

FIGURE 25.8

Exposure and landmarks for identification of the main trunk of the facial nerve.

The key step in parotid surgery is the identification of the main trunk of the facial nerve. In modern parotidectomy, the nerve is identified at the trunk level, and the branches followed forward in the glandular parenchyma. Useful landmarks for the facial nerve trunk include

- The *"cartilaginous pointer"* or *"tragal pointer,"* which is actually the anterior tip of the tragus portion of the external ear cartilage (Fig. 25.8). The main trunk is said to be 1 cm deep and 1 cm inferior to the pointer.
- The *posterior belly of the digastric muscle* and its insertion on the mastoid process, which is slightly lateral to the stylomastoid foramen.
- The *tympanomastoid suture,* which can be identified by palpation. The main trunk is said to be 6 to 8 mm from the "inferomedial end of the suture"; unfortunately, some controversy exists on what represents the end of the suture.
- The *stylomastoid artery* running with its vein a few millimeters lateral to the facial nerve. The stylomastoid artery arises from branches of the external carotid and follows the facial nerve in the stylomastoid foramen.
- The *styloid process,* which is located deep to the facial nerve. It can be palpated, but its visualization before identification of the nerve usually means that the nerve has been injured.

Of these anatomical landmarks, the tympanomastoid suture is probably the most useful because it is a bony landmark and the least subject to variation in location. The tympanomastoid suture is formed by edge of the tympanic bone lying on the mastoid bone. It starts at the posterior edge of the bony external auditory canal to extend on to the undersurface of the temporal bone. It terminates by the stylomastoid foramen, through which the facial nerve exits the skull. As pointed out earlier, the parotid fascia inserts on the tympanomastoid suture. According to Robertson, the fissure can be followed safely until this fascial layer, which is often quite tough. The fascia needs to be divided close to the temporal bone, and the dissection should proceed with gentle spreading of the tissues in the direction of the facial nerve trunk, using a fine mosquito forceps. The nerve appears as a white cord-like structure. Usually, the stylomastoid artery is coagulated with bipolar forceps prior to identifying the facial nerve trunk.

The nerve must be identified with certainty. One way to identify the facial nerve is to dissect the length of the trunk, until the bifurcation is clearly visualized. This dissection should be very cautious because accessory facial nerve trunks (actually a facial nerve that has bifurcated in the mastoid canal) have been described. Once the bifurcation is identified, try to selectively stimulate each division branch, that is, when the cervicofacial division is stimulated, the eyelids should not twitch and vice versa.

Another way is to use a facial nerve stimulator using the lowest possible electric current, in order to avoid nerve damage and fatigue. With modern monitoring devices, the minimal amount of current necessary to elicit nerve stimulation, ideally without facial muscle contraction, should be used: one gets an EMG response but not muscle twitching. Bipolar stimulating electrode is more selective, uses less current for stimulation, and is therefore preferred. The use of "nerve pinching" as nerve stimulation technique is to be discouraged, although a comparative trial of these two techniques has not been carried out.

Sistrunk, as well as Adson and Ott, proposed to identify the marginal mandibular branch and follow it by retrograde dissection to the main trunk of the facial nerve. State identified buccal branches anteriorly in the parotid gland and used retrograde dissection to find the main trunk of the facial nerve. Bailey identified temporal facial nerve branches, as they cross the zygomatic arch. While the routine use of these methods has been abandoned, they remain useful in reoperations of the parotid gland where the scar tissue renders identification of the main trunk both rather tedious and with a certain element of danger. A few authors still favor the identification of a peripheral branch (usually the marginal mandibular nerve) and its dissection back to the main trunk of the facial nerve. The branches, the least difficult to identify, are the temporal and the marginal mandibular because they are often away from the field of dissection and also because they exhibit the least variation. Finally, in difficult cases, the mastoid tip can be removed and the facial nerve identified in the descending mastoid segment.

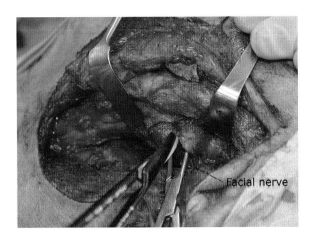

FIGURE 25.9 Dissection of facial nerve branches during superficial parotidectomy.

Once the main trunk is identified, the facial branches are dissected. The usual method is to dissect directly on top of a branch with fine hemostats or scissors (Fig. 25.9). The spreading action is in the direction of the "facio-venous plane," which is almost horizontal in supine position. During spreading, the superficial lobe parenchyma is then lifted and sectioned. This section should be performed with the dissected branch clearly in view. The instrument most often used is a no. 12-scalpel blade or more rarely scissors.

The dissection proceeds through the parenchyma of the gland and usually results in some bleeding that needs to be controlled with a bipolar electric coagulator. A preferred option is to coagulate the parotid tissue prior to cutting. Fee and Handen have advocated the use of the Shaw hemostatic scalpel, but this device has been associated with higher postparotidectomy facial nerve paresis in other hands. Bipolar electrocoagulator forceps are often used. I have found that bipolar scissors have been extremely helpful in preventing bleeding by providing vessel coagulation while cutting. Despite the close presence of nerve branches, no facial muscle movement or evoked EMG in the nerve monitor has been detected. Irrespective of the electrocoagulation device used, it is important that the tissue coagulated/sectioned is lifted from the underlying branch of the nerve since electric current does not spread well through air.

The dissection usually follows one branch and its tributaries to the anterior edge of the parotid gland. Then, the next branch is followed and so on. Some surgeons begin the dissection with the marginal mandibular and cervical branches and proceed in a superior direction, others begin with the superior division, and some start at both ends to finish in the middle of the gland. Actually, the dissection is greatly determined by the position of tumor. Although the facial nerve comes first, I try as much as possible to remove the superficial lobe and the tumor in monoblock and thereby obtain tumor-free deep margins.

During this dissection, no traction is applied to the facial nerve and its branches. For a superficial parotidectomy, the branches are left attached to the underlying parenchyma, thereby preserving their blood supply (Fig. 25.10). Coagulation is performed with a bipolar coagulator, after reduction of the electric current power. Usually, unless the bleeding is right on a branch of the nerve, no facial nerve paresis results from bipolar coagulation. In cases of a bleeding very close to the nerve, a sponge soaked in adrenaline can be used.

Peripheral branches of the facial nerve rapidly become superficial at the anterior border of the gland. Special attention should also be paid in large tumors, which tend to displace the branches, making them deeper and more superficial and splaying them.

After the delivery of the superficial lobe specimen, it should be inspected for exposed tumor surface (bare capsule). Because of the proximity of the branches of the facial nerve, this cannot be always avoided, but it might require an extra resection of deep lobe parenchyma, masseter muscle, or other important tissues.

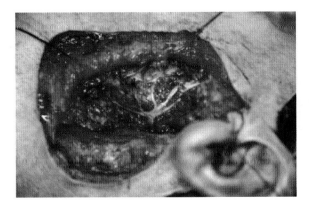

FIGURE 25.10 The operative field at the end of superficial parotidectomy.

Usually, there should be no good reason to see exposed tumor inferiorly, laterally, and even superiorly, since SMAS, skin, and SCM muscle are nonessential tissues.

During the entire dissection, it is important that the traction applied to the resected tissue, and thus, the tumor is not excessive. Larger and cystic tumors tend to rupture under too much traction or compression resulting in spillage of the tumor contents in the surgical bed, which is thought to be a major cause of recurrence, especially for pleomorphic adenoma. As soon as a breach in the tumor capsule is detected, I advise the use of a rhinology type of suction tip and to carefully insert it through the opening in the tumor capsule in order to aspirate the liquid content and to somewhat decompress the tumor. The opening is then sutured and the instruments used in this maneuver discarded as contaminated. The wound should be copiously irrigated with saline.

The handling of Stensens duct is variable: some ligate it, others do not even look for it, and finally, other surgeons think that it should be left in place to drain the wound in the mouth to preserve the function of the remaining deep lobe and prevent the development of postparotidectomy fistula. I never look for it.

Any lesion of the parotid gland should be excised with a margin of healthy salivary gland tissue, but the extent of parotidectomy should probably be adapted to the degree of malignancy of the lesion. Usually, frozen sections are relied upon to determine the extent of the procedure, although the reliability is not absolute and neither the main trunk of the facial nerve nor its branches should be sacrificed based on the results of the frozen section. A recent meta-analysis found that frozen sections are associated with 10% false-negative rates for malignancy. The rates for the correct diagnosis of the specific histologic cancer subtype are even lower. Nevertheless, frozen sections are recommended to diagnose pleomorphic adenoma and cancer.

In cancer of the parotid gland and some pleomorphic adenomas at greater risk for recurrence (large size, young patients, and stroma-rich histology), a total parotidectomy should be considered if the deep margin appears to be positive. In addition, during the wait for frozen section analysis, a selective neck dissection of levels II and III in the N0 neck is performed. For the N+ neck, a comprehensive neck dissection is necessary.

At the end of the resection, the hemostasis is checked again and remaining bleeders coagulated, usually with a bipolar coagulating forceps, taking extreme care when coagulating near branches of the facial nerve. Ties might be preferable close to the facial nerve, but this is sometimes limited by the small size of the vessels. Alternatively, pledgets soaked in adrenaline could be used to stop any oozing.

Considering the nightmare of revision parotidectomy, it is useful to take a picture of the disposition of facial nerve branches prior to closure (Fig. 25.10). This might also have some medicolegal value, demonstrating the anatomical integrity of the facial nerve.

Some form of Frey syndrome prevention barrier is then placed, usually the SMAS flap developed prior to resecting the tumor. It is mobilized as described before and put under tension by suturing it to the lateral aspect of the auricular cartilage. If excess SMAS is available, it is plicated and used to fill the parotidectomy defect. If part of the SMAS is resected to obtain sufficient later margins, the remainder is mobilized at sutured together. If there is insufficient SMAS, a Gore-Tex graft is used (Fig. 25.11).

The wound is then irrigated, preferably with warm saline, and a suction drain inserted in the retroauricular skin and placed in the inferior aspect of the resection, away from the branches of the facial nerve. Other surgeons do not use closed suction drains or do not drain at all, relying instead on pressure dressings.

The wound is closed in two layers, paying attention to correctly positioning the lobule of the ear. I routinely resect a portion of redundant skin from the posterior aspect of the anterior skin flap. The cosmetic value of this remains to be proven.

POSTOPERATIVE MANAGEMENT

The dressing is removed on the first postoperative day and the wound inspected. The drain is removed when drainage is below 20 mL/day, usually on the second postoperative day. The patient may be discharged at

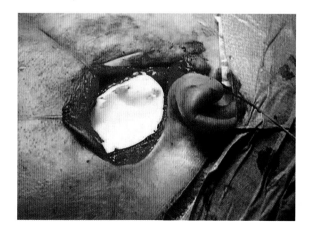

FIGURE 25.11

SMAS defect covered with a Gore-Tex implant in order to prevent Frey syndrome.

that point. Parotidectomy usually does not require antibiotics. If antibiotics are used, only a single dose is given, 1 hour prior to skin incision. Gram-positive aerobic bacteria should be covered, with first-generation cephalosporins being an excellent choice.

COMPLICATIONS

Besides the usual surgical wound problems, such as hematoma or infection, the specific complications of parotidectomy include facial palsy, Frey syndrome, anesthesia of the skin, retromandibular depression, and salivary fistula. While recurrence of a malignant tumor might not be seen as a complication, recurrence of benign neoplasms and specially pleomorphic adenoma should be considered as such.

Recurrence of Pleomorphic Adenoma

The incidence of recurrence of pleomorphic adenoma in earlier publications ranged from 20% to 40%. With present techniques of parotidectomy, the recurrence rate should remain below 2%. Problems of recurrent pleomorphic adenoma include the multicentricity of the recurrence; the increased incidence of facial paralysis, both temporary and permanent during revision parotidectomy; the increased incidence of a second recurrence; and the increased incidence of malignant transformation. Numerous reasons advanced for the recurrence of pleomorphic adenoma can be grouped into pathology related (thinness or lack of capsule, pseudopodia, satellite nodules, multicentricity) and surgery related (rupture of the tumor, spillage of tumor contents, insufficient margins of resection because of nerve branches, inadequate excision related to the type of surgery). The role of rupture has not been studied thoroughly, and until recently, publications were inconclusive. Although tumor spillage seemed always more frequent in the group that recurred (Table 25.2), the difference did not reach the significance level, except in recent studies.

Postparotidectomy Facial Paralysis

Postparotidectomy facial paralysis can be temporary or permanent and can involve the entire face or localized to a portion of the face. Temporary facial paralysis resolves in weeks to months postoperatively. In my opinion, permanent facial paralysis results from the section of the nerve or its branches.

The etiology of temporary facial paralysis has remained elusive, and a thorough discussion of potential causes concluded that nerve stretching during parotidectomy was the most probable origin. Ischemia, nerve cooling, and nerve compression are unlikely, based on animal experiments. Overzealous electric stimulation is unlikely in view of experimental and clinical data with various functional electric stimulating implants. The only remaining possible etiology is damage from electrocoagulators or other hemostatic devices.

An increased incidence of facial paralysis has been associated with (1) previous parotid surgery, that is, more paralysis in recurrent cases; (2) more extensive surgery, that is, more facial nerve deficits with total versus superficial parotidectomy; (3) malignant tumors; (4) size of the tumor; (5) inflammatory conditions; (6) patient's age, with less optimal results in older patients; (7) longer operating time; and (8) length of the dissected branch of the nerve. Most of these factors are disputed and beyond the control of the surgeon. Therefore, it is difficult to give a precise estimate overall, and data quoted to potential patients should come from the surgeon's own experience.

Because tumors of the parotid gland often involve the branches of the lower division of the nerve and the removal of the tumor requires the dissection of a rather long branch of the nerve, the marginal mandibular nerve is often the branch with the highest risk of injury. As discussed previously, even sectioning of small peripheral midface branches tends to recover, while lesions to the zygomatic and marginal mandibular branches are less forgiving.

Frey Syndrome

Frey syndrome (gustatory sweating and flushing) is characterized by sweating and flushing of the facial skin during eating. There is no direct relation with chewing. Once present, the gustatory sweating and flushing remain unchanged, that is, there is no spontaneous resolution, even after many years.

Frey syndrome is thought to result from an aberrant innervation of the sweat glands of the skin and vessels after parotidectomy by the parasympathetic neurons from the auriculotemporal nerve. The traumatized fibers lose their parotid targets and regenerate to innervate the vessels and sweat glands of the overlying skin. The regular function of the parotid parasympathetic fibers is to increase salivary secretion during eating; their activation following aberrant regeneration produces an activation of the new targets during meals, resulting in a local vasodilatation (gustatory flushing) and localized sweating (gustatory sweating).

The reported incidence of gustatory sweating after parotidectomy is highly variable and depends on the diligence with which it is sought and the time interval after surgery. Frey syndrome seemed "an unavoidable sequel of parotidectomy" that is not overtly symptomatic in all patients. The incidence of clinical (patient is

TABLE 25.2   Pathologic and Surgical Variables Related to Recurrence of Pleomorphic Adenoma

Author	Year	Pathologic Variables						Surgical Variable		
		Lack of Capsule	Pseudopodia	Satellite Nodules	Multicentricity	Exposed Capsule	Gross Specimen Damage	Tumor Puncture[a]	Tumor Spillage[a]	Margins (mm)[a]
Naiem	1976	22%/69%								
Danovan	1984	21%				40%	27%			
Lam	1990	33%			0%	100%	27%			
Buchman	1994								0% vs. 10%	
Natvig	1994					36%			33% vs. 2%	
Henriksson	1998		11%						22% vs. 12%	
Stennert	2001	11%/71%	28%							
Webb	2001	34%/74%	12%		0%	81% (62%)	9.5%			
Paris	2004		72%		0%					
Zbären	2007	14%/47%	40%	13%	0%	80%				
Orita	2010			3%	1%					
Riad	2011							27% vs. 0%	80% vs. 2%	1.3 vs. 6.0
Park	2012	29%/67%	54%	15%					30% vs. 4%	

Lack of capsule in some parts of the specimen (hypercellular/hypocellular subtype).
Gross specimen damage = surgical breaching of the tumor, enucleation, or piecemeal resection.
Exposed capsule = bare capsule macroscopically observed on the pathologic specimen. In parenthesis, more than 50% of the tumor capsule is bare.
(a) For surgical variable, the first number is the incidence (in %) in the group with recurrence, and the second number is the incidence (in %) in the group without recurrence.

symptomatic and consults for the problem) and objective (discovered only during testing) gustatory sweating following parotidectomy is respectively 40% and 90%. Because of these high numbers, some form of prevention during parotidectomy seems necessary.

In a prospective study, it was demonstrated that Frey syndrome was preventable with an impermeable, nondegradable barrier, although the material (Gore-Tex) resulted in high incidence of salivary fistula. A recent meta-analysis confirmed that Frey syndrome after parotidectomy is preventable.

Other possible means of preventing Frey syndrome include the SCM muscular rotation flap, the SMAS flap, different dermal or adipose tissue grafts, and synthetic implant sheets. While the SCM flaps probably have some merit in filling the retromandibular depression, their role in preventing Frey syndrome has been inconclusive when the results are assessed objectively. The SMAS technique is probably the most innocuous and seems to result in a decrease of Frey syndrome, although few studies have evaluated this objectively and especially in a randomized way. Only few publications have objectively evaluated dermal or adipose tissue graft. The various implant sheets are usually associated with a higher incidence of salivary fistula. Therefore, at the present time, the SMAS technique is my preferred method for prevention and has resulted in a low incidence of clinical Frey syndrome.

Retromandibular Depression

The depression observed after radical resections is rarely present solely after superficial parotidectomy. There is usually little need of extensive reconstructions with free flaps. The SMAS flap by itself provides an excellent mean of filling and/or covering the defect. The remaining question is whether supplementary local pedicled flaps are necessary. The issue is compounded by (1) the lack of precise objective measurements, (2) the absence of subjective blinded evaluation, and (3) the concomitant use of the SMAS flap in these reconstructions.

We have found little convincing evidence that the SCM rotation flap improves the esthetic outcome compared to the SMAS flap and do not routinely use it.

Different techniques have been described in which the parotid bed (mostly after total parotidectomy) is filled with adipose tissue, taken as a nonvascularized tissue from the abdominal wall, as a lipoaspirate, or rarely as a pedicled flap.

Anesthesia of the Skin

The handling of the greater auricular nerve has been the subject of much debate. It is my impression that the posterior branch of the great auricular nerve can be preserved in most cases. In addition, the lobular branch could be preserved with some careful dissection between the uppermost part of SCM and the ear lobule. The problem is that it is unclear if this makes any difference in the long run. Even when the entire trunk of the greater auricular nerve is cut, there is almost no difference in tactile and pain sensation 1 year after parotidectomy when comparing to the normal contralateral side. In this context, the use of posteriorly pediculated SMAS flap to encompass the anterior branch of greater auricular nerve seems difficult to recommend.

Hematoma, Infection, and Salivary Fistula

Hematoma is uncommon (3%) after parotidectomy and results from incomplete hemostasis and/or blood pressure elevation during extubation. Hematoma may also occur in patients who did not discontinue ingestion of aspirin or other anticoagulants. Unless minor, reoperation under general anesthesia is required for evacuation of the hematoma and identification and cauterization of the bleeding vessels.

Infection of the parotidectomy wound is rare (1%) even without perioperative antibiotics. Treatment requires antibiotics against gram-positive cocci and drainage in case of abscess.

Salivary fistula or sialocele occurs in about 5% of parotidectomies. Different sorts of implants placed in the wound are associated with an increased incidence. Sialoceles result from the accumulation of saliva from the remaining parotid tissue that collects beneath the skin flap. Treatment aims to avoid spontaneous drainage through the incision by repeated needle aspirations and pressure dressings. Anticholinergic patches or botulinum toxin injections can be used to reduce the amount of salivation.

External otitis can occur as a result of the accumulation of blood in the external auditory meatus. It can be prevented by placing a petroleum gauze pack in the canal. Treatment consists of cleansing and antibiotic ear drops.

Necrosis of the distal skin flap is also rare (<1%) and seems related to smoking, diabetes, prior radiation, as well as a narrow but long postauricular flap. Treatment is based on local wound care and debridement of necrotic tissue.

Mild trismus can occur after parotidectomy probably when the resection involves the masseter muscle. First bite syndrome might occur after total parotidectomy but has not been described after superficial parotidectomy.

RESULTS

For the majority of parotid lesions, appropriate parotidectomy is curative. Some inflammatory parotid conditions (e.g., Sjögren's) represent systemic diseases, and further medical treatments might be necessary. Parotid surgery for chronic sialadenitis, although reserved for cases refractory to other treatments, usually resolves the infectious symptomatology.

For cystic conditions and benign tumors, the recurrence is rare, except for HIV-related parotid cysts. The recurrence of pleomorphic adenoma has been a subject of debate throughout the history of parotid surgery and should remain around 2%. However, a delay of 5 to 10 years being the norm for the diagnosis of pleomorphic adenoma recurrence, improvements in surgical technique for the individual surgeon remain problematic. Because of the morbidity associated with operations for recurrent pleomorphic, adequate initial surgery is paramount.

Parotid cancers are rarely treated with superficial parotidectomy. A preoperative diagnosis of a benign condition warranting a superficial parotidectomy is sometimes diagnosed as a malignancy on final pathology. Usually, the pathology is one of the less aggressive parotid cancers, such as acinic cell carcinoma or low-grade mucoepidermoid carcinoma, and the oncologic outcome is excellent, providing that the tumor has been completely removed with negative margins.

PEARLS

- Try to obtain the diagnosis prior to surgery.
- Use facial nerve monitoring, and use the lowest possible electric current for nerve stimulation.
- Use a cosmetic incision for parotidectomy.
- Try to preserve the posterior and lobular branches of the great auricular nerve.
- Prepare the SMAS flap for esthetics and prevention of Frey syndrome.
- The posterior belly of the digastric muscle is at the same depth as the facial nerve.
- Use the tympanomastoid suture to find the facial nerve.
- Try to obtain a dry and bloodless operating field prior to searching for the facial nerve.
- In case of rupture of the tumor, use suction to decrease tumor size and suture the puncture site closed.
- The position and direction of the facial nerve are fairly constant.
- In dissecting branches of the facial nerve, lift the tissue so that air serves as an electric isolation between the parotid tissue to be cut and the branches of the nerve.
- Fill the parotid defect with autologous adipose tissue, fascia, or muscle in order to prevent depression of the retromandibular area.

PITFALLS

- Minimize the traction applied on the specimen by assistants to avoid rupture of the tumor and spillage into the wound.
- Without a barrier, Frey syndrome is likely to result, though the extent and severity are variable.
- Frozen sections should not be relied upon to sacrifice any branches of the facial nerve.
- Cutting structure(s) in the direction of the main trunk of the facial nerve may lead to facial nerve injury. Always achieve selective electric stimulation of the temporofacial and cervicofacial divisions.
- Avoidance of rupture of the tumor capsule is crucial since small pleomorphic adenomas in young patients might recur.
- At the anterior end of the parotid gland, facial nerve branches rapidly become superficial.
- Section of the midfacial branches could recover, but frontal and marginal mandibular branches will not.

INSTRUMENTS TO HAVE AVAILABLE

- Nerve monitor
- Bipolar scissors
- Fine mosquito dissection clamps
- Narrow but long retractors (Langenbeck)

SUGGESTED READING

Davis RA, Anson BJ, Budinger JM, et al. Surgical anatomy of the facial nerve and parotid gland based upon a study of 350 cervicofacial halves. *Surg Gynecol Obstet* 1956;102:385–412.

Robertson MS, Blake P. A method of using the tympanomastoid fissure to find the facial nerve at parotidectomy. *Aust N Z J Surg* 1984;54:369–373.

Dulguerov P. Parotidectomy complications. New techniques for their objective evaluation, prevention and treatment. Thesis Geneva University; 1999. Available at: http://archive-ouverte.unige.ch/unige:22052

Zbaren P, Stauffer E. Pleomorphic adenoma of the parotid gland: histopathologic analysis of the capsular characteristics of 218 tumors. *Head Neck* 2007;29:751–757.

Dulguerov P. Treatment of Frey's syndrome. In: Myers E, Ferris RL, eds. *Salivary Gland Disorders*. New York: Springer, 2007:111–126.

Park GC, Cho KJ, Kang J, et al. Relationship between histopathology of pleomorphic adenoma in the parotid gland and recurrence after superficial parotidectomy. *J Surg Oncol* 2012;106(8):942–946.

26 EXTRACAPSULAR DISSECTION OF PAROTID TUMORS

Heinrich Iro

INTRODUCTION

The majority of tumors of the parotid gland are benign neoplasms with the pleomorphic adenoma, the most frequently encountered histologic type followed by Warthin tumor and then other less-frequent entities. The treatment of choice for these tumors is complete surgical removal. Besides the prospect of slow but constant tumor growth, two specifics have additionally to be taken into account in the case of the pleomorphic adenoma: the risk of malignant degeneration into a *carcinoma ex pleomorphic adenoma* with a reported frequency between 3% and 15% and the rare phenomenon of dissemination by developing benign distant (e.g., pulmonary) metastases documented by a number of case reports in the literature in recent years.

Therefore, the complete removal of the tumor to prevent recurrence as the objective of surgical treatment is without disagreement. However, the required scope of surgical resection has been the subject of controversy during the last several decades: proponents of the standardized surgical techniques of superficial and total parotidectomy base their arguments mainly on a supposedly raised level of recurrence after less-invasive resection procedures. Those who favor extracapsular dissection (ED) and other partial parotidectomies claim a lower rate of postoperative complications for this approach, in particular a lower risk of facial nerve paresis.

The controversy about ED of parotid tumors is understandable in light of the historical development of parotid surgery during the last century. In the first half of the 20th century, benign parotid tumors were often treated by (intracapsular) enucleation, that is, the tumor was exposed, the capsule was intentionally opened, and the contents were shelled out leaving the capsule in situ. The rate of tumor recurrence was high, reaching rates of 20% to 45% in different reports. The relationship of these tumors to the facial nerve was not recognized, so no effort was made to identify it. This led to a high association of the removal of parotid tumor with facial paralysis. Over the following decades, the technique of parotidectomy became refined in the sense that the tumor was removed in toto with surrounding glandular tissue and that the facial nerve was fully dissected and preserved. Since the 1950s, the consistent use of either a superficial or a total parotidectomy led to a dramatic reduction in the recurrence of pleomorphic adenomas resulting in numerous reports with recurrence rates of 0% to 5%.

However, the dissection of the facial nerve and its branches together with the removal of large parts of the parotid gland can lead to significant postoperative complications. The rates of temporary and permanent facial nerve paresis are reported to be 15% to 25% and 5% to 8%, respectively, after superficial parotidectomy and as high as 20% to 50% and 5% to 10%, respectively, after total parotidectomy. There is also a risk of developing Frey syndrome, the incidence of which has been reported by some authors to be over 10% after superficial parotidectomy and over 30% after total parotidectomy. Moreover, doing a total parotidectomy will usually result in a visible cosmetic defect.

In view of these complications and the benign nature of the tumors, more conservative techniques have evolved over the past 20 years. These include partial resection of the parotid gland where less than the entire superficial lobe of the gland is removed and the facial nerve is dissected only in part or not at all. The introduction of more conservative procedures has resulted in markedly lower rates of facial nerve paresis and Frey syndrome. At the same time, the first published long-term observations show no increase in recurrence after circumscribed resections (ED) of this type. Unfortunately, the descriptions of the surgical technique used for partial resection of the parotid gland vary greatly and consequently are confusing.

Classification of Parotidectomies

As the descriptions of the different surgical techniques of parotidectomy vary greatly in the literature, we propose the consistent use of a five-stage classification system based on the exposure of the main trunk of the facial nerve and the extent of the resection:

1. An *extracapsular dissection (ED)* is defined as the removal of a tumor from the parotid gland without exposure of the main trunk of the facial nerve.
2. Whenever the main trunk is exposed, the procedure is designated as a *partial parotidectomy* because parts of the superficial or deep lobe of the gland are left in place.
3. Removal of the entire superficial lobe defines a *superficial lobe parotidectomy*.
4. Removal of the entire gland is a *total parotidectomy*.
5. A *radical parotidectomy* implies resection of the entire parotid, surrounding tissue including the facial nerve or parts of it, which may become necessary in surgery of malignant tumors.

On no account should the term "enucleation" be used nowadays to refer to a partial resection, since this will cause confusion with the historical and obsolete technique of opening and shelling out the tumor. The general lack of acceptance of ED for the treatment of pleomorphic adenomas is sometimes based on the supposedly higher recurrence rates resulting from the inexact differentiation of the different surgical techniques and especially of equation of the historical enucleation and the contemporary ED.

HISTORY

The patient's history usually suggests a benign neoplasm of the parotid gland in case of a painless swelling of the cheek or the mandibular angle persisting for several months or years showing slow growth and lacking any impairment of function of the facial nerve.

PHYSICAL EXAMINATION

The clinical examination includes a complete examination of the head and neck including endoscopy but focuses on bimanual palpation of the tumor in order to thoroughly appreciate the size, location within the gland, consistency, and mobility. Facial nerve function is assessed in detail and recorded in the patient's record along with the characteristics of the mass.

INDICATIONS

The surgical technique to be performed in an individual case is defined in a two-stage process: First, the preoperative clinical and sonographic findings suggest a potential approach. For example, patients can be scheduled for ED in case of a single and mobile tumor located superficially within the superficial lobe of the parotid gland. On the contrary, a total parotidectomy should be planned for a lesion lying in the deep lobe of the gland or in case of multifocality. However, the final decision about the surgical procedure and especially about preparation of the main trunk of the facial nerve is always made intraoperatively: a supposedly superficial mobile tumor can turn out to extend deeper into the gland or to be located in close proximity to the facial nerve—preparation of the nerve and performance of a conventional parotidectomy are mandatory in this situation. Thus, the surgeon has to be capable of switching between ED and the different forms of parotidectomies at any time during the operation.

CONTRAINDICATIONS

Any suspicion of malignancy by clinical or sonographic findings is a clear contraindication for ED; the patient has to be scheduled for total parotidectomy and neck dissection in this case. Moreover, if multiple lesions are present within the gland or if the lesion extends into the deep lobe, a parotidectomy will be necessary.

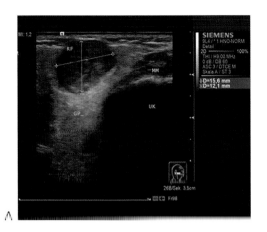
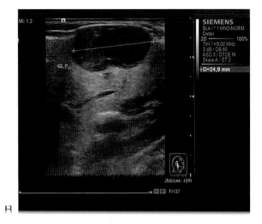

A   B

FIGURE 26.1
B-mode sonography of a benign tumor (oncocytoma) located in the inferior part of the right parotid gland in the transverse **(A)** and longitudinal **(B)** plane.

PREOPERATIVE PLANNING

Imaging is indispensable for the preoperative evaluation of tumors of the parotid gland and for further planning. Ultrasound is the imaging modality of choice as it is frequently available without a waiting period and as neither exposure to radiation nor contrast enhancement is necessary. Because of the excellent accessibility of the parotid gland, tumors can be examined in detail sonographically with regard to their shape, echotexture, perfusion, and exact localization within the gland (Fig. 26.1). If ultrasound is not available, additional investigations such as computed tomography (CT) and magnetic resonance imaging (MRI) may be used instead. CT especially is carried out in the case of suspected invasion of the mandible, whereas MRI is the modality of choice to evaluate deep lobe involvement of a tumor. However, tumors scheduled for ED will neither expand into the deep retromandibular part of the parotid gland nor raise any suspicion of bone invasion.

Fine needle aspiration cytology can be performed preoperatively depending on local standards and conventions. Another possibility to exclude malignancy during the operation is the use of frozen sections, especially if ED is performed.

SURGICAL TECHNIQUE

The surgical preparations do not differ between ED and conventional parotidectomy. Injection of a solution of 1:200,000 adrenaline in a local anesthetic is recommended prior to draping the patient because it provides an excellent bloodless field of dissection. The skin incision (according to Blair) is conducted curvedly around the ear lobe starting at the tragus and ending in a skin fold in the neck; in contrast to conventional parotidectomy, the length of the incision and the resulting flap size in ED may be adapted to the size and location of the tumor. After dissection of the subcutaneous tissue, the sternocleidomastoid muscle, and the greater auricular nerve, the skin flap is raised, and the "shining" capsule of the parotid gland is thus exposed. Before the capsule is opened, the tumor is once again palpated. If the exact position of the tumor cannot be determined, an ultrasound scan can be performed intraoperatively. The capsule of the parotid gland is now incised and the dissection extended toward the tumor; however, the tumor capsule itself is never opened. Blunt dissection is now extended through the healthy glandular tissue around the tumor so as to gradually separate it, care being taken at all times to dissect away from the tumor (Figs. 26.2 and 26.3). With this technique, a small rim of healthy glandular tissue is left on the tumor, without damaging the facial nerve (Fig. 26.4). Direct retraction of the tumor by instruments should be avoided in order to

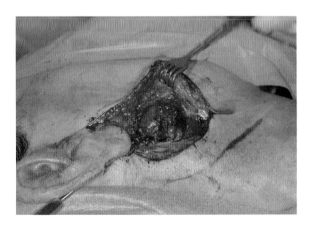

FIGURE 26.2 ED of the tumor shown in Figure 26.1. The capsule of the parotid gland is opened, and the mass is mobilized, always covered by a rim of healthy glandular tissue.

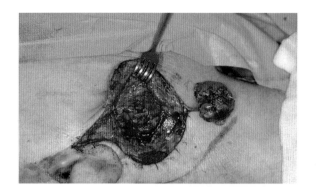

FIGURE 26.3
Intraoperative view of the parotid gland after removal of the tumor before closing the wound.

reduce the risk of rupture of the capsule; however, the covering parenchyma can be grasped gently. After the tumor has been removed, the defect within the parenchyma is checked for bleeding and then irrigated several times. The remnants of the edges of the parotid fascia are sutured back together, or in case of a defect that cannot be closed primarily, it may be sutured to the anterior border of the sternocleidomastoid muscle. A rubber drain is inserted, and subcutaneous and skin sutures are applied. Finally, a pressure dressing may be applied.

Neuromonitoring and neurostimulation consisting of an electrical bipolar stimulating probe and two electrodes for conducting the action potentials of the orbicularis oculi and orbicularis oris muscles are mandatory. In ED, it is especially important to identify and protect then-on visible branches of the facial nerve. Care has to be taken that no long-lasting muscle relaxants are used during anesthesia. In the beginning, stimulation is carried out with a maximum current of 5 mA. As soon as a branch of the facial nerve is identified by positive stimulation, the stimulating current is reduced to 1 to 2 mA. After exposure of a branch of the nerve, the current is reduced further to 1 mA or less. Branches of the nerve are exposed only if they are situated close to the tumor and their definite identification is considered desirable before further dissection. The main trunk of the facial nerve, on the other hand, is never exposed during ED—in cases where this is done, the procedure changes to at least a partial parotidectomy (see definition above).

POSTOPERATIVE CARE

A pressure dressing is applied immediately after the operation and is kept in place for several days in order to avoid formation of a salivary fistula or sialocele. The dressing is changed daily in order to check the wound for signs of inflammation or abnormal swelling. In the case of a suspected accumulation of fluid, ultrasound can be performed to verify the presence of a seroma or hematoma and to estimate its extent. This fluid usually has to be aspirated two to three times until it resolves. Systemic antibiotic therapy is not given routinely but reserved for selected cases.

After the patient's discharge, a regular follow-up should be performed comprising at least an annual clinical and sonographical examination in order to detect late complications and especially recurrent tumors at an early stage.

COMPLICATIONS

Regarding the spectrum of potential complications, ED does not differ from the parotidectomies: An acute swelling can occur caused by a hematoma, seroma, or sialocele. The rate of such a fluid accumulation following ED accounts for <5%, but opening and drainage of the wound can become necessary. The consistent use of a pressure

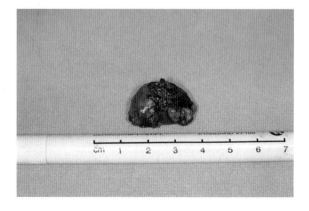

FIGURE 26.4
Benign tumor of the parotid gland (cf. Fig. 26.1) removed by ED (cf. Figs. 26.2 and 26.3).

dressing for at least 3 to 5 days is to reduce the risk of accumulation of blood, seroma, or saliva. Since the fascia of the parotid gland is opened during ED but the parenchyma is predominantly left in situ, a sialocele or salivary fistula develops more frequently than after total parotidectomy. In addition to the pressure dressing, transdermal application of scopolamine can benefit the wound healing by reducing the secretion of saliva. In cases of a prolonged salivary fistula, application of botulinum toxin into the parotid gland parenchyma can be considered.

Paresthesia around the skin incision, namely, the cheek and the ear lobe, is encountered rather frequently after both ED and the different forms of parotidectomy, due to injury of the greater auricular nerve. A persisting paresthesia (>6 months) is described in about 10% after ED; however, the majority of patients do not feel impaired. An advantage of ED is a shorter skin incision and less-invasive dissection so that the great auricular nerve can usually be preserved from injury.

The most severe complication after parotidectomies, including ED, feared by both patients and surgeons is facial nerve paresis. In due consideration of the current literature and my own experiences, it can be summarized that as the surgical procedure becomes more invasive, the frequency of both temporary and a permanent facial nerve pareses increases. Reviewing the current literature, the rate of temporary paresis of the facial nerve is reported as 15% to 25% after superficial parotidectomy and 20% to 50% after total parotidectomy, while the rate of permanent facial nerve paresis is reported as 5% to 10%. Temporary facial nerve paresis is therefore to be expected in about one-fifth of patients after superficial parotidectomy and in one-third to one-half of patients after total parotidectomy. However, there is evidence in the literature to suggest that the risk of facial nerve paresis is significantly less after more conservative procedures such as ED and partial parotidectomy: temporary paresis is reported in only 10% to 15% and permanent paresis in 2% to 5% of patients; moreover, these impairments are mostly classified as House-Brackmann HBI II, and impairments of higher degree do occur rarely.

Like facial nerve paresis, Frey syndrome (gustatory sweating) also occurs far less commonly after ED (0% to 5%) than after superficial or total parotidectomy (25% to 50%). The lower incidence of gustatory sweating after ED is presumably due to the fact that with this technique, less glandular tissue is disrupted and, in addition, the parotid fascia can be closed over the parotid gland at the completion of the procedure to prevent the ingrowth of parasympathetic fibers from the sweat glands in the skin.

RESULTS

During the last 20 years, ED has proven to be a less invasive technique in removing benign parotid tumors than superficial or total parotidectomy, resulting in low rates of postoperative complications, a markedly reduced risk of facial nerve paresis and Frey syndrome, and a better cosmetic result contributing to a high degree of patient satisfaction (Fig. 26.5).

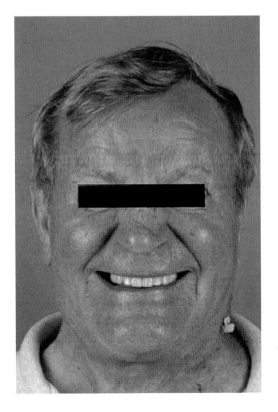 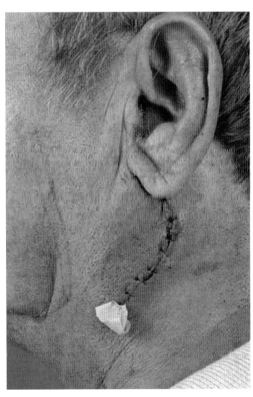

FIGURE 26.5

Photograph of a patient on the first day following ED of a benign tumor of the left parotid gland; the facial nerve's function is unimpaired (HBI I).

TABLE 26.1	Nonstandardized Approach to Surgery of Benign Parotid Tumors: Appropriate Surgical Techniques Depend on Tumor Characteristics			
Number of lesions	Single	Single	Single	Multiple
Localization of tumor	Superficial	Superficial	Deep	Irrelevant
Mobility of tumor	Mobile	Fixed	Irrelevant	Irrelevant
Surgery of choice	**Extracapsular dissection**	**Partial/superficial parotidectomy**	**Total parotidectomy**	**Total parotidectomy**

The evaluation of ED with respect to its long-term performance substantially depends on the prevention of recurrent pleomorphic adenomas. The main argument often used against ED in the literature is a postulated higher risk of recurrence. It was already mentioned that the modern technique of ED is frequently confused with the historical technique of enucleation (see above) when quoting recurrence rates. Thus, importance should always be attached to the correct description and nomenclature. Keeping this confusion in mind, the high 20% to 40% rates of recurrence reported for enucleation and other partial resections seldom represent substantive information. There are, on the other hand, numerous studies demonstrating that the risk of a recurring tumor is no higher with ED than with superficial or total parotidectomy, namely, 0% to 5%. For example, as early as 1996, McGurk et al. reported on a recurrence rate for pleomorphic adenomas of 2% after an average follow-up observation period of 12.5 years, following both ED ($n = 380$) and superficial parotidectomy ($n = 95$). Our own experiences after more than 10 years of regularly performing ED confirm these figures as we have not encountered a case of a recurrent pleomorphic adenoma following primary ED.

Nevertheless, revision surgery may become necessary after any kind of parotidectomy including ED as the risk of recurrence of a pleomorphic adenoma can be summarized with 2% to 5% independent of the surgical procedure applied. ED proves to be advantageous in these cases too, because it provides better conditions for revision than the conventional parotidectomies. If the main trunk of the facial nerve is dissected during the first operation, scarring will have taken place, and dissecting the nerve again at the time of revision surgery will present a higher risk of damaging the nerve and, thus, of temporary and permanent paresis. In contrast, as the main trunk is not dissected during ED, the conditions in case of a required revision surgery are considerably better as no scarring complicates dissection of the facial nerve.

I recommend the following individual approach toward surgery of benign parotid tumors (Table 26.1):

1. Treatment of choice for a single, mobile benign tumor located superficially within the superficial lobe should be an ED. Facial nerve neuromonitoring is indispensable here.
2. If the tumor lies superficially, but during surgery is found to be fixed to the facial nerve, then the conservative technique can be abandoned, and the surgeon reverts to a partial or lateral parotidectomy.
3. For multiple tumors and tumors lying within the deep lobe of the gland, a total parotidectomy should be employed.

In summary, head and neck surgeons have to be able to reliably identify situations in which they have to convert from an ED to some form of conventional parotidectomy, and they have to be familiar with the entire spectrum of parotid surgery in order to do so. It is not a procedure for the beginning surgeon.

PEARLS

- ED is the optimum surgical technique for single, mobile, and superficial tumors of the parotid gland.
- Expect a low rate of postoperative complications with ED, especially facial nerve paresis and Frey syndrome.
- Recurrence rate of pleomorphic adenoma is identical to other forms of parotidectomies (2% to 5%).
- Better surgical conditions in case of required revision

PITFALLS

- An ED cannot performed if facial nerve monitoring is not available. Neuromonitoring is a *condition sine qua non*.
- Switching from ED to conventional parotidectomy has to be possible at any time intraoperatively.
- The capsule of the tumor must not be injured during dissection as this might result in a higher risk of tumor recurrence.
- In case of an unexpected malignancy diagnosed postoperatively, a second surgical intervention will become necessary (completion of parotidectomy combined with ipsilateral neck dissection).

INSTRUMENTS TO HAVE AVAILABLE

- Neuromonitoring with bipolar stimulation probe
- Special dissection clamp with an angled fine tip

SUGGESTED READING

Ghosh S, Panarese A, Bull PD, et al. Marginally excised parotid pleomorphic salivary adenomas: risk factors for recurrence and management. A 12.5-year mean follow-up study of histologically marginal excisions. *Clin Otolaryngol Allied Sci* 2003;28(3):262–266.

McGurk M, Thomas BL, Renehan AG. Extracapsular dissection for clinically benign parotid lumps: reduced morbidity without oncological compromise. *Br J Cancer* 2003;89(9):1610–1613.

Klintworth N, Zenk J, Koch M, et al. Postoperative complications after extracapsular dissection of benign parotid lesions with particular reference to facial nerve function. *Laryngoscope* 2010;120(3):484–490.

Albergotti WG, Nguyen SA, Zenk J, et al. Extracapsular dissection for benign parotid tumors: a meta-analysis. *Laryngoscope* 2012;122(9):1954–1960. doi: 10.1002/lary.23396.

Iro H, Zenk J, Koch M, et al. Follow-up of parotid pleomorphic adenomas treated by extracapsular dissection. *Head Neck* 2013;35(6):788–793. doi: 10.1002/hed.23032.

TOTAL PAROTIDECTOMY

David W. Eisele

INTRODUCTION

Total parotidectomy describes removal of the entire parotid gland. From a practical standpoint, total parotidectomy is a difficult operation as removal of all parotid tissue with facial nerve preservation is challenging. The benefits of complete removal of all parotid tissue must be weighed against potential morbidity. Total parotidectomy is described. Less extensive resection of the gland may be appropriate based on tumor extent, type, and location.

HISTORY

A thorough history is obtained prior to consideration for surgery. Most patients with parotid neoplasms note a progressively enlarging asymptomatic mass. Pain can be associated with some neoplasms but is not a reliable indicator of malignancy. Symptoms of sensory loss, trismus, and facial weakness are worrisome for local invasion by a malignant neoplasm. A past medical history should include information regarding any prior cutaneous lesions or malignancies. In addition, the patient should be queried about any prior radiation exposure to the head and neck including multiple dental radiographs. Smoking is associated with Wharthins tumor and, therefore, should be investigated.

PHYSICAL EXAMINATION

All patients should have a complete examination of the head and neck. Cranial nerve function should be examined, and facial nerve function should be evaluated carefully. Facial weakness may be subtle, or facial muscle fasciculation may be noted. Facial nerve paralysis is usually an indication of nerve invasion by a malignant tumor. Fixation to the skin, decreased mobility, and associated cervical lymphadenopathy are other signs consistent with malignancy.

INDICATIONS

The most common indications for this operative procedure are a malignant neoplasm involving the entire parotid gland, metastases to parotid lymph nodes, recurrent multifocal neoplasm, and chronic parotid sialadenitis refractory to medical and sialendoscopic management.

CONTRAINDICATIONS

Total parotidectomy is a major operation. Significant medical comorbidities, limited life expectancy, bleeding disorders, and anticoagulated states represent contraindications.

PREOPERATIVE PLANNING

Fine Needle Aspiration Biopsy

Fine needle aspiration (FNA) biopsy is an accurate and useful investigation for the diagnosis of a parotid mass. FNA allows for improved patient selection for surgery since it can identify conditions such as reactive lymph nodes or cysts that might clinically mimic parotid neoplasms. The information gained by FNA is useful for patient counseling, surgical timing and planning, and guidance of preoperative consultations.

Imaging Studies

Imaging studies are helpful to assess malignant neoplasms or neoplasms that are large, have diminished mobility, or have suspected local invasion or deep extension. In general, magnetic resonance imaging is the preferred imaging study for parotid neoplasms.

SURGICAL TECHNIQUE

Total parotidectomy is performed under general anesthesia. Long-term paralytic agents are avoided to allow for facial nerve monitoring and stimulation. After the induction of general anesthesia, the endotracheal tube is positioned in the contralateral oral cavity and secured by tape only on the contralateral face. A modified Blair incision is planned in a preauricular crease coursing around the ear lobule and then into an upper neck crease (Fig. 27.1). The ipsilateral face is prepared with an antiseptic solution, and nerve electrodes are placed in the ipsilateral facial muscles if intraoperative electrophysiologic facial nerve monitoring is planned. The surgical field is then draped with a transparent adhesive sterile drape to allow intraoperative visualization of facial motion and maintenance of a sterile operative field.

The skin incision is made with a scalpel and carried down through the subcutaneous tissues and platysma muscle inferiorly. Care is taken to avoid division of the greater auricular nerve. An anterior flap is elevated superficial to the greater auricular nerve and the parotid fascia (Fig. 27.2). Elevation of a thick flap is desirable to reduce the occurrence of Frey syndrome. As the flap is elevated toward the anterior aspect of the gland, the peripheral facial nerve branches are carefully avoided. A posterior–inferior flap is also elevated to expose the tail of the parotid gland. After elevation, the flaps are retracted with silk sutures or self-retaining hooks. The flaps are kept moist during the procedure to prevent tissue desiccation.

The tail of the parotid gland is dissected from the sternocleidomastoid muscle by dissecting deep to the posterior branch of the greater auricular nerve, if preservation of this nerve is feasible based on tumor location. Next, the posterior belly of the digastric muscle is exposed with further elevation of the tail of the parotid gland. During elevation of the tail of the parotid, the posterior facial vein is divided and ligated with silk ligatures.

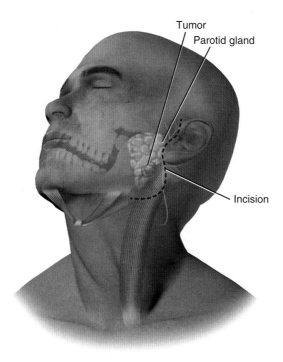

FIGURE 27.1
Modified Blair incision along a natural skin crease.

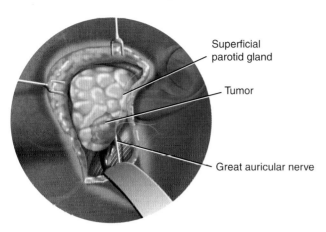

Superficial
parotid gland

Tumor

Great auricular nerve

FIGURE 27.2 Flap elevated to expose the parotid gland.

The preauricular space is opened by division of parotid gland attachments to the cartilaginous external auditory canal with blunt and sharp dissection. A wide plane of dissection from the zygoma to the digastric muscle is created to facilitate exposure of the facial nerve. Hemostasis is assured with bipolar electrocautery as indicated.

The parotid gland is carefully retracted anteriorly. This exposes the operative field for identification of the facial nerve. The facial nerve is identified using anatomic landmarks, which include the posterior belly of the digastric muscle, the tragal pointer, and the tympanomastoid suture. Of these, the tympanomastoid suture is most consistent. Frequently, they are all used to some degree to "triangulate" the facial nerve. If the proximal segment of the facial nerve is obscured, retrograde dissection of one or more of the peripheral facial nerve branches may be necessary. In select cases, the facial nerve can be identified in the mastoid bone by mastoid-ectomy and followed peripherally. Also, some deep lobe neoplasms may distort the course of the nerve, and the surgeon should be aware of potential anatomic alterations in the course of the facial nerve.

Once the facial nerve is identified, the parotid gland superficial to the facial nerve is divided carefully, preserving the integrity of the nerve. A McCabe dissector is used for dissection of the proximal facial nerve. The dissector is passed along the facial nerve, lifted, and then gently spread. The gland superficial to the exposed segment of the facial nerve is then carefully divided. Anatomic distortion particularly superficially by a neoplasm or operative manipulation must be considered. Division of the glandular tissue is performed with the Hemostatix scalpel. Any bleeding that occurs is carefully controlled with the Hemostatix scalpel or bipolar electrocautery. The facial nerve is followed peripherally, and the gland is dissected from successive facial nerve branches (Fig. 27.3).

The facial nerve is preserved except in cases of confirmed malignancy invading the nerve. In instances of facial nerve invasion by carcinoma, facial nerve resection is performed. Proximal and distal nerve resection margins are examined histologically by frozen section to ensure clear surgical margins. Immediate nerve recon-struction by a nerve interposition graft is performed if the facial nerve is resected.

After the facial nerve is dissected completely and the superficial lobe removed, the facial nerve and its branches are exposed. Careful circumferential dissection of the facial nerve is then undertaken to free the branches of the facial nerve completely from the remaining deep lobe gland tissue. Blunt and sharp dissection is used to dissect the nerve with care to avoid traction on the nerve.

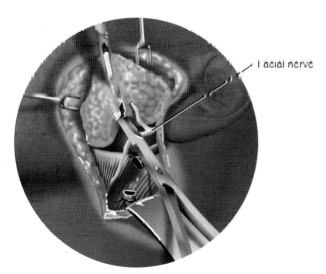

Facial nerve

FIGURE 27.3 Facial nerve dissection and division of the glandular tissue.

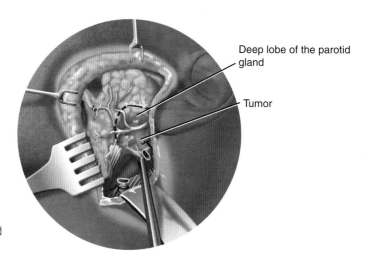

Deep lobe of the parotid
gland

Tumor

FIGURE 27.4
Deep lobe neoplasm exposed
with planned resection.

Once the facial nerve is mobilized from the main trunk to the peripheral branches, the deep lobe tissue is freed with dissection in planes deep to the parotid tissue over the fascia of the masseter muscle from anterior to posterior, over the digastric muscle and stylohyoid muscle from inferior to superior, and over the temporomandibular joint and mandibular condyle from superior to inferior (Fig. 27.4). Arteries that supply the parotid gland including branches of the external carotid artery, the posterior auricular artery, the superficial temporal artery, the internal maxillary artery, and the transverse facial artery must be divided and ligated. In addition, the associated veins are divided and ligated. Hemostasis of the pterygoid venous plexus may be difficult and may require bipolar electrocautery and/or packing with a hemostatic material such as Avitene (collagen topical). Once mobilized, the deep lobe is carefully delivered en bloc or in segments from beneath or between the branches of the facial nerve.

The wound is carefully inspected, and bleeding sites are controlled with bipolar electrocautery or ligatures. The integrity of the facial nerve is confirmed by visual inspection and by electrical stimulation of the main trunk of the facial nerve. If any facial nerve branches are identified to be injured, they are repaired immediately using a microscopic repair technique.

The wound is realigned and closed in layers over a closed-suction drain, which is brought out through an opening in the postauricular crease. Bacitracin ointment is applied to the wound and drain site.

POSTOPERATIVE MANAGEMENT

The patient is instructed in routine wound care with application of antibiotic ointment to the wound twice daily. The drain is removed when its output is <30 mL/day, and the skin sutures are removed within 1 week.

If there is postoperative facial nerve paresis, strict eye care is undertaken. This consists of frequent instillation of moisturizing eye drops during the day and eye protection with ophthalmic ointment application and eyelid taping or use of an eye moisture chamber during the night. Ophthalmologic consultation is needed should any signs or symptoms of corneal desiccation or visual impairment occur.

COMPLICATIONS

There are both early and late complications and sequelae of total parotidectomy, and the patient should be informed of them and how they differ.

Facial nerve paresis or paralysis can occur as an early complication. Temporary facial nerve paralysis involving all or just one branches of the nerve occurs in 10% to 30% of parotidectomies. Permanent facial nerve paralysis occurs in <1% of parotidectomies. The nerve at most risk for injury during parotidectomy is the marginal mandibular branch of the facial nerve. Temporary facial nerve paresis usually resolves from weeks to months postoperatively. Complete nerve transection during surgery requires immediate microsurgical repair.

Hemorrhage or hematoma is an uncommon early complication of parotidectomy and is usually related to incomplete hemostasis during the procedure. Treatment consists of evacuation of the hematoma and surgical control of any identified bleeding vessels.

Infection is uncommon after parotidectomy and is avoided by the use of aseptic technique and careful handling of tissues. The rarity of infection is probably related to the rich vascular supply to the parotid region. Treatment of infection consists of appropriate antibiotics. Abscess formation is rare and requires surgical drainage and antibiotics.

TABLE 27.1 Complications of Total Parotidectomy	
Early	**Late**
Bleeding/hematoma	Frey syndrome
External otitis	Hypertrophic scar or keloid
Facial nerve paresis or paralysis	Recurrent tumor
First bite syndrome	Soft tissue deficit
Infection	
Necrosis of the skin flap	
Salivary fistula/sialocele	
Sensory loss	
Seroma	
Trismus	

External otitis can occur postoperatively and may be related to an intraoperative collection of blood in the external auditory canal. A petrolatum gauze pack placed in the external auditory canal can prevent blood entry during the procedure. Treatment of external otitis consists of cleaning the auditory canal and instillation of antibiotic ear drops.

Necrosis of the skin flap is an uncommon complication. When it occurs, it is usually located in the distal tip of the postauricular skin flap. Care must be taken to avoid compromise of the vascular supply to this portion of the skin flap. Smoking, prior radiation therapy, and diabetes mellitus may contribute to this complication due to impairment of the blood supply to the flap. Treatment of flap necrosis consists of conservative debridement of necrotic tissue and local wound care.

Mild trismus may occur following parotidectomy and may be related to inflammation and fibrosis of the masseter muscle. This complication usually resolves with range of motion exercises of the jaw.

Salivary fistula or sialocele can occur in approximately 10% of cases of partial parotidectomy. This problem is a result of leakage of saliva from remaining salivary gland tissue that collects beneath the flap or drains from the wound. This complication is usually mild and self-limited. Treatment of a sialocele consists of repeated needle aspiration. A salivary fistula is managed with local wound care. A chronic salivary fistula is rare.

Frey syndrome, or gustatory sweating, is a relatively common long-term sequela of parotidectomy. This complication is thought to be related to aberrant regeneration of nerve fibers from the postganglionic secretomotor parasympathetic innervation of the parotid gland to the severed postganglionic sympathetic fibers that supply the sweat glands of the skin of the face. As a result, sweating with or without a dermal flush occurs during salivary stimulation. If objective testing is performed, Frey syndrome occurs in the majority of patients undergoing parotidectomy. Only about 10% of patients, however, complain of symptomatic Frey syndrome. Most patients with Frey syndrome do not seek therapy. Medical treatment of symptomatic Frey syndrome includes topical application of antiperspirant, topical anticholinergics (1% glycopyrrolate), or injections of botulinum toxin.

First bite syndrome results from interruption of the sympathetic innervation of the parotid gland with denervation supersensitivity of myoepithelial cell receptors. This problem manifests with recurrent severe pain with initial oral intake that subsides with successive bites. The severity of this condition usually diminishes over time. Severe cases may benefit from botulinum toxin injection of residual gland tissue.

RESULTS

A higher incidence of temporary facial nerve paresis occurs following total parotidectomy compared to partial parotidectomy. In addition, a more significant facial contour deformity results after total parotidectomy compared to partial parotidectomy. Therefore, consideration should be given to defect reconstruction to improve the cosmetic outcome.

Benign neoplasm recurrence is unusual unless the tumor is removed incompletely or ruptured. Malignant tumor control depends on completeness of resection, tumor type and extent, and adjuvant therapy.

PEARLS

- Counsel the patient preoperatively regarding sequelae and potential complications.
- Have imaging studies available for intraoperative review.
- Ensure adequate exposure of the operative field.
- Minimize facial nerve manipulation and traction forces.
- Keep the operative field and flaps moist throughout the case.
- Ensure complete removal of the tumor.

PITFALLS

- Plan operative time accordingly.
- Do not rush, particularly dissecting near the facial nerve.
- Avoid tumor rupture as this is a major risk factor for multifocal tumor recurrence of pleomorphic adenoma.
- Institute immediate proper eye care if postoperative facial paresis occurs.

INSTRUMENTS TO HAVE AVAILABLE

- Head and neck set with hook retractors, McCabe dissector, and fine dissecting clamps
- Hemostatix scalpel, no. 15 and no. 12 blades
- Fine bipolar electrocautery forceps
- Nerve monitor and electrodes
- Clear adhesive drape
- 7-mm Jackson-Pratt drain

SUGGESTED READING

Moore EJ, Olsen KD. Total parotidectomy. In: Myers EN, Ferris RL, eds. *Salivary Gland Disorders.* Heidelberg, Germany: Springer Verlag, 2007:248–266.

Wang SJ, Eisele DW. Superficial parotidectomy. In: Myers EN, Ferris RL, eds. *Salivary Gland Disorders.* Heidelberg, Germany: Springer Verlag, 2007:237–246.

Gillespie MB, Eisele DW. Complications of surgery of the salivary glands. In: Eisele DW, Smith RV, eds. *Complications in Head and Neck Surgery.* 2nd ed. Philadelphia, PA: Elsevier, 2008:221–239.

Eisele DW, Wang SJ, Orloff LA. Electrophysiologic facial nerve monitoring during parotidectomy. *Head Neck* 2010;32: 399–405.

Wang SJ, Eisele DW. Parotidectomy—anatomical considerations. *Clin Anat* 2012;25:12–18.

28 MINIMALLY INVASIVE VIDEO-ASSISTED PAROTIDECTOMY

Mu-Kuan Chen

INTRODUCTION

A wide variety of tumors occur in the parotid gland. Thus, parotidectomy requires a precise preoperative evaluation. A detailed history, clinical examination, and imaging studies are essential in defining the location and extent of these tumors, and fine needle aspiration biopsy (FNAB) may also provide important diagnostic information. Most of the lesions in the parotid space originate in the gland itself, and about 80% of parotid tumors are benign. However, other types of benign and malignant tumors may appear in this area (Table 28.1). Surgical treatment of the parotid gland is a challenging undertaking, due primarily to the intraparenchymal course of the facial nerve.

HISTORY

A mass within the parotid space poses a diagnostic problem, since it may represent inflammatory disease, glandular lesion, lymph node, primary or metastatic tumor, connective tissue tumor, vascular lesion, neural tumor, or other miscellaneous disease. The history, clinical examination, and imaging studies may suggest a specific etiology. The final diagnosis of a lesion in the parotid space may be elusive and, in these situations, relies on pathologic evaluation of the parotidectomy specimen.

PHYSICAL EXAMINATION

A lesion in the parotid space should be inspected carefully and should be evaluated by bimanual palpation; the dimensions and the location of the lesion should be measured and recorded. Detailed inspection of facial nerve function should be performed. Any sign of weakness of the facial nerve branch(es) should be recorded. Fixation of the skin, facial weakness, and pain without other infectious signs strongly suggest the presence of a malignant tumor.

INDICATIONS

Indications for endoscopic parotidectomy include chronic sialadenitis and benign neoplasms located in the tail of the parotid gland.

CONTRAINDICATIONS

Suspected cases of a malignant parotid tumor, sialadenitis during acute inflammation, tumors too large to extract through the surgical wound, and revision surgery are relative contraindications to this technique through an endoscopic approach.

TABLE 28.1   Lesions Reported in the Parotid Space

Glandular	Vascular	Lymph Node	Connective	Inflammatory	Neural	Miscellaneous
Acinic cell carcinoma	Hemangioma	Benign reactive node	Fibrosarcoma	Actinomycosis	Neurofibroma	Cat scratch fever
Adenocarcinoma		Lymphoma	Lipoma	Inclusion disease	Schwannoma	Hepatic cell carcinoma
Adenoid cystic carcinoma		Lymphosarcoma	Rhabdomyosarcoma	Kimura disease		Kussmaul disease (sialodochitis fibrinosa)
Branchial cleft cyst		Squamous cell carcinoma		Mumps		Necrotizing sialometaplasia
Lymphoepithelial cyst				Sarcoidosis		Pneumoparotitis
Monomorphic adenoma				Sialadenitis		Sialolithiasis
Mucoepidermoid carcinoma				Sjögren syndrome		
Oncocytoma				Tuberculosis		
Parotid duct tumor						
Pleomorphic adenoma (benign and malignant)						
Retention cyst						
Squamous cell carcinoma						
Undifferentiated carcinoma						
Warthin tumor						

PREOPERATIVE PLANNING

Imaging Studies

Imaging studies provide valuable information that can help in the differential diagnosis of a mass in the parotid gland. Both computed tomography (CT) and magnetic resonance imaging (MRI) may be used in evaluating the mass in the parotid gland. While the CT scan is specific in defining the anatomic localization and extent of a mass in the parotid gland, it has limited value in differentiating benign from malignant tumors. The sensitivity, specificity, and accuracy for detecting malignant parotid tumors are approximately 87%, 94%, and 93%, respectively, for MRI scanning. The reliability and associated anatomic information of MRI in parotid gland tumor diagnosis may make MRI the radiographic test of choice although cost and feasibility vary by clinical site. High-resolution ultrasonography (US) may be useful, if available, and may also assist in FNAB.

Fine Needle Aspiration Biopsy

FNAB is a noninvasive, and quick examination which may be useful information for the assessment of parotid lesions. However, the diagnostic utility of FNAB in guiding the extent of surgery remains a matter of controversy.

In my opinion, morbidity, such as hemorrhage, facial nerve damage, and introduction of infection after FNAB, can be minimized using US guidance. Technical factors may reduce the accuracy of diagnosis if the FNAB is not under US image guidance. Misdiagnoses could also result from relatively inexperienced FNAB technique by the pathologist or even the radiologist. Nonetheless, FNAB is a precise, less invasive tool with which to diagnose a mass in the parotid.

Regardless of the cytologic diagnosis, complete excision with definitive pathologic analysis based on permanent section histopathology still provides the most accurate diagnosis. Most of these lesions are benign, and complete excision is both diagnostic and therapeutic and thus should be curative.

SURGICAL TECHNIQUE

A parotidectomy can be conventionally classified in terms of the extent of resection as conservative, superficial, or total. A conservative parotidectomy is defined as any procedure that is less than a superficial parotidectomy and where all facial nerve branches are not dissected. Due to the minimal invasiveness, reduced tissue damage, improved cosmetic appearance, fewer wound-related complications, and short recovery time, minimally invasive endoscopic surgery has in recent years emerged as the standard and most frequently preferred technique in a number of surgical disciplines, including urologic, general, and orthopedic surgery. However, such operations are not yet a standard procedure in the head and neck because of the anatomic complexity of this region. The head and neck applications have largely been limited to endoscopic sinus surgery, endoscopic cosmetic surgery, and endoscopic thyroidectomy. With the advancement of instruments and endoscopic techniques, since 1999, I have applied the strictly endoscopic or endoscope-assisted surgery to sinonasal, skull base, and head and neck surgery. I have recently reported several advanced techniques for endoscopic surgery for sinonasal malignancies with or without skull base invasion, advanced nasopharyngeal angiofibromas, recurrent nasopharyngeal carcinoma, excision of submandibular glands, parotidectomy, and miscellaneous other diseases including parotidectomy.

Description of Technique

All operations are done under general anesthesia with the patient supine. No paralytic agent is given. A 20- to 35-mm skin incision is made using a postauricular skin crease. The skin flap is undermined sharply off the superficial lobe of the parotid gland using a Metzenbaum scissor, and the surgical plane is dissected under the 4-mm diameter, 0-degree angle endoscope (Karl-Storz, Tuttlingen, Germany)

After dissection between the skin flap and the superficial lobe of the parotid gland, the main trunk of the facial nerve is identified by using an intraoperative nerve stimulator or Medtronic-ENT nerve integrity monitoring system (NIM-2.0 or NIM-3.0, Medtronic, USA). The main landmark that I use to identify the main trunk of the facial nerve is the tympanomastoid fissure. When using the intraoperative nerve stimulator, the facial nerve stimulation is performed at 0.5 to 1 mA per stimulus. The stimulator is grounded in the sternocleidomastoid muscle, and the exposed nerve is stimulated. Stimulation is verified by observing gross movement in the involved facial musculature. In the last 5 years, with the advancement of the intraoperative nerve integrity monitor, I routinely use the facial nerve integrity monitor during the whole procedure in every case.

The surgeons should listen for subtle signals to minimize nerve damage due to surgical manipulation. To minimize the possibility of damage to individual branches of the facial nerve, after identification of the main trunk and with the assistance of the 4-mm diameter, 0-degree and 30-degree angle endoscope (Karl-Storz) and harmonic scalpel (Ethicon EndoSurgery, Cincinnati, OH) at a power level of 3, the peripheral branches of the facial nerve are dissected by dividing the glandular tissue.

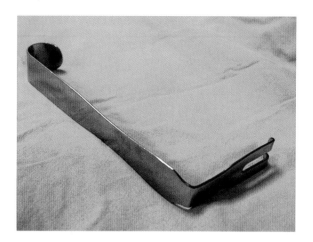

FIGURE 28.1
A special retractor with a groove to avoid facial nerve damage.

Due to the endoscopic magnification, the branches of the facial nerve can be identified clearly. The main task of the first assistant is to keep the endoscope in the correct position during the procedure. The second assistant provides working space by holding the retractor to lift the tissue up and away from the skin. I designed a special retractor with a groove that could help to avoid damage to the facial nerve (Fig. 28.1). Using the endoscope, for visualization, the lower pole of the tumor is carefully dissected from the circumferential tissue in the neck space avoiding a large cervical skin incision. Subsequently, the tumor is excised (conservative parotidectomy) and removed through the surgical wound. For histologic examination, the specimen is sent for frozen section. The wound is then closed by using subcuticular suture with 4-0 Dexon, and a small Hemovac drain is placed into the wound. The small operative scar is concealed in the postauricular area resulting in improved cosmetic results (Fig. 28.2). The key procedure is demonstrated in Video 28.1.

POSTOPERATIVE CARE

Proper functioning of the Hemovac must be monitored by the nursing staff. The drain is removed on the first or second postoperative day, and the patient is discharged.

COMPLICATIONS

Complications of the two surgical approaches, conventional (open) or minimally invasive video-assisted parotidectomy, are similar and are listed in Table 28.2. Management of the mass in the parotid gland has evolved with advances in technology. Despite painstaking efforts to minimize the risk of facial paresis during parotidectomy, an incidence of early transient facial paresis ranging from 9.3% to 64.6% may be expected, which carries a significant risk of corneal exposure and potential loss of sight. In addition, an incidence of permanent total paralysis ranging from 0% to 0.9% has been reported in patients who received conventional parotidectomy. In our series, six patients (9.7%) had transient grade II paresis, eight patients (12.9%) developed postoperative sialocele, and one case (1.6%) had postoperative bleeding who was sent to operation room to recheck bleeding. All patients who experienced temporary weakness of the facial nerve or developed a sialocele resolved

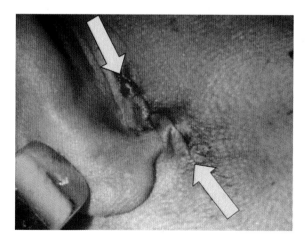

FIGURE 28.2
The small operative scar (*arrows*) is almost invisible due to the concealed location in the postauricular area.

TABLE 28.2   Complications Associated with Parotidectomy
• Facial nerve paresis (temporary or permanent)
• Fistula
• Frey syndrome
• Hematoma and seroma
• Hypesthesia of the cheek or ear lobe
• Postoperative hemorrhage
• Postoperative sialocele

spontaneously. Facial nerve damage can be minimized by identifying the main trunk of the facial nerve using endoscopic magnification of the branches of facial nerve with meticulous dissection.

RESULTS

The preoperative diagnosis of a tumor in the tail of the parotid gland is an essential criterion for selection of appropriate candidates for minimally invasive video-assisted parotidectomy. Clinical examination and radiologic correlation provide valuable information regarding the location and extent of these tumors. FNAB may also provide additional preoperative information. The video-assisted parotidectomy can magnify the branches of the facial nerve; thus, meticulous dissection and protection of the branches of the facial nerve are possible. In my experience, the minimally invasive video-assisted parotidectomy is feasible for both inflammatory diseases and benign tumors located in the tail of the parotid, with or without parapharyngeal space extension. In cases with parapharyngeal space extension, the advantage of this new approach is obvious due to the concealed scar without cervical skin incision.

From year 2002 to June 2010, 62 operations were performed via the minimally invasive video-assisted parotidectomy. Most of them were pleomorphic adenoma, followed by Warthins tumor and sialadenitis. All operations were successfully performed via the endoscope, with one conversion to conventional procedure due to the frozen section which revealed a malignant tumor. Of these cases, only one case (1.6%) had a recurrence of the tumor. The advantages of minimally invasive endoscope-assisted parotidectomy include superior visualization, magnification of key structures, and concealment of the scar in the postauricular skin crease.

PEARLS

- Preoperative rigorous evaluation including imaging studies is essential.
- Educating the patient regarding the risk of postoperative facial paresis (transient or permanent) and possible complications is critical. Compared with the conventional open procedure, the minimally invasive procedure provides better cosmetic results although the procedure may be riskier and time-consuming especially in the surgeon's early cases.
- Do not use long-term paralyzing anesthetics to ensure proper intraoperative nerve stimulator or monitor.
- Bloodlessly undermine in the plane between the skin flap and the superficial lobe of the parotid gland with the assistance of the endoscope.
- Identify the main trunk of the facial nerve using the facial nerve integrity monitor or nerve stimulator and trace the branches of the facial nerve.
- Dissect the facial nerve away from the tumor in order to excise the tumor without injury to the nerve.

PITFALLS

- Lack of experience in identifying the main trunk of facial nerve from the small incision wound and limited surgical field may lead to damage to the facial nerve.
- The primary challenge for the change from open to endoscopic surgery is the endoscope itself. The head and neck surgeon may be not familiar with operating using an endoscope, or its two-dimensional, flat view on the screen.

INSTRUMENTS TO HAVE AVAILABLE

- Basic head and neck surgery instruments
- Endoscope (4-mm diameter, 0-degree angle Karl-Storz, Tuttlingen, Germany)
- Intraoperative nerve stimulator or Medtronic-ENT nerve integrity monitoring system (NIM-2.0 or NIM-3.0, Medtronic, USA)

SUGGESTED READING

Reilly J, Myssiorek D. Facial nerve stimulation and postparotidectomy facial paresis. *Otolaryngol Head Neck Surg* 2003;128:530–533.

Chen MK, Su CC, Tsai YL, et al. Minimally invasive endoscopic resection of the submandibular gland: a new approach. *Head Neck* 2006;28:1014–1017.

Chen MK, Chang CC. Minimally invasive endoscope-assisted parotidectomy: a new approach. *Laryngoscope* 2007;117: 1934–1937.

Myers EN, ed. *Operative Otolaryngology—Head and Neck Surgery*. Philadelphia, PA: Saunders/Elsevier, 2008.

Carrillo JF, Ramirez R, Flores L, et al. Diagnostic accuracy of fine needle aspiration biopsy in preoperative diagnosis of patients with parotid gland masses. *J Surg Oncol* 2009;100:133–138.

29 EXCISION OF TUMORS OF THE PRESTYLOID PARAPHARYNGEAL SPACE

Kerry D. Olsen

INTRODUCTION

Tumors of the prestyloid parapharyngeal space are uncommon but challenging due to the variety of lesions encountered and the complex anatomy of the involved area. Fortunately, these tumors are generally benign, and therefore, they bring expectations from the patient and the physician that excision should lead to low morbidity and very low mortality. Since patients rarely die of these tumors, the goal of management should be to perform the operation safely with complete removal of the tumors to minimize the risk of recurrence and to preserve surrounding structures.

The prestyloid portion of the parapharyngeal space is actually a potential space. It contains adipose tissue, a portion of the deep lobe of the parotid gland (the retromandibular portion), minor salivary glands, and scattered vessels and nerves (Table 29.1). Tumors of salivary gland origin in the pharyngeal space have the same distribution as those in the parotid gland, that is, 80% to 90% are benign and 10% to 20% are malignant. The majority are pleomorphic adenomas. The challenge to the surgeon is understanding tumor behavior and appropriate preparation to manage the simple and complex tumors that are encountered in this area.

It is essential that the surgeon is familiar with the anatomy. The prestyloid space superiorly is contained by fascial areas that direct tumor growth. The parapharyngeal space itself is divided into the pre- and poststyloid areas by the fascia of the styloid process that connects to the tensor veli palatini muscles and its surrounding fascia (Fig. 29.1). Another important structure is the stylomandibular ligament that forms part of the boundary of the stylomandibular tunnel. The stylomandibular ligament unites the fascia of the styloid process to the angle of the mandible. It can be thinned by tumors but is always present, and its division insures adequate opening of the parapharyngeal space and successful subsequent tumor removal. It is also a structure where constriction can occur as tumors grow between the mandible and this ligament. This leads to the classic "dumbbell" tumors that extend from the tail of the parotid gland into the parapharyngeal space. Table 29.2 lists the anatomic boundaries of the prestyloid space.

HISTORY

Most tumors of the prestyloid space are benign and, as such, have a slow growth rate and generally are asymptomatic. The majority are discovered on routine physical examination when a physician, or the patient, notices a bulging or displacement of the nonrigid portions of the parapharynx: generally the medial surface, the displacement of the constrictor muscles, or the inferior soft border near the inferior aspect of the parotid gland or digastric muscle. For prestyloid tumors, displacement of the lateral pharyngeal wall usually occurs in the region of the tonsil or soft palate or anterior tonsillar pillar (Fig. 29.2). Eventually, as the tumors enlarge, they will displace the entire tonsil and lateral pharynx up to the nasopharynx. One may notice tumors in the deep lobe of the parotid that also extend through the stylomandibular tunnel and present as a swelling or mass in the pretragal area, as well as the pharynx. It is common today to discover prestyloid lesions on routine imaging—CT or MRI scans—done for other indications.

TABLE 29.1   Structures Contributing to Tumors of the Prestyloid Parapharyngeal Space
Adipose Tissue Deep lobe of the parotid gland Minor salivary glands and ectopic salivary rests Muscles Nerves Vessels

As these tumors extend superiorly, the muscles of the eustachian tube can be compressed, causing a feeling of fullness and pressure in the ear. Eustachian tube dysfunction can also lead to middle ear effusion with decreased hearing. Involvement of the medial pterygoid muscle can lead to trismus, which is more common with malignant tumors. As the tumor enlarges, it displaces the pharynx and interferes with eating, speech, and especially sleep. Some of the early symptoms are snoring or symptoms of obstructive sleep apnea. This occurs before these tumors impact eating and phonation.

There are several cases of prestyloid parapharyngeal lesions that were untreated in elderly sick individuals that enlarged to the point where they caused significant dysphagia, inanition, respiratory distress, and death. It is also not uncommon for lesions of the prestyloid parapharyngeal space to be confused with pathology of the tonsil, such as infection, enlargement, or tumors. Pain is not a common finding, but if it is present, one must be concerned about a malignant lesion. Other symptoms of malignancy, of course, include the presence of facial nerve involvement and regional adenopathy.

PHYSICAL EXAMINATION

Small tumors, due to their location in the prestyloid parapharyngeal space, cannot be detected on physical examination. A tumor must be >3 cm to cause displacement of the surrounding structures before it can be seen or felt. Early tumors are detected only serendipitously on a prior imaging study. It is important to carefully inspect the pharynx and the parotid gland and palpate both intraorally and bimanually. A palpable deep parotid mass that is immobile and of indeterminate deep extent may extend into the parapharyngeal space. One must assess the function of the seventh cranial nerve and palpate the parotid and neck carefully for any enlarged nodes. In a

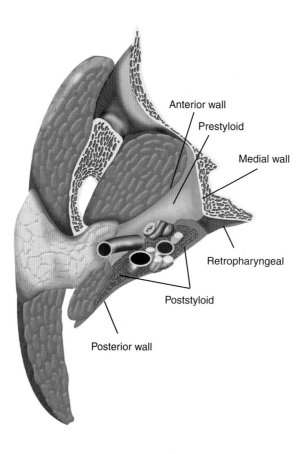

FIGURE 29.1

Division of the parapharyngeal space into prestyloid and poststyloid compartments.

TABLE 29.2	Anatomic Boundaries of the Prestyloid Parapharyngeal Space
Superior	Fascial junction of the medial pterygoid and tensor veli palatini fascia
Superior medial	Fascia from the tensor veli palatini muscle to the spine of the sphenoid
Medial	Superior constrictor muscles
Inferior medial	Fascia of the constrictor muscles joins the fascia of the styloglossus and stylopharyngeus muscles
Superior lateral	Fascia of the medial pterygoid muscles and ramus of the mandible
Lateral	Retromandibular portion of the deep lobe of the parotid gland
Inferior lateral	Fascia extension that forms the stylomandibular ligament
Inferior	Posterior belly of the digastric muscle

series from Mayo Clinic of almost 200 parapharyngeal tumors, an intraoral mass alone occurred in 63%, an external mass in the parotid region was present in 58%, and both findings were found in only 28% of the cases.

INDICATIONS

- Parapharyngeal deep lobe benign parotid tumors
- Parapharyngeal deep lobe malignant parotid tumors
- Mesenchymal tumors located in the prestyloid space

CONTRAINDICATIONS

As with any mass of the parotid gland, the decision to operate must take into consideration the patient's age, the patient's health, his or her wishes, and the surgeon's experience. In addition, one should have available key colleagues, including pathologists, to complete the procedure as dictated by the pathologic findings.

The final recommendation for surgery is always individualized based upon the patient, the history, the examination, and the evaluation. The discussion about removing a benign pleomorphic adenoma from the parapharyngeal space is vastly different than that of an obvious malignant tumor in this region.

PREOPERATIVE PLANNING

Management of a prestyloid parapharyngeal tumor is approached similar to any mass discovered in the parotid gland on physical examination. Whether it is felt on clinical examination or noted on imaging studies, the evaluation is the same. Since prestyloid tumors are usually of salivary gland origin, awareness of a mass will lead to a recommendation for removal—for diagnosis, to prevent growth, and to prevent malignant degeneration.

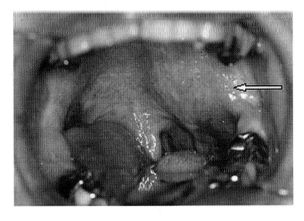

FIGURE 29.2 Typical displacement of the anterior tonsil region from a mass in the parapharyngeal space (arrow).

TABLE 29.3 Tumors of the Prestyloid Parapharyngeal Space	
Benign	**Malignant**
Pleomorphic adenoma	Mucoepidermoid carcinoma
Warthin tumor	Adenocarcinoma
Oncocytoma	Acinic cell carcinoma
Benign lymphoepithelial lesion	Adenoid cystic carcinoma
Hemangioma	Carcinoma ex pleomorphic
Branchial cleft cyst	adenoma
Venous malformation	Hemangiopericytomas
Fibroma	Variety of sarcomas
Schwannoma	
Neurofibroma	
Rhabdomyoma	
Hibernoma	

The most common tumors extend from the retromandibular portion of the deep lobe of the parotid gland. As such, they grow into the space and generally have a round or irregular shape. The dumbbell shape is rarer and occurs when tumors extend through the stylomandibular tunnel. Other sources of salivary gland tumors include the extraparotid minor salivary gland tissue that can occur when minor salivary glands are found lateral to the superior constrictor muscles. These tumors, if <4 cm, can be detected as minor salivary gland in origin on imaging study by the finding of preservation of the adipose tissue plane between the tumor and the deep lobe of the parotid gland. The presence of adipose tissue in the parapharyngeal space aids in removal, as the majority of the tumors have to be removed by finger capsular dissection. Dissection is further aided as the capsule of a pleomorphic adenoma in the parapharyngeal space appears to be thicker on histologic study than many of the pleomorphic adenomas found within the superficial or deep portion of the parotid gland. Table 29.3 lists the tumors and lesions found in the prestyloid parapharyngeal space.

After the history and physical examination are completed, the key steps include accurate imaging to assess the extent and characteristics of the tumor. One can gain additional information regarding the possible tumor histology and involvement of surrounding structures. An MRI scan with gadolinium is most helpful as it provides triplanar information to determine the tumor's extent, its relationship to surrounding structures, and relationship to key vasculature. If an MRI scan is contraindicated, then a high-resolution CT with contrast is indicated.

The findings of a prestyloid mass with discreet borders and generally low-signal T1 and bright T2 are often indicative of a pleomorphic adenoma. Generally, no further study is necessary. It is important to remember, however, that a pleomorphic adenoma in the parapharyngeal space can be predominately cystic and over time may even cause erosion of surrounding bony structures such as the pterygoid plates and still be benign.

Fine needle aspiration (FNA) biopsy, either transorally or directed with CT or ultrasound, can accurately identify pleomorphic adenomas. This rarely is done as it does not usually change the recommendation for removal. However, one should never perform a transoral or open biopsy of a parapharyngeal mass as the subsequent capsular rupture can lead to scarring and increased risk of tumor recurrence.

Imaging characteristics of low-grade carcinomas are difficult to distinguish from benign lesions. That is why the availability of pathologic assistance and frozen section evaluation is so helpful at the time of surgery.

If there is concern of malignancy based upon history, physical examination, and imaging, then an FNA may be helpful for operative planning and in the preoperative discussion with the patient. One must remember, however, the difficulty in accurately diagnosing any salivary gland neoplasm on the basis of a FNA. There remains a high incidence of false positives and false negatives.

Once a tumor of the parapharyngeal space is identified, the discussion with the patient as to why it should be removed includes the following: to make a diagnosis, to avoid growth, to eliminate the risk of malignant degeneration, and to appropriately treat it if it is malignant. If the pathologist notes malignancy, the histology may warrant cervical nodal removal, removal of the entire parotid gland to remove intraparotid nodes, or removal of involved surrounding structures such as bone, vessels, and nerves. One must be prepared to perform the necessary reconstruction in these situations. The full complement of risks, benefits, and potential complications is always discussed with the patient preoperatively.

SURGICAL TECHNIQUE

Multiple surgical approaches have been described to remove masses from the prestyloid parapharyngeal space. These include a cervical approach, a transparotid approach, a submandibular approach, a transoral approach, and a cervical–parotid approach. Mandibulotomy can also be combined with these approaches for a variety of tumors. However, in most cases, mandibulotomy is not indicated except for extremely large or select malignant tumors.

The variety of tumors encountered includes the challenge of removing a 1-cm tumor high in the superior aspect of the prestyloid parapharynx, as well as a 13-cm lesion that involves a massive amount of the parapharyngeal space.

For a description of the surgical technique, it is most helpful to assume that the tumor is the most common one, a pleomorphic adenoma arising from the retromandibular portion of the deep lobe of the parotid. This is the classic prestyloid lesion, and if it is managed successfully, one can then approach other tumors in this area using minor variations in this technique.

I use the cervical–parotid approach, which has proved safe, effective, and versatile. This approach provides the basic framework for surgical excision of tumors in this area. It also provides flexibility to alter the approach based upon size, pathologic findings, and surgical findings. If there is involvement of surrounding structures, additional surgery can be done. A retroauricular incision is added to access tumors that involve or extend into the skull base or posterior fossa. A mandibulotomy approach with parasymphyseal swing is used for select malignancies, superiorly based small lesions, or massive tumors in the prestyloid space. A mandibulotomy, however, is necessary in <5% of all prestyloid tumors.

The transoral approach can be performed for highly select tumors, especially extraparotid salivary lesions when imaging studies show a benign appearance and there is a clear separation of the tumor from the deep lobe and from the surrounding vessels. This approach can also be used for rare, select neurogenic tumors. A transoral removal is done through or adjacent to the tonsil bed. Several authors suggest that these should be removed using a transoral robotic approach as opposed to conventional instrumentation. The main disadvantage of the robotic approach is the lack of tactile feel and the risk of rupture of the tumor capsule with retraction. If there is tumor rupture, oftentimes recurrence will not be noted for up to 10 or 20 years, and one may get a false sense of security. If a transoral approach is used in the wrong individual, there can be incomplete removal, damage to vessels and nerves, capsular rupture, and subsequent tumor recurrence.

For safety, control, and adequate removal of the lesion, I generally recommend the cervical–parotid approach for most cases of prestyloid parapharyngeal lesions. This approach allows for short hospitalization, minimal morbidity, safety, and proven efficacy.

Description of Technique

Universal protocol confirms the correct identification of the patient and the operative site. Using general anesthesia without paralysis, the is prepped and draped to expose the hemiface, neck, entire ear, and the corner of the mouth and the eye. A pen is used to mark the incision in front of the ear and extended into a natural skin crease beneath the mandible. The skin incision is then made with a 15-blade, and the flaps are raised over the parotid fascia to expose the upper neck using a scalpel and Jones scissors. The parotid gland is then separated from the anterior border of the sternocleidomastoid muscle and from the cartilaginous ear canal. Kocher clamps are placed on the edge of the gland to retract the gland. If one can preserve the posterior branch of the great auricular nerve, this is done. The anterior branch is divided. The gland is then separated from the superior border of the posterior belly of the digastric muscle. The main trunk of the facial nerve is then identified, and the postauricular artery is ligated. The lower division and lower branches of the facial nerve are followed out to the level of the submandibular gland (Fig. 29.3). At this point, the stylomandibular fascia that separates the submandibular gland from the tail of the parotid gland is divided freeing the submandibular gland to allow for anterior retraction of this gland. A block of upper deep jugular nodes are removed after elevating the fascia from the sternocleidomastoid muscle and are sent to pathology. The removal of these nodes allows exposure of cranial nerves X, XI, and XII; the internal jugular vein; and the internal and external carotid arteries (Fig. 29.4). The posterior belly of the digastric muscle and the stylohyoid muscles are then isolated and divided near the mastoid tip and retracted medially. This gives further exposure of the vascular structures, nerves, and the styloid process. The external carotid artery is now easily seen as it passes between the stylohyoid and stylopharyngeus muscle. This artery is divided (Fig. 29.5). A ribbon retractor is then placed on the angle of the mandible to retract it medially. This makes identification of the stylomandibular ligament easier. This dense, connective tissue band extends from the styloid process to the angle and a portion of the ramus of the mandible. It can be quite thinned by very large tumors, and one must be careful to ensure the ligament and not cut the tumor. In most cases, however, the ligament can be easily isolated and divided with scissors (Fig. 29.6). The mandible can then be further retracted anteriorly, opening the parapharyngeal space. At this point, the surgeon generally gets the first view of the tumor (Fig. 29.7). With the mandible retracted and with finger dissection, a plane is then established along the styloglossus and submandibular gland inferiorly and continues anteriorly to the mass. I establish a plane superiorly along the medial pterygoid muscle and medially along the constrictor muscles (Fig. 29.8). Next, I identify the site of attachment of the tumor to the deep lobe of the parotid gland. It is helpful to know the exact location of the main trunk of the facial nerve as you can be surprised by the proximity of the tumor to the facial nerve and the often superior extension in the deep lobe of a parapharyngeal lesion above the level of the facial nerve. If the styloid process is impinging on the surface of the tumor and if there is any risk for potential rupture of the tumor capsule with inferior displacement of the tumor by finger dissection, the styloid process can be removed (Fig. 29.9). This occurs when a long, thin, or sharp styloid compresses the tumor capsule. The portion of the deep lobe around the tumor attachment site from the retromandibular portion of the deep lobe of the parotid gland is isolated (Fig. 29.10). Knowing the position of the facial nerve and the external

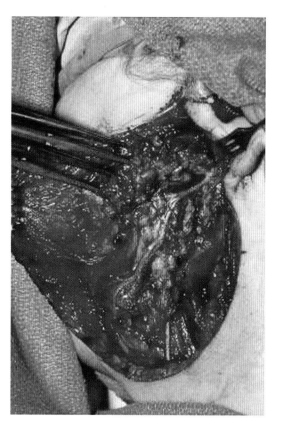
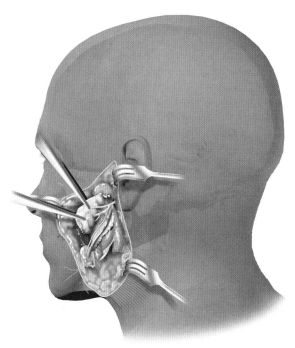

FIGURE 29.3 Isolation of the lower division and main trunk of the facial nerve.

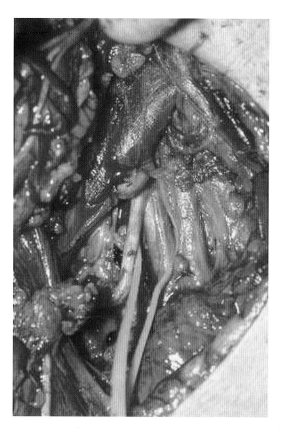
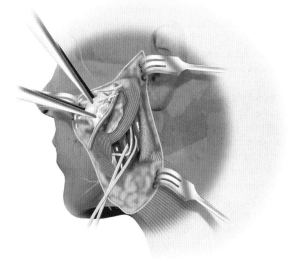

FIGURE 29.4 Exposure of the neurovascular components of the upper neck.

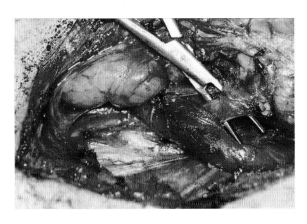

FIGURE 29.5 Isolation and division of the external carotid artery as it passes above the stylohyoid muscle.

carotid vessels and associated veins is essential in this step and allows for removal of a portion of the gland with avoidance of tumor rupture. The tumor is then easily delivered into the surgical field and removed (Fig. 29.11).

Hemostasis is obtained with bipolar cautery, a Hemovac drain is placed, and the Hemovac is put on suction for 2 days. The digastric and stylohyoid muscles are sutured. The superficial portion of the parotid gland is repositioned and sutured to the sternocleidomastoid muscle. The incision is then closed using chromic sutures and 5-0 fast-absorbing chromic in the skin. A parotid and neck dressing is then applied.

Reconstruction is generally not necessary. If there is a malignancy that requires removal of the entire parotid gland and surrounding adjacent structures, I have to individualize the need to follow the operative bed for recurrence versus the desire to reconstruct the soft tissue defect.

POSTOPERATIVE CARE

Hemovac drains are kept on continuous suction for 48 hours to collapse the dead space and lessen the risk of infection, seroma, or hematoma. For very small tumors, this can be done overnight. Antibiotics are given for 24 hours to prevent infection, as there is a large dead space after tumor removal. The parotid and neck dressings are removed the following day and reapplied for one further day for additional pressure and hemostasis.

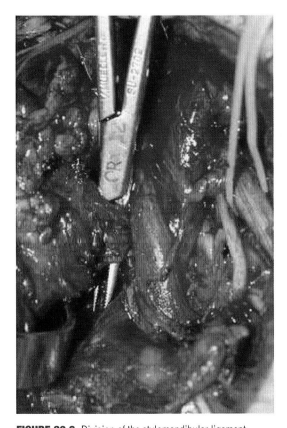

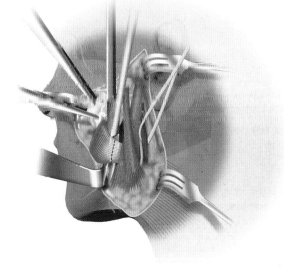

FIGURE 29.6 Division of the stylomandibular ligament.

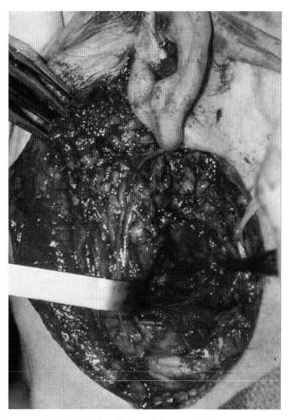

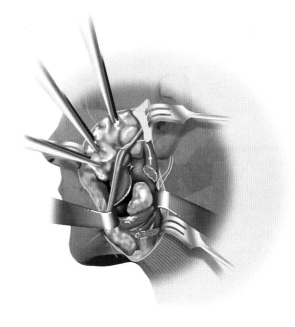

FIGURE 29.7 Early visualization of the prestyloid mass.

The patient is hospitalized until the drains are removed, generally within 48 hours after surgery. For wound care, antibiotic ointment or Vaseline is applied to the incision site until the sutures dissolve or fall out. Patients are allowed to shower 48 hours following their operation.

COMPLICATIONS

Complications generally occur because of poor knowledge of regional anatomy, an incomplete preoperative assessment, performing the wrong operation, or an inexperienced surgeon. One must individualize the approach and operative extent based upon the surgical findings. The complication to avoid is rupture of the tumor capsule

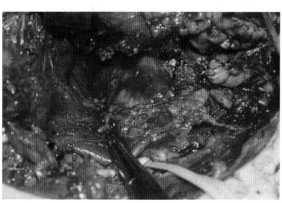

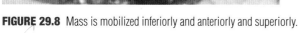

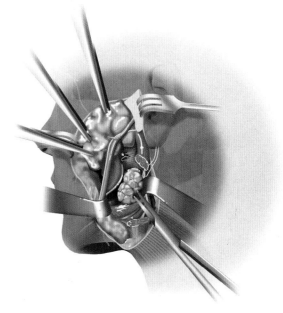

FIGURE 29.8 Mass is mobilized inferiorly and anteriorly and superiorly.

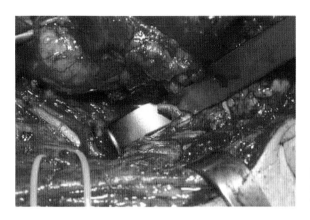

FIGURE 29.9 Styloid process can be removed in certain cases to assist in exposure or lessen risk of tumor capsule rupture.

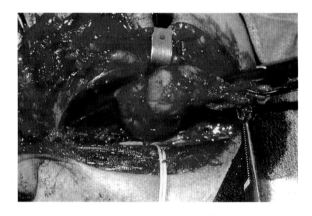

FIGURE 29.10 Removal of the deep lobe portion of the parotid gland at the site of the tumor origin.

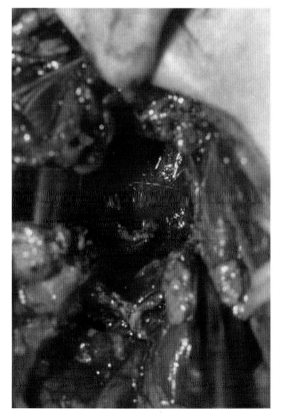

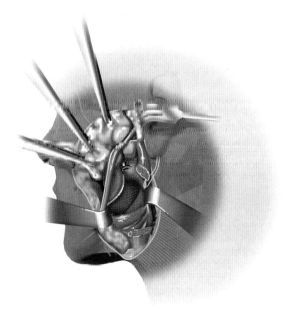

FIGURE 29.11 Tumor has been removed with exposure of the constrictor muscle and remaining tumor cavity.

and tumor spillage. Incomplete removal, especially with pleomorphic adenomas, will likely lead to tumor recurrence and the need for subsequent treatment. Subsequent surgery in the parapharyngeal space is much more difficult. There are often multiple tumors, and a long-standing problem begins with managing recurrent pleomorphic adenomas. Rupture of the tumor capsule can occur even with wide exposure. The thickness of the tumor capsule can be quite variable depending upon whether the tumor is mesenchymal or glandular. The glandular areas are often softer and easier to rupture. Rupture can occur due to inadvertent pressure of the tumor against the mandible, the styloid process, and the pterygoid plates or from failure to adequately remove a portion of the deep lobe near the site of the attachment point of the tumor. One must maximize exposure before any manipulation of the tumor is done.

If rupture does occur, one should remove all gross tumor and then thoroughly irrigate the wound. Even with rupture, it has been reported that recurrence occurs in only 10% of patients, but it can take 10 to 20 years to detect, and therefore, these numbers may rise with time.

Injury to the facial nerve is one of the most feared complications and should not occur if the surgeon knows where the nerve is located. If you know the location of the nerve, you should not injure it. It is often not appreciated how close the deep lobe component of the parapharyngeal tumor is to the main trunk of the facial nerve. Temporary mild paresis of the lower face can occur from mobilization of the marginal branch of the facial nerve, but this generally resolves in a short period of time.

First bite syndrome is a common occurrence with mobilization or division of the inferior portion or tail of the parotid gland. The exact etiology of this is indeterminate. First bite pain lasts for several seconds and then is gone. It may occur with only certain foods or beverages. Starting the meal with another type of food may prevent the pain. First bite pain generally lessens over time and is gone by 1 year.

Numbness of the ear lobe as a result of cutting the greater auricular nerve always occurs. However, in one year's time, secondary to an ingrowth of additional sensory nerves, the main area of numbness is the lobule of the ear. Hematomas, seromas, and infections are all lessened by meticulous hemostasis, antibiotics, Hemovac drains, and pressure dressings.

Damage to the carotid artery is rare with prestyloid lesions, but one has to be aware of the potential risk to the internal carotid artery in elderly individuals. Tortuous carotid arteries can extend to or through the floor of the parotid bed and contact the capsule of prestyloid tumors. Injury, in these cases, is possible. Hematoma and postoperative bleeding with parapharyngeal lesions can cause significant airway obstruction requiring emergency tracheostomy and necessary reexploration of the surgical site. Therefore, surgical care and attention to detail is mandatory.

Removal of a malignant prestyloid tumor with its attendant expanded excision and, when necessary, removal of surrounding structures, nerves, bone, muscle, vessels, and lymphatics all increase the risk of potential morbidity. The biggest risk remains tumor recurrence.

RESULTS

Prestyloid tumors that are benign have a low risk of recurrence if the exposure and principles described in the cervical–parotid approach are followed. Detection of recurrence, however, can be challenging, and patients have to be followed with yearly and then every other year imaging studies. A report detailing results in 68 patients with pleomorphic adenomas of the parapharyngeal space showed recurrences in only three patients. In cases in which the tumor was ruptured, recurrence may be detected over many years. For all cases of parapharyngeal lesions that were benign, in one reported series, time of recurrence was noted from 2 to 23 years with a median of 7 years. Factors associated with recurrence included prior open biopsies, tumor rupture, and incomplete removal. There clearly are unique challenges removing certain prestyloid lesions such as lymphovascular lesions and, of course, malignancies.

Patients with malignant tumors of the prestyloid parapharyngeal space generally do poorly, and their ultimate outcome is primarily determined by the histology and extent of the tumor. In one series of 35 cases of malignant tumors of the prestyloid space, recurrence or persistence was noted in 27, and ultimately, 63% died of their tumor. When recurrence does occur, death is likely in over 80%. In this series, only five patients were alive without disease at the time of last follow-up indicating the problems with late diagnosis, tumor extent, and significant morbidity with malignant lesions of the prestyloid space.

PEARLS

- For large tumors, maximizing the space to work in when mobilizing a tumor will reduce the risk of capsular rupture by retraction of the mandible, medialization of the lateral aspect of the submandibular gland, division of the stylomandibular ligament, division of the external carotid artery, division and reflection of the posterior belly of the digastric and stylohyoid muscle, and removal of a prominent styloid process.
- For dumbbell tumors that are palpable as a parotid mass and displace the facial nerve, the superficial lobe can be reflected anteriorly to isolate the nerve and then replaced after tumor resection.

- For most prestyloid tumors, only a small portion of the deep lobe of the parotid needs to be removed.
- Identification of the facial nerve will avoid injury to this structure.
- Always individualize the approach to the surgery in this area based upon the clinical behavior, size, imaging studies, and operative findings.
- In elderly patients, the internal carotid artery can be quite tortuous and extend through the floor of the parotid musculature and fascia of the prestyloid space to lie in close contact to the tumor. Careful review of imaging will aid avoidance of carotid injury to the carotid artery.
- The cervical–parotid approach can be extended retroauricularly for patients with skull base extension from involvement of the poststyloid portion of the parapharyngeal space. Further exposure of the parapharyngeal space can be done with a combined parasymphyseal mandibulotomy through a lip split incision.
- For small tumors, removal of the upper jugular nodes and isolation of the vessels are not necessary.
- Keep a Hemovac drain in place for 2 days to collapse dead space and reduce the risk of hematoma or infection.
- If a plane is not established easily around the borders of the tumor, with the exception of the attachment portion to the deep lobe, you should be concerned about malignancy or prior transoral biopsy.
- Treat a prestyloid parapharyngeal tumor like one would manage a palpable mass in the parotid gland.
- Awareness of the facial nerve will aid in removing the necessary deep lobe parotid tissue with the tumor.
- Frozen section pathology will aid in performing additional surgery, that is, a parotidectomy or neck dissection. This discussion should occur preoperatively with the patient. Additional surgery is easier to do at the time of the first operation than later.

PITFALLS

- Not identifying the facial nerve could lead to injury of this structure.
- Failure to always individualize the approach to the surgery in this area based upon the clinical behavior, size, imaging studies, and operative findings
- In elderly patients, the internal carotid artery can be quite tortuous and extend through the floor of the parotid musculature and fascia of the prestyloid space to lie in close contact to the tumor. Careful review of imaging will aid avoidance of injury to the carotid artery.
- Not keeping a Hemovac drain in place for 2 days to collapse dead space may increase the risk of seroma, hematoma, or infection.
- Biopsy of a tumor via an incisional transoral approach as opposed to a FNA may lead to the recurrence of the tumor.

SUGGESTED READING

Olsen KD. Tumors and surgery of the parapharyngeal space. *Laryngoscope* 1994;104:1–28.
Hughes KV, Olsen KD, McCaffrey TV. Parapharyngeal space neoplasms. *Head Neck* 1995;17:124–130.
Moore EJ, Olsen KD. Complications of surgery of the parapharyngeal space. In: Eisele DW, Smith RV, eds. *Complications in Head and Neck Surgery*. Philadelphia, PA: Mosby/Elsevier, 2009:241–250.
Bradley PJ, Bradley PT, Olsen KD. Update on the management of parapharyngeal tumours. *Curr Opin Otolaryngol Head Neck Surg* 2011;19:92–98.

EXCISION OF THE MASS IN THE BUCCAL SPACE

Eugene N. Myers

INTRODUCTION

Masses arising in the buccal space or in the accessory lobe of the parotid gland are uncommon and may present as a visible mass in the cheek or as a mass distorting the buccal mucosa. Since a wide variety of tumors arise in this area, a precise diagnosis is often difficult to make. A detailed history, clinical examination, and imaging studies are essential in defining the location and extent of these tumors. Although fine-needle aspiration biopsy (FNAB) may provide important diagnostic information, only complete excision of the mass with histopathologic evaluation will provide a definitive diagnosis.

Most of the tumors in the buccal space are benign and are of salivary gland origin. However, other types of benign as well as malignant tumors and other histologic types may arise in this area. Rarely, cancer metastatic from a distant site will present a challenge in diagnosis and management. Table 30.1 lists the lesions from our own experience and those reported in the literature. The operative techniques for removal of these tumors are challenging because the technique must provide good exposure for tumor removal in order to prevent damage to the facial nerve and Stensens duct and to assure a good cosmetic outcome.

HISTORY

The finding of a mass within the substance of the cheek poses a diagnostic problem since this may arise from many types of tissues present in the buccal space or may be metastatic from a distant site. A detailed history, clinical examination, and imaging studies are important in arriving at a specific diagnosis. However, the final diagnosis is often elusive and must be confirmed by surgical excision and histopathologic evaluation. Obviously, pain, infiltration of the overlying facial skin, and facial weakness suggest malignancy.

A mass in the buccal space presents in a unique fashion. These are readily apparent because they may be seen just deep to the skin of the cheek or in the buccal mucosa. The typical history encountered in such patients is that of a slowly growing, painless mass in the cheek, which disturbs facial symmetry. The mass is usually nontender and rarely is pain or facial nerve paralysis noted at the time of presentation. The mass may lie closer to the buccal mucosa so that the patient may discover the intraoral mass by feeling it with their tongue. In some patients, the mass interferes with their dentures fitting properly.

PHYSICAL EXAMINATION

A mass in the buccal space, which presents externally, should be inspected carefully, and the dimensions of the lesion should be measured and recorded. These lesions are typically nontender and should be evaluated by bimanual palpation. Stensens duct should be identified and an attempt should be made to express saliva from the duct. Detailed inspection of facial nerve function must be carried out. Any sign of weakness of the

TABLE 30.1 Lesions Reported in the Buccal Space

Glandular	Vascular	Lymph Node	Connective	Muscular	Inflammatory	Neural	Miscellanous
Accessory parotid or aberrant salivary gland tumors	False Aneurysm	Benign reactive lymph node	Alveolar soft part sarcoma	Masseteric hypertrophy	Abscess	Neurofibroma	Clear cell carcinoma metastatic from kidney
Acinic cell carcinoma	Hemangioma	Calcified lymph node	Fibroma	Myositis ossificans	Aspergilloma	Neuroma	Foreign body granuloma, for example, paraffinoma
Adenoid cystic carcinoma	Hyalinized thrombus	Lymphangioma	Fibromatosis		Polymorphous low-grade adeno-carcinoma		Kimura disease
Carcinoma ex pleomorphic adenoma	Recurrent juvenile nasopharyngeal angiofibroma	Lymphoma	Fibrosarcoma		Sarcoidosis		
Chronic sialadenitis		Lymphosarcoma	Lipoma		Tuberculous granuloma and adenoid cystic carcinoma presenting as a single mass in the buccal space		
Minor salivary gland calculus		Metastatic lymph node involvement	Liposarcoma				
Mixed tumors (benign and malignant)			Nodular fasciitis	Masseteric hypertrophy			
Mucoepidermoid carcinoma (low- and high-grade)			Pseudoherniation of buccal fat pad				
Oncocytoma			Rhabdomysarcoma				
Papillary cystadenoma lymphomatosum			Solitary fibrous tumor				
Parotid duct tumor or calculus			Spindle cell lipoma				
Sebaceous adenoma							

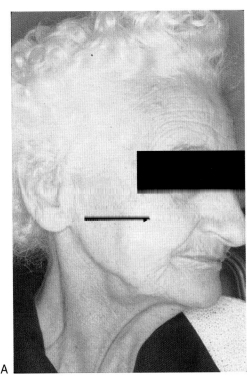
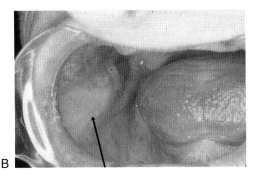

FIGURE 30.1 A: External view of a mass in the right buccal space mass. **B:** Note the intraoral bulge produced by the mass.

facial nerve should be recorded since this will have an impact on the plan for surgical management. Fixation of the skin, obstruction of Stensens duct, facial weakness, and pain are suggestive of a malignant tumor. In some instances, particularly in very thin individuals, the mass may be visible both externally and internally (Fig. 30.1).

INDICATIONS

A mass arising in the buccal space should be removed for definitive pathologic diagnosis. Removal of a mass in the buccal space should be considered an excisional biopsy, but, as such, the approach must be thorough since most of these lesions are benign and complete excision is both diagnostic and therapeutic and should be curative. Simply exposing the tumor and taking a biopsy only invites spillage of tumor into the wound and sets the stage for seeding of the wound and potential recurrence.

CONTRAINDICATIONS

There are no contraindications to surgery based upon the local factors; however, comorbidities, such as severe cardiovascular disease, markedly debilitated or demented patients, or patients with end-stage renal or pulmonary disease, will probably not benefit by excision of these tumors. If the tumor involves the skin or buccal mucosa or facial nerve, malignancy would be suspected, and in such cases, ultrasound-guided FNAB may help in achieving a diagnosis necessary to plan for palliative treatment.

PREOPERATIVE PLANNING

Imaging Studies

Imaging studies should be carried out because often times they provide valuable information that can help in the differential diagnosis of a mass in the buccal space. Both CT and MR scanning are used in the evaluation of the mass in the buccal space. Detailed studies by Kurabayashi et al. evaluated a large series of patients by CT and MR. The CT images were assessed for the number, location, internal architecture, and margin of the lesions and their relationship to surrounding structures. Their study concluded that while CT was useful in demonstrating the presence and location of the mass in the buccal space, it had limited value in differentiating benign from malignant tumors. Only 7 out of 11 malignant tumors in their study were correctly identified. Kurabayashi et al.

also studied a series of 30 patients with benign and malignant lesions in the buccal space using MRI. The authors concluded that MRI was useful in demonstrating the extent of lesions in the buccal space because of its excellent soft tissue contrast; however, the sensitivity of predicting malignancy was only 29%.

PET–CT scan can also be useful in defining the location of the lesions and in forming the differential diagnosis and, in the case of malignant tumors, can also aid in demonstrating distant metastases. No large series of cases evaluated by PET–CT scanning exists.

Fine-Needle Aspiration Biopsy

The role of FNAB in the evaluation of a mass in the cheek is another tool in the evaluation of a mass in the buccal space. While some authors have found it useful, it may also be misleading and have certain disadvantages. Several disadvantages have been pointed out such as possible damage to the facial nerve, hemorrhage, introduction of infection, and scarring of tissue planes around the facial nerve, thereby increasing the chances of damage to the facial nerve during surgery. The complications can be minimized using image guidance for this procedure. Under no circumstance should a core biopsy be taken due to the potential for damage to the facial nerve.

I do not advocate routine FNAB in the evaluation of a mass in the buccal space since it really does not alter the management. Complete excision with definitive diagnosis based upon permanent section histopathology should be the standard approach.

SURGICAL TECHNIQUE

Many external surgical approaches to tumors of the buccal space have been described. However, the most commonly used approach to the lesion is a direct intraoral, transmucosal incision with dissection and removal of the mass. This approach is appealing because the bulging of the tumor into the intraoral area would seem to lend itself to easy excision and eliminates an external scar. However, while this may seem advantageous and is quicker owing to less dissection, it does not provide adequate exposure of the branches of the facial nerve and Stensens duct and is to be discouraged. Complications arising from intraoral excision include temporary or permanent facial nerve weakness or paralysis and a sialocele resulting from transection of Stensens duct.

There is no need to identify the main trunk of the facial nerve, dissect each branch, or do a parotidectomy since these masses are located anterior to the anterior border of the parotid gland. I have designed the extended parotid submandibular incision approach to remove tumors of the buccal space and accessory lobe of the parotid gland. This approach eliminates the problems found with previously described incisions. It also provides excellent exposure and minimizes the risk of the most common complications such as injury to Stensens duct and the facial nerve. I have found that this technique also provides an excellent cosmetic result because most of the incision is placed in natural skin folds. For those patients who desire almost complete camouflage of the excision, a modified rhytidectomy incision can be used. Following the doctrine of informed consent, the operation is described to and discussed with the patient prior to surgery, and I explain that the buccal branch of the facial nerve is usually incorporated into the capsule of the tumor or lies adjacent to the tumor and is therefore vulnerable to intraoperative injury with postoperative weakness or paralysis possible due to direct injury or stretching of the nerve during the dissection. I use an intraoperative facial nerve stimulator, which facilitates the accurate identification of the facial nerve and its branches. The surgeon should have a detailed knowledge of the anatomy of the buccal space, the contents of which include the branches of the buccal branch of the facial nerve, Stensens duct, the facial artery and vein, and the lymphatic structures (Fig. 30.2).

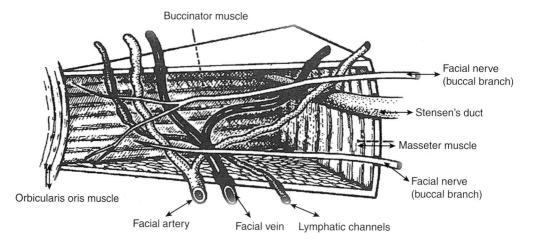

FIGURE 30.2

Schematic illustration in oblique lateral view of the left buccal space and its contents.

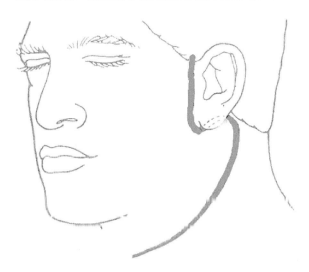

FIGURE 30.3 Extended parotid–submandibular incision.

Description of Technique

The patient is placed under general endotracheal anesthesia without paralytic agents. The endotracheal tube is secured in the oral commissure contralateral to the side of surgery. The patient is prepped and draped with the hemiface exposed. Ointment is placed in both eyes and the eyelids contralateral to the surgical site are taped shut. No sutures or tape is placed on the eye in the operative field. I do not usually use facial nerve monitoring since only branches of the buccal branch of the facial nerve are at risk and can readily be identified.

The incision is the usual parotidectomy incision modified only by extending it approximately 2 cm superiorly and 2 to 3 cm anteriorly in the submandibular skin crease. Extending the skin incision in this manner allows dissection more anteriorly than would be possible with the usual incision. The incision is placed in natural skin folds to camouflage the scar (Fig. 30.3). To make the incision, I use a needle tip electrocautery set on coagulation, which provides a dry field. Skin hooks are inserted and the skin is undermined sharply off the superficial musculoaponeurotic system (SMAS) using a no. 15 blade staying in a plane between the subcutaneous tissue and the SMAS. Bleeding is rarely encountered. As the dissection proceeds anteriorly, right angle retractors are used to retract the skin anteriorly in order to identify the mass. Dissection is carried to the anterior border of the mass. Once the anterior border of the mass has been reached, a nerve stimulator is used to locate the buccal branches of the facial nerve. There are usually two branches associated with the mass, which may be incorporated into the capsule of the tumor (Fig. 30.4) or may be located either superior or inferior to the mass. After the nerve is identified with the nerve stimulator, the soft tissue surrounding the nerve is dissected off the mass with a small blunt tip scissors. The nerve is skeletonized anteriorly and posteriorly and mobilized off of the tumor.

Once mobilization of the nerve(s) is complete, sharp and blunt dissection is used with the blunt tip scissors to separate the capsule of the tumor from the surrounding soft tissues. A small nerve retractor is used to retract the nerves off the tumor and arterial loops are placed around them. The nerves are mobilized. Stensens duct is medial in the buccal mucosa and is not identified with this approach. Once the tumor has been mobilized from the surrounding soft tissue, it is removed, and before the specimen is sent to pathology, a suture is placed in the mass for orientation. The nerves are returned to their normal anatomic position.

Removal of the tumor leaves a noticeable defect in the facial contour, which I eliminate by approximating the SMAS over the defect. Hemostasis is obtained. The wound is irrigated and closed in layers over a Hemovac drain brought out just adjacent to the postauricular aspect of the incision. I use 3-0 chromic catgut subcutaneous and 6-0 fast-absorbing catgut in the skin. Steri-Strips are applied to support the wound. A gauze pressure dressing is applied.

Rhytidectomy Approach

Mitz and Peyronie, in 1976, described the rhytidectomy approach and how this technique allows for reconstruction of the contour defect associated with tumor extirpation using the SMAS interposition. The incision employed in these cases is the one used for cosmetic rhytidectomy (Fig. 30.5). The incision begins at the temple and continues in a preauricular crease and then along the posterior aspect of the tragus. The incision is carried inferior to the ear lobe and up to the level of the posterior auricularis muscle and posteriorly into the hairline. The skin is undermined anterior to the tumor, mobilized, and retracted away from the tumor.

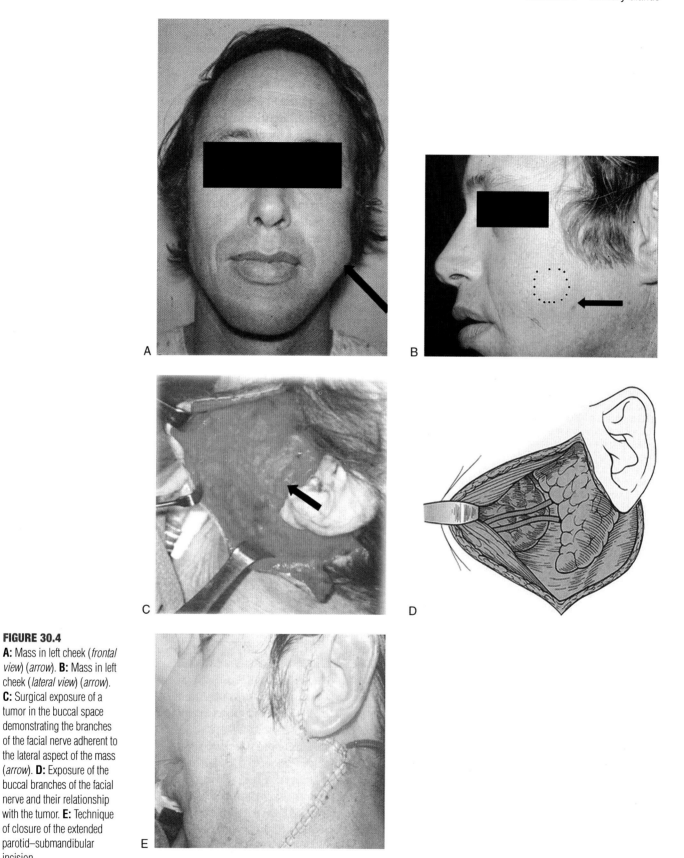

FIGURE 30.4
A: Mass in left cheek (*frontal view*) (*arrow*). **B:** Mass in left cheek (*lateral view*) (*arrow*). **C:** Surgical exposure of a tumor in the buccal space demonstrating the branches of the facial nerve adherent to the lateral aspect of the mass (*arrow*). **D:** Exposure of the buccal branches of the facial nerve and their relationship with the tumor. **E:** Technique of closure of the extended parotid–submandibular incision.

The tumor is then excised as described above. After removal of the tumor, the SMAS is closed directly to give sufficient support to the cheek to avoid deformity. Rotation of a flap of SMAS has been recommended for defects that are too large for direct closure or advancement closure. This technique distributes the volume defect over a wider area and makes the depression less noticeable. Postoperative care is the same as for the parotid submandibular approach.

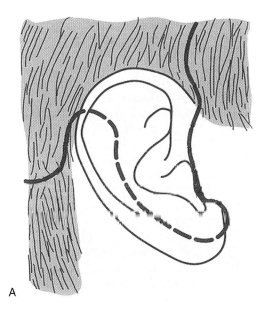

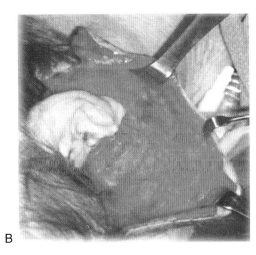

A

B

FIGURE 30.5
A: Standard rhytidectomy incision. **B:** Skin flap elevated to the anterior border of the mass.

POSTOPERATIVE CARE

The Hemovac is attached to suction. Proper functioning of the Hemovac must be monitored by the nursing staff. The pressure dressing and drain are removed on the first postoperative day, and the patient is discharged. Steri-Strips and sutures are removed in 5 to 7 days.

COMPLICATIONS

The most common perioperative complication is a hematoma occurring with a frequency of 1% to 15%. I have had one hematoma in our series of cases. Other important potential complications include injury to the facial nerve, parotid gland, or Stensens duct, which may result in facial asymmetry, parotid sialocele, or parotid fistula. Care must be taken in undermining the superior aspect of the flap because the zygomatic branch of the upper division of the facial nerve is superficial in this area and the branch could be injured with resultant facial nerve paralysis.

Complications can be minimized by excellent exposure, meticulous dissection, and identification of important structures, which is exactly why I use the parotid–submandibular approach. My motivation to design the extended parotid–submandibular incision to provide excellent exposure resulted from an experience I had of providing postoperative care for a patient who had a buccal space mass removed through an incision in the buccal mucosa, sustaining injury to the facial nerve and developing a sialocele in the buccal space due to inadvertent injury to Stensens duct, all of which took several months to resolve. The resultant technique prevents such an injury.

RESULTS

Masses arising in the buccal space are usually common tumors that present in an unusual site. Clinical examination and radiologic correlation provide valuable information regarding the location and extent of these tumors. FNAB may provide additional information in certain cases. However, the only way to characterize these masses is by excision and pathologic evaluation. Surgery is both diagnostic and usually curative with these tumors. The parotid–submandibular technique is a systematic, versatile, and cosmetically acceptable approach that provides excellent exposure to the buccal space and allows identification and protection of the branches of the facial nerve. I have had no recurrences or serious complications in our two series.

Two patients are worthy of mention. One patient had a lymphoma. She was referred to medical oncology for further evaluation and treatment. The second patient presented with a mass in the cheek. MRI revealed a well-circumscribed mass in the accessory lobe of the parotid. Excision of this mass through the parotid–submandibular approach was uneventful. However, the pathology report indicated that this was metastatic renal cell carcinoma. MRI of the abdomen revealed the primary tumor in the kidney, which was subsequently removed surgically.

PEARLS

● Rigorous evaluation and treatment planning including imaging studies are essential prior to surgical management.
● Educating the patient regarding postoperative appearance and possible complications is critical.
● Undermine in the plane between the subcutaneous tissue and the SMAS.
● Begin to look for the branches of the buccal branch of the facial nerve once the soft tissues have been undermined to the anterior border of the parotid gland.
● Identify the branches of the facial nerve using the nerve stimulator and dissect them off of the tumor.
● Retract the branches of the nerve away from the tumor in order to excise it without injury to the nerve.
● Closing the SMAS will prevent an unsightly depression in the cheek.

PITFALLS

● Lack of exposure of the mass of the buccal branch of the facial nerve may lead to permanent damage to the facial nerve.
● Damage to Stensens duct will result in sialocele.

INSTRUMENTS TO HAVE AVAILABLE

● Standard parotidectomy tray
● Small sharp/blunt Senn retractors
● Nerve retractors
● Facial nerve stimulator

SUGGESTED READING

Gallia L, Rood SR, Myers EN. Management of buccal space masses. *Otolaryngol Head Neck Surg* 1981;89:221–225.
Rodgers GK, Myers EN. Surgical management of the mass in the buccal space. *Laryngoscope* 1988;98:749–753.
Madorsky SJ, Allison GR. Management of buccal space tumors by rhytidectomy approach with superficial musculoaponeurotic system reconstruction. *Am J Otolaryngol* 1999;20:51–55.
Kurabayashi T, Ida M, Tetsumura A, et al. MR imaging of benign and malignant lesions in the buccal space. *Dentomaxillofac Radiol* 2002;31:344–349.
Kim HC, Han MH, Moon MH, et al. CT and MR imaging of the buccal space: normal anatomy and abnormalities. *Korean J Radiol* 2005;6:22–30.
Walvekar RR, Myers EN. Management of the mass in the buccal space. In: Myers EN, Ferris RL, eds. *Salivary Gland Disorders*. Springer, Heidelburg 2007;17:281–294.

31 EXCISION OF THE SUBMANDIBULAR GLAND

Randal S. Weber

INTRODUCTION

The principal reasons for excision of the submandibular gland are the presence of refractory sialadenitis or the concern for neoplasia. Prior to embarking upon excision of the submandibular gland, it is incumbent upon the surgeon to ascertain the diagnosis of the salivary gland pathology present so that the surgery may be tailored appropriately. Submandibular sialadenitis may be idiopathic or secondary to chronic sialolithiasis. Neoplasia, on the other hand, comprises a wide spectrum of heterogeneous tumors that may be benign or malignant.

A detailed history and physical examination are important for differentiating chronic inflammatory disease from a neoplasm. Preoperative imaging studies and the use of fine-needle aspiration biopsy will provide diagnostic information for achieving the appropriate preoperative diagnosis.

The surgical approach is quite different depending upon whether the surgeon is dealing with a chronic inflammatory process or neoplasia. To avoid inappropriate or inadequate surgery, the surgeon must achieve a working diagnosis prior to excision. Table 31.1 displays our experience with tumors of the submandibular gland and the histologic spectrum of malignancy. Benign neoplasms include pleomorphic adenoma, monomorphic adenoma and benign lymphoepithelial lesion.

For a chronic inflammatory process, an extracapsular dissection and a capsular excision of the submandibular gland is adequate, whereas for suspected neoplasia, the minimal surgical procedure should be a complete dissection of levels IA and IB. Thus, appropriate preoperative planning and differentiating between sialadenitis and neoplasia of the submandibular gland are critical to avoid an inadequate operation should a neoplasm be the underlying pathology.

HISTORY

A complete history will assist the clinician in achieving the correct diagnosis. For patients with chronic sial adenitis, typical symptoms includes intermittent swelling of the submandibular gland often exacerbated by eating or drinking. Over time, the gland may become firm, fibrotic, and chronically painful. There may be a history of sialoliths that have been removed transorally. In severe cases of sialadenitis, abscess formation may have occurred in the past. Conversely, in patients with submandibular gland neoplasia, gradual enlargement is typical. For instance, in patients with a pleomorphic adenoma of the submandibular gland, enlargement may have occurred over several years. For those with malignant tumors, progressive enlargement generally occurs over a shorter interval. Pain may be a symptom in patients with an acute relapse of sialadenitis. For patients with benign neoplasms of the submandibular gland, pain is an uncommon symptom. In up to 20% of patients with malignant tumors of the submandibular gland, pain may be constant and progressive. Cranial nerve palsies, including weakness of the lower lip, numbness of the tongue or paresthesias, and paralysis of the hemitongue, may occur in patients with malignant tumors. Inquiry into the presence or absence of these symptoms is important.

TABLE 31.1 Histologic Distribution of Submandibular Gland Carcinomas

N = 82 patients	
Histology	**Number**
Adenoid cystic	49/82 (59.8%)
Mucoepidermoid	13/82 (15.9%)
Adenocarcinoma	5/82 (6.1%)
Squamous cell	1/82 (1.2%)
Undifferentiated	3/82 (3.7%)
Acinic cell	1/82 (1.2%)
Lymphoepithelioma	1/82 (1.2%)
Carcinoma ex pleomorphic adenoma	1/82 (1.2%)
Other	2/82 (2.4%)

PHYSICAL EXAMINATION

Physical examination for patients with submandibular gland enlargement should include inspection and palpation of the neck as well as the oral cavity. The size and consistency of the gland should be documented, as should the presence or absence of tenderness and whether or not the gland is mobile. The important cranial nerves assessed include the marginal mandibular branch of the facial nerve; the lingual nerve, which provides sensation to the ipsilateral oral tongue; and the hypoglossal nerve, which provides motor innervation. Involvement of the hypoglossal nerve may be manifest by atrophy of the hemitongue, fasciculations, or deviation on protrusion of the tongue to the side of the paralysis. The presence or absence of trismus should be assessed and, if present, is indicative of invasion of the medial pterygoid muscle. With the mouth open, the submandibular gland should be palpated and massaged to determine if saliva can be expressed from the Wharton duct. Bimanual palpation of the floor of the mouth and submandibular gland is important and may indicate the presence of a stone in the submandibular duct. Bimanual palpation will also provide an estimate as to the size of the gland, an indication as to fixation of the gland to the mandible or surrounding structures. Palpation for enlarged lymph nodes is critical and, if adenopathy is present, supports the presence of malignancy. The presence of lymphadenopathy in the upper neck should raise a concern that one is dealing with a malignant tumor of the submandibular gland, especially if present in level I along with enlargement of the gland.

INDICATIONS

Surgery for excision of the submandibular gland has two broad indications. The first is for chronic inflammatory disease that includes certain patients with sialoliths, and the second is for suspected neoplasia. In patients with chronic inflammatory disease, repeated painful swelling of the gland during stimulated salivation is usually not alleviated by medical treatment, and surgical excision should be considered. These patients may or may not have sialoliths. Occasionally salivary stones are in the most proximal portion of the Wharton duct and are not amenable to removal with sialendoscopy or sialodochotomy. In these cases, excision of the gland and the proximal portion of the duct harboring the stone is indicated. For patients with a history of submandibular gland infection and abscess, excision should be performed following an interval to allow the acute inflammation to subside.

Patients with suspected neoplasia should be considered for surgery. The minimal surgery for a neoplasm of the submandibular gland is a level I dissection that removes the gland and the facial lymph nodes. Enucleation of the gland should be avoided in these cases to avoid incomplete excision of tumor.

CONTRAINDICATIONS

A contraindication to surgical removal of the submandibular gland for patients with either salivary stone or chronic inflammatory disease is lack of adequate conservative therapy. Stone removal by endoscopic or transoral procedures should be performed as a first step when feasible. For recurring sialadenitis, hydration, oral antibiotics, and sialogogues should be given a trial to alleviate symptoms. When neoplasia is suspected, the principal contraindication to surgical removal would be the patient's inability to tolerate general anesthesia.

PREOPERATIVE PLANNING

Imaging Studies

Imaging studies may be performed prior to excision of the gland. A computed tomography (CT) scan with contrast will provide information regarding involvement of the mandible, the presence or absence of pathologic lymphadenopathy, and the local extent of the tumor. Submandibular sialoliths are radiopaque in 80% of patients when present. The gland may demonstrate enlargement and diffuse enhancement in cases of chronic inflammatory disease. As with parotid neoplasms, imaging lacks specificity for differentiating benign from malignant tumors. Magnetic resonance imaging (MRI) scanning will provide soft tissue detail superior to CT scans and may demonstrate enhancement of the lingual or hypoglossal nerves or enlargement of the neural structures that would raise suspicion for malignancy. At times, both modalities may be helpful when evaluating a patient with a malignant tumor.

Fine-Needle Aspiration Biopsy

Fine-needle aspiration biopsy is a useful tool for differentiating chronic inflammatory disease from neoplasia. In patients with chronic sialadenitis, cytologic examination will typically demonstrate the presence of acute and chronic inflammatory cells. In contrast, however, fine-needle aspiration for patients with neoplasms will demonstrate the presence of neoplastic cells, but differentiating benign from malignant tumors is more difficult. Nevertheless, an experienced cytopathologist will accurately differentiate inflammation from neoplasia in 85% to 90% of cases. Ultrasound-guided fine-needle aspiration biopsy should be employed when anatomic imaging demonstrates areas of heterogeneity in the gland suspicious for neoplasia. This will improve the accuracy and the diagnostic utility of fine-needle aspiration biopsy. Finally, if enlarged lymph nodes were present, fine-needle aspiration biopsy may confirm the presence of regional metastasis.

Table 31.2 provides an algorithm for differentiating benign inflammatory conditions from a neoplastic process.

Informed Consent

Prior to embarking on surgery, the risks of the procedure should be carefully explained to the patient. The usual risk factors include general anesthesia, bleeding, and infection. Due to the proximity of important cranial nerves in the operative field, the patient should be apprised of the possibility of weakness of the lower lip, numbness of the tongue, or paralysis of the tongue on the operated side due to injury to the marginal mandibular, lingual, and hypoglossal nerves, respectively.

SURGICAL TECHNIQUE

The surgical approach differs depending upon the diagnosis of sialadenitis versus neoplasia. The former requires a limited incision and essentially an extracapsular removal of the submandibular gland with preservation of all nerves in the region. Conversely if one is excising either a benign or malignant neoplasm,

TABLE 31.2 Differentiating Neoplasia From Chronic Sialadenitis		
	Neoplasm	**Sialadenitis**
Swelling	Progressive (slow/rapid)	Intermittent
Fever	None	Acute suppurative
Lymphadenopathy	20%–30% (malignant only)	Rare (reactive)
Pain	Malignant tumors (20%)	With infection/during meals
Cranial nerve deficits	Lingual/hypoglossal nerves	None
Plain radiographs	Intraglandular calcifications (pleomorphic adenoma)	Sialoliths (80% radiopaque)
CT/MRI	Mass/soft tissue extension, bone, nerve involvement, poorly defined margins	Enlarged gland w/o mass
Fine-needle aspirate	Positive or suspicious for tumor	Negative for tumor

the incision should be more generous, since the basic surgical procedure is a dissection of level I. In an operation for chronic sialadenitis, it is important to remove the entire gland, including any sialoliths that may be present in the submandibular duct, and all adjacent nerves should be preserved. When operating for neoplasia, all uninvolved nerves should be spared; however, the lymph nodes in levels IA and IB and the entire submandibular gland should be removed. The anatomic boundaries of the level I dissection are from the medial edge of the contralateral anterior belly of the digastric muscle anteriorly including the submental lymph nodes. The inferior limit of the dissection is the digastric tendon. Posteriorly the limit extends to the posterior belly of the digastric muscle. Within level IA, the facial lymph nodes as well as lymph nodes anterior to the mylohyoid muscle that drain the floor of the mouth should be included along with submandibular gland.

Gland Excision for Chronic Sialadenitis

General anesthesia is used without paralytic agents. The patient is placed on a transverse shoulder roll to extend the neck and to facilitate dissection. The ipsilateral neck is prepped and draped including the entire submental region with the corner of the mouth exposed. For chronic sialadenitis, the entire submandibular gland is removed in an extracapsular plane without the need for lymphadenectomy. The appropriate incision is made two fingerbreadths below the angle of the mandible in a natural skin crease and approximately 4 to 5 cm in length. The skin may be infiltrated with 1% Xylocaine 1–100,000 epinephrine for hemostasis. The skin incision is deepened through the platysma muscle. The superior skin flap is elevated to the edge of the mandible with care being taken to avoid incising the superficial layer of the deep cervical fascia. By leaving the fascia undisturbed, the marginal mandibular nerve will be protected. The inferior flap is elevated below the inferior edge of the submandibular gland. Next, at the inferior edge of the submandibular gland, the superficial layer of the deep cervical fascia is incised. The fascia is elevated to the superior edge of the submandibular gland and just below the inferior border of the mandible. At the superior edge of the submandibular gland, adipose and areolar tissue are present. Within this adipose tissue lies the marginal mandibular nerve, the facial artery and vein, and lymph nodes. The facial artery and vein are ligated close to the superior aspect of the gland with care being taken not to injure the marginal mandibular nerve, which lies more superiorly and has been elevated within the superficial layer of the deep cervical fascia. Once the facial vessels are ligated, the gland is dissected inferiorly exposing the mylohyoid muscle. The inferior edge of the mylohyoid muscle is retracted anteriorly in order to identify the lingual nerve. The submandibular ganglion is identified, isolated, clamped, and ligated just inferior to the lingual nerve. Just anterior to the ganglion and coursing from inferior to superior toward the floor of the mouth is the submandibular duct. This structure should be carefully palpated to exclude the presence of sialoliths. If these are present, they should be stripped inferiorly before ligating the duct. The duct is ligated as close to the floor of the mouth as possible. Just deep to the submandibular duct and anterior to the hyoglossus muscle is the hypoglossal nerve. Prior to ligating the duct, the nerve is identified, but the venae comitantes that course with the hypoglossal nerve should be avoided to prevent troublesome bleeding. The gland is now free of its attachments and can be reflected posteriorly. At the posterior inferior edge of the gland, the facial vein may be encountered and may be retracted or ligated as necessary. The main trunk of the facial artery will be found at the superior edge of the posterior belly of the digastric muscle where branches enter the submandibular gland. At times, the main trunk of the facial artery is intimately associated with the submandibular gland. The main trunk of the facial artery is ligated with a 2-0 silk suture proximal to where the vessel enters the substance of the gland. The gland is removed and sent for pathologic analysis. The wound is carefully inspected for any bleeding, hemostasis is obtained, and the wound is thoroughly irrigated. A small suction drain is placed through a separate stab wound inferior to the inferior aspect of the incision. The incision is closed by first approximating the platysma muscle with 3-0 Vicryl interrupted sutures, and then the skin is closed with a subcuticular absorbable monofilament suture. The suture line is reinforced with Steri-Strips oriented in a vertical fashion. The patient can be discharged home with the drain, which should be removed the following day.

Gland Excision for Neoplasia

The minimal procedure for excision of the submandibular gland when a neoplasm is suspected is a level IA and IB dissection. This procedure is analogous to superficial parotidectomy as the minimal procedure for tumors of the parotid gland. Shelling out the submandibular gland when a neoplasm is present risks leaving gross disease or a microscopically positive margin, thus requiring additional surgery or postoperative radiation for malignant tumors and a higher risk for recurrence in cases of pleomorphic adenoma.

The following is a description of the surgical technique for excision of a submandibular gland neoplasm. The patient is supine, placed under general anesthesia with a transverse shoulder roll present to extend the neck. The neck and face are prepped and draped in the usual fashion with the neck, submental area, and

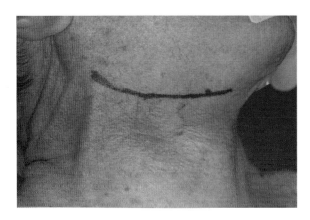

FIGURE 31.1 Transverse incision below the horizontal ramus of the mandible.

corner of the mouth exposed. A 6- to 7-cm incision is marked out in a natural skin crease extending from the anterior border of the sternocleidomastoid muscle to the submental region (Fig. 31.1). The incision is placed at least two fingerbreadths below the edge of the mandible. The skin and platysma are incised, and the flap is elevated superiorly to the inferior border of the mandible (Fig. 31.2). The inferior flap is elevated below the submandibular gland. If the platysma is infiltrated by tumor, the flaps should be elevated in the subcutaneous plane with sacrifice of the platysma muscle. Once the flaps are elevated and secured, the marginal mandibular branch of the facial nerve is identified and elevated superiorly with gentle traction to just above the inferior edge of the mandible (Fig. 31.3). The facial lymph nodes, which lie at the inferior border of the mandible, will be included in the dissection. Next, the facial artery and vein are identified, clamped, cut, and ligated just inferior to the marginal mandibular nerve (Figs. 31.4 and 31.5). The lateral aspects of the submandibular gland, the facial vessels, and the facial lymph nodes are reflected inferiorly with skeletonization of the mylohyoid muscle to its inferior edge just above the digastric tendon (Fig. 31.6). All of the adipose and areolar tissue should be included so that the muscle is visible.

The submental region is dissected next by first skeletonizing the medial edge of the contralateral anterior belly of the digastric muscle. The submental lymph nodes are reflected inferiorly from the lower edge of the mentum exposing the underlying mylohyoid muscle in the submental triangle. The specimen is reflected toward the ipsilateral anterior belly of the digastric that is also skeletonized. The level IA specimen is dissected posteriorly and kept in continuity with the level IB tissue. Once this is completed, a Richardson retractor is used to retract the mylohyoid muscle superiorly and anteriorly, exposing the lingual nerve and the deeper portion of the submandibular gland. If nerves or muscles are infiltrated or encased by tumor, they should be resected en bloc with the gland. With the lingual nerve exposed, the submandibular ganglion is clamped, cut, and ligated. If perineural invasion is suspected, the ganglion can be sent for frozen section to exclude the presence of tumor infiltration. The submandibular duct is then identified and followed anteriorly and superiorly. The duct is ligated and the surrounding portion of the submandibular gland is reflected inferiorly with the attached specimen (Figs. 31.7 and 31.8). Prior to ligating the duct, the hypoglossal nerve should be identified deep to the duct and preserved if uninvolved by tumor (Fig. 31.9). The specimen is now reflected posteriorly, where it remains tethered by the proximal portion of the facial artery. The artery is cross-clamped, cut, and ligated. The wound is copiously irrigated and a suction drain is placed. The wound is closed in multiple layers (Figs. 31.10 and 31.11). Pressure dressings should be avoided since they can mask an expanding hematoma and are of dubious value in preventing postoperative bleeding.

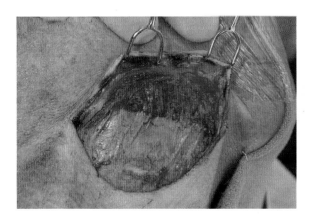

FIGURE 31.2 Subplatysmal flap elevation. The superficial layer of the deep cervical fascia remains intact.

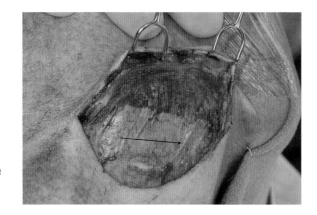

FIGURE 31.3
The arrow indicates the marginal mandibular nerve that is visible just deep to the superficial layer of the deep cervical fascia.

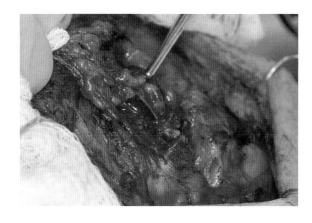

FIGURE 31.4
The facial artery is ligated at the inferior edge of the mandible.

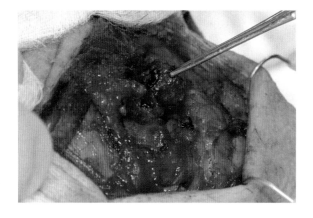

FIGURE 31.5
The facial lymph nodes are reflected inferiorly with the lateral portion of the submandibular gland.

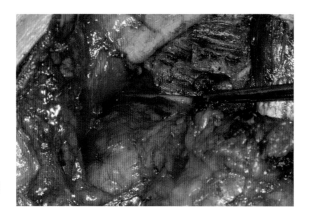

FIGURE 31.6
The anterior belly of the digastric muscle and the mylohyoid muscle are skeletonized. The nerve to the mylohyoid muscle is indicated by the tip of the forceps.

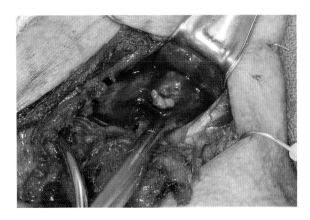

FIGURE 31.7 The submandibular duct has been ligated. The submandibular ganglion is indicated by the tip of the clamp.

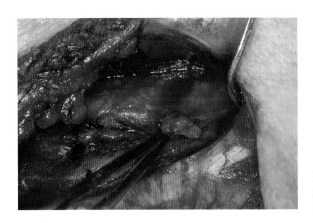

FIGURE 31.8 The submandibular duct and the ganglion have been ligated. The lingual nerve is visible coursing from posterior to anterior.

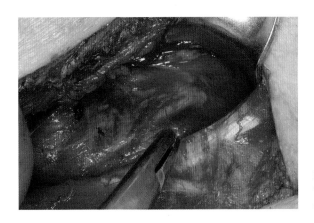

FIGURE 31.9 The hypoglossal nerve is visible on the surface of the hyoglossus muscle. The nerve is deep to the submandibular duct that has been ligated.

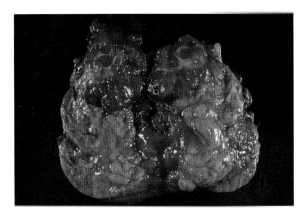

FIGURE 31.10 The gland has been removed and bisected demonstrating the neoplasm on the superior aspect of the gland.

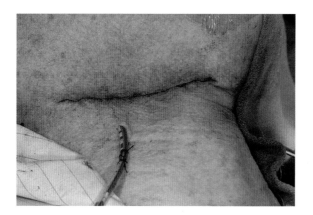

FIGURE 31.11
The wound has been closed
with a subcuticular suture,
and the drain is brought
out through a separate stab
wound.

POSTOPERATIVE CARE

If the patient is kept overnight, the suction drain may be removed the next morning and the patient discharged home. The patient is seen in the office 1 week later, and the pathology report is discussed. Should the pathologic analysis identify a malignant process, the need for radiation or other adjunctive therapy versus observation is discussed at that time.

COMPLICATIONS

Complications of this procedure are rare but include hemorrhage, infection, and nerve injury. Bleeding may be secondary to a branch of the facial artery that was not ligated adequately or may be of venous origin. Arterial bleeding can result in swelling of the floor of the mouth and airway obstruction. Patients with an early postoperative hematoma should be returned to the operating room immediately for exploration of the neck and identification of the bleeding source. Weakness of the lower lip may occur due to neuropraxia of the marginal mandibular nerve but should resolve spontaneously if the nerve is anatomically intact. Inadvertent injury of the lingual or hypoglossal nerves is rare, provided that the nerves are properly identified and protected when the gland is excised.

RESULTS

A good outcome is expected following gland excision for sialolithiasis or chronic inflammatory disease. A recurrent problem is encountered when the surgeon fails to remove a distal portion of the submandibular duct that contains a stone. Subsequent abscess can occur in this setting and may require a transoral incision of the duct, abscess drainage, and stone removal. For benign salivary gland tumors completely excised, tumor recurrence is rare unless spillage has occurred at the time of resection. Local regional control among patients with malignant disease is determined by factors such as: margin status, tumor grade, lymph node metastasis, extraglandular spread, and perineural invasion. With adequate surgery and appropriate use of adjuvant radiation, local-regional failures are rare and occur in <10% of patients. In patients with adenoid cystic carcinoma, local-regional control is excellent, but patients may develop distant metastasis 5 to 10 years after initial treatment.

PEARLS

- The history and physical examination are critical for differentiating chronic sialadenitis versus neoplastic disease arising within the submandibular gland. The former is chronic and progressive, associated with sialolithiasis, and exacerbated by meals, while the latter is progressive glandular enlargement. Hallmarks of malignant disease include pain, skin fixation, cranial nerve involvement, and lymphadenopathy.
- Preoperative imaging is a critical adjunct to physical examination. A neoplasm will often be heterogeneous and may demonstrate normal-appearing gland with a tumor arising from the gland parenchyma.
- Ultrasound-guided fine-needle aspiration biopsy provides accurate cytologic evidence for neoplasia in 85% to 90% of cases, but final diagnosis always requires histologic confirmation.
- Extracapsular dissection of the gland for chronic sialadenitis is an adequate procedure. The marginal mandibular branch of the facial, lingual, and hypoglossal nerves is routinely preserved.

- Analogous to superficial parotidectomy for parotid tumors, in cases of neoplasia, the minimum procedure for neoplasms arising within the submandibular gland is dissection of levels IA and IB to include the gland and adjacent lymph nodes. "Shelling out" the gland in these cases is discouraged, and it risks leaving gross disease or a microscopically positive margin, requiring additional surgery or postoperative radiation.
- Invasion of adjacent muscles or cranial nerves in cases of malignant disease mandates resection of these structures. Every attempt should be made to excise all gross disease.

PITFALLS

- Failure to preoperatively differentiate inflammatory disease from neoplasia can lead to an inappropriate surgical strategy.
- While extracapsular dissection is adequate for chronic sialadenitis, when neoplasia is suspected, the minimum surgical procedure should be dissection of level I to include the entire gland and facial lymph nodes.
- Variably a lymph node exists on the lateral aspect of the mylohyoid muscle, just posterior and inferior to the attachment of the anterior belly of the digastric muscle to the lower edge of the mandible. This is a primary echelon lymph node for submandibular gland malignancies and should be included in a complete level I dissection.
- Inadequate surgery for a submandibular gland malignancy where gross disease is left behind will increase the patient's risk for local failure and decreased survival.

INSTRUMENTS TO HAVE AVAILABLE

- Fine mosquito clamps
- McCabe dissector
- Small Richardson retractor
- DeBakey forceps

SUGGESTED READING

Weber RS, Byers RM, Petit B, et al. Submandibular gland tumors. Adverse histologic factors and therapeutic implications. *Arch Otolaryngol Head Neck Surg* 1990;116(9):1055–1060.

Garden AS, Weber RS, Morrison WH, et al. The influence of positive margins and nerve invasion in adenoid cystic carcinoma of the head and neck treated with surgery and radiation. *Int J Radiat Oncol Biol Phys* 1995;32(3):619–626.

Stewart CJ, MacKenzie K, McGarry GW, et al. Fine-needle aspiration cytology of salivary gland: a review of 341 cases. *Diagn Cytopathol* 2000;22(3):139–146.

Kaszuba SM, Zafereo ME, Rosenthal DI, et al. Effect of initial treatment on disease outcome for patients with submandibular gland carcinoma. *Arch Otolaryngol Head Neck Surg* 2007;133(6):546–550.

Preuss SF, Klussmann JP, Wittekindt C, et al. Submandibular gland excision: 15 years of experience. *J Oral Maxillofac Surg* 2007;65(5):953–957.

32 ENDOSCOPIC NASOPHARYNGECTOMY

Sheng-Po Hao

INTRODUCTION

Nasopharyngeal carcinoma (NPC) is a common cancer among the Chinese people. NPC is a squamous cell carcinoma that originates from the epithelial lining of the nasopharynx. Thus, the definition of NPC strictly excludes all the other nasopharyngeal malignancies arising from lymphoid tissue or connective tissue, such as lymphomas or sarcomas.

Currently available therapeutic modalities for NPC are radiation therapy (RT), chemotherapy, or a combination of both. NPC is highly radiosensitive, and patients presenting with a limited-stage cancer have a high possibility for cure after RT. The treatment of NPC with current techniques of RT can achieve more than 80% local control rate. Concurrent cisplatin-based chemoradiotherapy with or without neoadjuvant chemotherapy has produced significant improvement in survival and is currently the standard treatment strategy for patients with advanced locoregional disease. Though NPC is usually a radiosensitive tumor, some do recur after RT. Local failure, either persistence or recurrence, in the nasopharynx, occurs in 10% to 30% of patients with NPC after initial RT.

HISTORY

NPC is diagnosed by clinical history, physical examination, and biopsy. A typical clinical history of NPC includes unilateral or bilateral enlarged painless lymph nodes in the superior aspect of the neck, blood-tinged rhinorrhea, conductive hearing loss, and headache.

PHYSICAL EXAMINATION

Physical examination of the nasopharynx is performed in the clinic with a mirror or fiberoptic nasopharyngoscope. A tumor mass can be visualized in the nasopharynx. These are usually exophytic with superficial ulceration. Biopsy is necessary to reach a definitive diagnosis.

Direct visualization with an endoscope is the most sensitive modality for demonstrating mucosal recurrence in the nasopharynx. However, postradiation mucositis or crusting may hinder endoscopic examination. Unfortunately, endoscopy may miss residual or recurrent carcinoma, especially when the tumor is primarily submucosal. In one report, 27.8% of deep-seated recurrent NPC detected by magnetic resonance imaging (MRI) were not detected by endoscopy.

INDICATIONS

Once NPC persists or recurs in the nasopharynx, salvage nasopharyngectomy should be the treatment of choice since there is no reason to believe that the NPC cells, which are resistant to a first course of RT, would respond to a second course of RT not to mention the risk of osteoradionecrosis (ORN) of the base of the skull, a recognized and potentially fatal complication of high-dose RT. The indication for endoscopic nasopharyngectomy for recurrent nasopharyngeal carcinoma (rNPC) includes lesions of the central roof or floor of the nasopharynx with minimal lateral extension.

CONTRAINDICATIONS

Involvement of the parapharyngeal space or bone of the skull base is a contraindication for endoscopic resection, and I recommend a facial translocation procedure or even a standard craniofacial resection for such recurrence. However, patients with extensive involvement of the parapharyngeal space or infratemporal fossa by rNPC are generally not good candidates for salvage skull base surgery, as it is difficult to achieve oncologically safe surgical margins in these areas.

PREOPERATIVE PLANNING

Imaging Study for Recurrent Nasopharyngeal Carcinoma

Imaging studies are required for the correct staging and treatment planning for rNPC. Computed tomography (CT) and MRI are recommended for the diagnostic evaluation of the extent of the cancer. MRI appears to be better than CT imaging for visualizing soft tissue invasion outside of the nasopharynx, demonstrating involved retropharyngeal nodes, and identifying skull base or intracranial involvement. MRI is also valuable in defining locally recurrent cancer. Both MRI and CT scans have a low sensitivity and moderate specificity for detecting rNPC and for distinguishing recurrence from postradiation changes. MRI is superior to CT in differentiating postradiation fibrosis from rNPC. Early recurrence is difficult to identify because immature scars and well-vascularized granulation tissues generally reveal contrast enhancement. Sophisticated nuclear medicine examination, such as positron emission tomography (PET) scans, appears promising for the detection of rNPC. Asymptomatic distant metastases are not rare at the initial presentation; thus, a pretherapeutic evaluation with positron emission tomography with [18F] fluoro-2-deoxy-D-glucose (FDG–PET) is recommended in the staging process. On PET scans, a viable tumor is seen as a focal area of increased FDG uptake due to its hypermetabolic activity, while radiation fibrosis is hypometabolic and appears as a focal area of decreased uptake. This technique may be superior to CT or MRI for detecting recurrent or residual disease. PET, however, cannot provide detailed anatomic information about the location of lesions, invasion of vascular and bony structures, and submucosal spread. False-positive results may also occur in PET because of hypermetabolic features seen in the inflammatory process.

Molecular Detection of rNPC

Differentiating between locally recurrent cancer, radiation-induced necrosis, and scarring in the nasopharynx by direct visualization with endoscopy or radiologic imaging is difficult until the tumor mass becomes grossly visible with ulceration or asymmetric change in the mucosa. It has been reported that the appearance of the mucosa of the nasopharynx does not necessarily correlate well with the occurrence of early NPC. Epstein-Barr virus (EBV) is a double-stranded DNA virus, which is closely related to NPC. The presence of EBV in NPC is well documented. Almost every NPC tumor cell carries clonal EBV genomes and expresses EBV proteins such as latent membrane proteins. Quantification of plasma EBV DNA is useful for monitoring patients with NPC and predicting the outcome of treatment. The detection of EBV genomic latent membrane protein 1 (LMP-1) using a nasopharyngeal swab technique has a sensitivity of 81.8% and a specificity of 98.3% for predicting mucosal recurrence of NPC. A recurrence in the mucosa should be strongly suspected if LMP-1 is present again in patients with treated NPC who had a latent disease remission of LMP-1 that exceeded 6 months, even if a nasopharyngoscopy revealed no abnormality. In such situations, further investigation by punch biopsy or imaging, such as MRI or PET scans, needs to be considered.

Undoubtedly, detection of EBV LMP-1 by PCR assay with nasopharyngeal swabbing should be incorporated as an important part of a follow-up investigation in all NPC patients treated with radiotherapy. The detection of LMP-1 again in NPC patients treated with radiation can enhance physicians' awareness and encourage physicians to shorten patient follow-up intervals, pay increased attention to changes in the nasopharynx, and even perform biopsies more frequently in suspicious areas of the mucosa in the nasopharynx. Thus, it is reasonable to expect that mucosal recurrence may be diagnosed earlier using detection of LMP-1 as one of the follow-up screening modalities. Moreover, salvage treatment can be more successful when rNPC is detected early.

The role of LMP-1 as a tumor marker to monitor local or residual cancer after RT has been established. In one report, of the 12 patients with local recurrence, 11 patients had positive LMP-1, including 2 cases with normal findings at nasopharyngoscopy. It suggests that nasopharyngeal swabs with LMP-1 detection could detect early recurrence, which, after salvage surgery, may actually improve local control and enhance survival. The detection of LMP-1 with subsequent verification of EBNA-1 from nasopharyngeal swabs in NPC patients treated with radiotherapy predicted local recurrence with a sensitivity of 91.7% and a specificity of 98.6%.

Nasopharyngeal swabs coupled with LMP-1 and EBNA-1 detection is simple and convenient, and it has proved to be a reliable method in detecting local recurrence in NPC patients after RT. The detection and removal of local recurrence in the early phases may improve local control as well as enhance patient survival.

SURGICAL TECHNIQUE

The nasopharynx occupies the most cephalic portion of the upper aerodigestive tract. It is a hollow cubic space located above the soft palate and posterior to the nasal cavity. It is located beneath the sphenoid sinus and superior aspect of the clivus, anterior to the inferior aspect of the clivus and the body of the first cervical vertebra, and medial to the medial pterygoid plate. The lateral wall of the nasopharynx is formed by the torus tubarius—the bulging cartilage of the medial end of the Eustachian tube. The nasopharynx is lined with pseudostratified ciliated columnar epithelium. Deep into the mucosal layer is the pharyngobasilar fascia, a tough fascia surrounding the superior posterior and lateral walls. The fascia originates from the pharyngeal tubercle of the occipital bone posteriorly and inserts into the posterior sharp end of the medial pterygoid plate anteriorly. It forms the posterior boundary of the nasopharynx and continues inferiorly as the buccopharyngeal fascia. The lateral wall of the nasopharynx is bounded by the medial pterygoid plate. It is formed by an incomplete cartilaginous ring that is deficient inferolaterally. The Eustachian tube and the tensor veli palatini muscle pierce through this natural defect, known as the sinus of Morgagni, on the lateral wall of the pharyngobasilar fascia to the middle ear space. As the pharyngobasilar fascia is tough and forms a good barrier, the NPC, which originates from the fossa of Rosenmüller, preferentially ascends and destroys the floor of the sphenoid sinus to involve the sphenoid sinus and skull base. More commonly, it invades laterally through the sinus of Morgagni, extends along the Eustachian tube to destroy the base of the pterygoid plate, and involves the parapharyngeal space and the area of the foramen ovale. When the cancer reaches the foramen lacerum laterally, it may encase the petrous internal carotid artery. In this case, it is almost impossible to achieve complete resection.

Salvage nasopharyngectomy has been the mainstay of treatment after RT failure. Surgical access to the nasopharynx has been a challenge to head and neck surgeons for years. Various surgical approaches to the nasopharynx have been developed, such as the transpalatal, transmaxillary, midline mandibulotomy, transpterygoid, facial translocation, and infratemporal fossa approaches. Minimally invasive endoscopic nasopharyngectomy has been reported to be a feasible treatment of a small mucosal recurrence. However, I am very cautious in endoscopic nasopharyngectomy as the role of endoscopic surgery for skull base malignancies remains to be determined. The indication of endoscopic nasopharyngectomy for rNPC includes lesions of the central roof or floor of the nasopharynx with minimal lateral extension.

All operations are performed under general anesthesia. The nasal cavity is decongested for 15 minutes with cotton plugs saturated with epinephrine 1:100,000. A careful inspection of the nasopharynx with a rigid endoscope is first performed (Fig. 32.1). Careful inspection of the entire tumor is mandatory to form a good surgical plan. One percent lidocaine and 1:80,000 epinephrine is used to infiltrate the mucoperichondrium of the nasal septum, middle and inferior turbinates, and operative field of the nasopharynx. A posterior septectomy is performed to allow a panoramic view of the nasopharynx and access by instruments via each nares. The ipsilateral middle and inferior turbinates are selectively removed to create a working space. The binostril technique with an endoscope through the contralateral nostril with the dissection or resection instruments working through the ipsilateral nostril avoids two instruments fighting for space and is crucial for a successful operation.

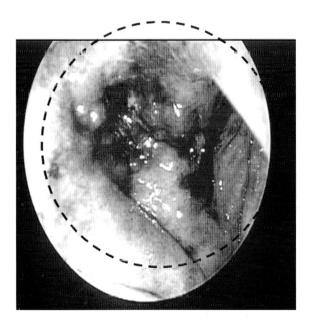

FIGURE 32.1 Recurrent NPC is detected in the right fossa of Rosenmüller. The *dotted line* presents the planned mucosal incision.

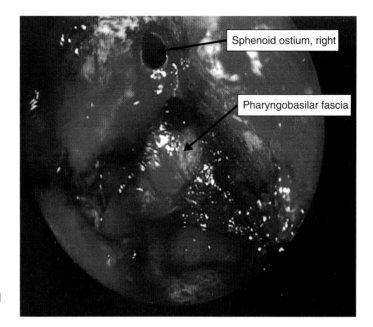

Sphenoid ostium, right

Pharyngobasilar fascia

FIGURE 32.2
The incision is made in the sphenoethmoid recess and connects with the right torus tubarius. The specimen is retracted to expose the ostium of the right sphenoid sinus and pharyngobasilar fascia.

The dissection can be carried out with electrocautery or laser. A continuous wave, contact type of Diomed 25 diode laser (Diomed Co., Cambridge, UK) can be used to achieve a bloodless surgical field. Under the 4-mm diameter, 0-degree, 30-degree, and 70-degree angle endoscopes (Karl-Storz, Tuttlingen, Germany), the widely exposed tumor can be removed with an adequate mucosal surgical margin (Video 32.1). The incision is usually started along the ipsilateral sphenoethmoidal recess. It should be made transversely across the roof of the nasopharynx down to the bone and connecting the septum and the ipsilateral fossa of Rosenmüller. The ipsilateral sphenoid sinus ostium is first identified and widened medially, and sphenoid incisions are connected in the midline. The rest of the face of the sphenoid sinus and the rostrum are removed. The mucosa is then elevated off of the face of the sphenoid sinus from a superior to inferior direction. The floor of the sphenoid sinus is then removed using a combination of Kerrison punches and cutting burrs. The mucoperiosteum is then elevated inferiorly to the sphenoclival junction, and the pharyngobasilar fascia is exposed. Electrocautery or laser is then applied to separate the tough pharyngobasilar fascia attachment from the bone and to use the fascia as the deep margin (Fig. 32.2).

The lateral margin of the tumor was first defined using diathermy along the posterior edge of the ipsilateral eustachian tube. The dissection is carried out laterally until the cartilaginous portion of the eustachian tube is encountered, and it is transected. The left lateral margin included excising the left Eustachian tube as laterally as possible. The mucosa is incised down to bone and then elevated medially. The lateral surgical margin should be assessed at this point. A vertical incision from the ipsilateral roof to the inferior border of the cancer is then carried out.

The medial and inferior mucosal incisions are carried out based on the extent of the cancer. The medial incision usually reaches the medial border of the orifice of the contralateral Eustachian tube. The inferior incision is usually made at the level of the superior surface of the soft palate to reach the left lateral wall of the nasopharynx.

Finally, the cancer is completely removed after careful dissection beneath the pharyngobasilar fascia (Fig. 32.3). This strong fascia often offers an effective barrier for tumor spread and can be used as a deep margin. A cutting burr is then used to drill the surface of the clivus and sphenoid ridge to obtain additional

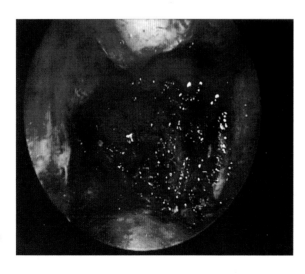

FIGURE 32.3
The tumor has been completely resected. The raw surgical defect includes the right fossa of Rosenmüller to the left torus tubarius and the sphenoethmoid recess down to the level of soft palate in the posterior pharyngeal wall.

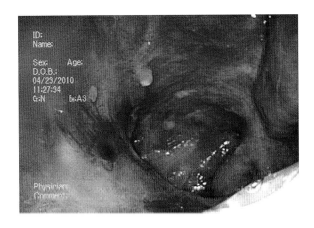

FIGURE 32.4 At follow-up nasopharyngoscopy 2 years after surgery, the defect is well epithelialized, and no local recurrence was identified

clear surgical margins. The bone of the base of the pterygoid plate can also be burred away for better exposure. The superior and medial portion of the pterygoid plate can also be removed for margin control. Frozen sections are obtained to ensure clear margins. Hemostasis is achieved with electrocautery.

The surgical margins are sent for frozen sections during nasopharyngectomy to evaluate the need for further resection. A nasoseptal flap based on the septal branch of the sphenopalatine artery can be raised and transferred to cover the surgical defect. It is extremely difficult to preserve the septal branch of the sphenopalatine artery when it is necessary to cut across the sphenoethmoidal recess. The flap, however, remains a good option for reconstruction if it is not involved by the tumor. The wound surface could also be covered with a free mucosal graft harvested from the inferior turbinate. Nasal pack and balloon-inflated Foley catheter are placed into the resected nasopharynx for 24 hours after the surgery.

POSTOPERATIVE MANAGEMENT

The patient is treated with antibiotics for at least 3 days. The nasal packing and Foley catheter are removed between 24 and 28 hours. The patient may be discharged within 3 days postoperatively. The patient is instructed to irrigate the nasal–nasopharyngeal space with warm saline every day. Endoscopic examination every week is critical until the wound is properly healed (Fig. 32.4).

COMPLICATIONS

Operative complications are rarely encountered in endoscopic nasopharyngectomy. In open nasopharyngectomy, the most common perioperative complication is bleeding, particularly from branches of the sphenopalatine artery. Wound infection might be encountered if there is too much crust accumulation, and thus, frequent self-cleaning by irrigation of the nasal–nasopharyngeal cavity or manual debridement of crusts by the surgeon is extremely important. Chronic wound infection in the form of ORN of the nasopharynx is not rare as the surgical bed has been heavily irradiated and there is no local well-vascularized flap outside the radiation field available to cover the surgical defect. The nasal septal flap is a good option, but the pedicle is difficult to preserve during the nasopharyngectomy, and it is also within the radiation field.

The management of ORN of the nasopharynx remains frequent cleaning, irrigation, debridement, and sequestrectomy. Hyperbaric oxygen therapy maybe indicated in some cases. Other complications include ascending meningitis and chronic headache, which are seldom seen.

RESULTS

Extreme care in patient selection is critical when considering a surgical approach to the nasopharynx. Ideal cases will be strictly limited to the lesions of the central roof. Some lateral extensions can also be managed using endoscopic nasopharyngectomy.

Eight rNPC cases were operated with endoscopic nasopharyngectomies on my service. In all of the cases, the surgical margins were clear; thus, there was no indication for immediate postoperative RT. Two patients developed recurrence in a retropharyngeal node and underwent subsequent chemoradiation therapy and remain free of the disease.

I further expanded the indications to include rNPC cases with skull base bone invasion and I now use navigation to facilitate endoscopic nasopharyngectomy.

From 2004 to 2010, 12 rNPC cases were operated with endoscopic nasopharyngectomy, which included 8 cases after one course and 4 cases after two courses of CRT. The preoperative clinical stage was rT1 in 9, rT2 in 1, and rT3 in 2. Endoscopic nasopharyngectomy was carried out with diode laser in most of the cases. Navigation assistance was applied in rT2 (1) and rT3 (2) cases.

The surgical margins in all the patients were clear; thus, there was no indication for immediate postoperative RT. They were followed up in the outpatient clinic for 9 to 50 months, mean 29.5 months. Two patients out of 4 rNPC after two courses of CRT recurred. One patient was salvaged with another endoscopic nasopharyngectomy and had still a third recurrence. The other patient had a recurrence over the hard palate and was salvaged with transoral palatectomy. The initial local control rate after first endoscopic nasopharyngectomy was 83.3%. Two patients developed recurrence in a retropharyngeal lymph node and underwent a second course of CRT; one remained disease free, but one died of distant metastasis. Eight patients developed ORN of the skull base including all the 4 patients with 2 courses of CRT. To date, 10 patients are alive without disease, while one is alive with disease. The overall survival rate at 2 years is 87.5%.

Minimally invasive endoscopic nasopharyngectomy is a feasible treatment for rNPC. With the aid of navigation, endoscopic nasopharyngectomy can also be a good surgical intervention in rNPC cases even with skull base bone involvement.

PEARLS

- Careful patient selection is the key to success. Ideal cases are lesions of the central roof with minimal lateral extension.
- Preoperative evaluation with MRI and PET is mandatory to define the extent of the tumor.
- Binostril technique, selectively removing the posterior part of the nasal septum, middle, and inferior turbinates to create adequate working space, is critical.
- Use pharyngobasilar fascia as a deep margin.
- Send surgical margins as with open nasopharyngectomy.
- Diligent postoperative cleaning of the nasal–nasopharyngeal space is mandatory and may be labor intensive.

PITFALLS

- Lack of meticulous surgical technique leads to recurrent cancer and complications.
- Need meticulous dissection under endoscopy
- Basic endoscopic dissection and resection skill needed
- Technically feasible, but no long-term results to justify the procedure

INSTRUMENTS TO HAVE AVAILABLE

- Continuous wave, contact type of Diomed 25 diode laser (Diomed Co., Cambridge, UK)
- 4-mm diameter, 0-degree, 30-degree, and 70-degree angle endoscopes (Karl-Storz, Tuttlingen, Germany)
- Nasal speculae of various lengths
- Endoscopic scissors (double action)
- 25-gauge spinal needle for injection of mucosa
- Cottle elevator
- Endoscopic bipolar cautery
- Kerrison punch (various diameter)
- Drill with cutting burrs
- Nasal packing (absorbable and nonabsorbable), inflatable nasal balloon

SUGGESTED READING

Fee WE, Gilmer PA, Goffinet DR. Surgical management of recurrent nasopharyngeal carcinoma after radiation failure at the primary site. *Laryngoscope* 1998;98:1220–1226.

Chang KP, Hao SP, Tsang NM, et al. Salvage surgery for locally recurrent nasopharyngeal carcinoma–a 10-year experience. *Otolaryngol Head Neck Surg* 2004;131:497–502.

Hao SP, Tsang NM, Chang KP, et al. Molecular diagnosis of nasopharyngeal carcinoma-detecting LMP-1 and EBNA by nasopharyngeal swab. *Otolaryngol Head Neck Surg* 2004;131:651–654.

Chen MK, Lai JC, Chang CC, et al. Minimally invasive endoscopic nasopharyngectomy in the treatment of recurrent T1-2a nasopharyngeal carcinoma. *Laryngoscope* 2007;117:894–896.

Hao SP, Tsang NM, Chang KP, et al. Nasopharyngectomy for recurrent nasopharyngeal carcinoma: a review of 53 patients and prognostic factors. *Acta Otolaryngol* 2008;128:473–481.

33 TRANSPALATAL ACCESS FOR NASOPHARYNGECTOMY

Alexander C. Vlantis

INTRODUCTION

A nasopharyngectomy is the surgical excision of the mucosa and adjacent soft tissues of the nasopharynx usually performed for surgical salvage of residual or recurrent nasopharyngeal carcinoma following primary radiotherapy. It can be done as (i) an endoscopic procedure; (ii) a minimally invasive procedure with or without the use of an endoscope, surgical navigation, and/or a surgical robot; or (iii) an open procedure. Open procedures use wide access to the surgical field for adequate visualization and protection of vital structures during tumor resection and are named according to the approach taken to the nasopharynx as anterior (transnasal), anterolateral (transmaxillary), lateral (infratemporal fossa), or inferior (transpalatal).

HISTORY

These patients have a history of nasopharyngeal carcinoma (NPC) treated with radiotherapy with or without chemotherapy. Symptoms suggestive of a residual or recurrent cancer include nasal obstruction, blood-stained nasal discharge, epistaxis, blood-stained saliva, hearing loss, and a mass in the neck. The patient may volunteer these symptoms at routine follow-up visits or present because of them.

PHYSICAL EXAMINATION

The nasopharynx is examined at each planned routine follow-up visit and at any other time when symptoms or investigations such as imaging or serology dictate. Any suspicious lesions seen are biopsied transnasally under topical anesthesia with the endoscope used to direct biopsy forceps to the lesion. Occasionally, a general anesthetic is needed if the lesion is deeper and is less accessible or an awake biopsy is contraindicated.

INDICATIONS

The surgical salvage of residual or recurrent rT1 or early rT2 NPC where the tumor does not abut the internal carotid artery (ICA) and hence clear margins of resection can be anticipated. Surgery avoids the significant morbidity and remote chance of cure associated with a second course of external beam radiotherapy.

CONTRAINDICATIONS

Residual or recurrent NPC abutting the ICA makes safe and complete resection unlikely. Involvement of the bone of the base of the skull (rT3), intracranial or cranial nerve involvement (rT4), or distant metastases (M1) are also contraindications.

PREOPERATIVE PLANNING

Following histologic confirmation of residual or recurrent cancer, an MRI with contrast is mandatory to delineate the extent of the cancer and to define its relationship to surrounding structures, especially the internal carotid arteries. The presence and position of any ectatic portion of the ICA must be noted.

A PET–CT is useful to exclude regional and systemic disease.

SURGICAL TECHNIQUE

Tracheostomy

A tracheostomy is done under local anesthesia in an awake patient or under general anesthesia after intubation.

Mandibulotomy and Mandible Swing in Patients with Trismus

In patients with significant trismus, a mandibulotomy and mandible swing is done to gain access to the palate for the transpalatal procedure.

Transpalatal Access

Lateral Transpalatal Access
The lateral transpalatal approach is used for unilateral lesions involving the posterior and/or lateral wall of the nasopharynx that do not extend into the contralateral pharyngeal recess. This approach is also suitable for unilateral cancers that extend to the inferior nasopharynx or superior oropharynx.

Palatal Incisions

Soft palate incision: The soft palate is divided from its junction with the lateral pharyngeal wall on the side of the cancer. A finger or instrument placed behind the soft palate to tense it enables the correct position of the lateral incision on the oral surface of the soft palate to be made with a scalpel. The incision is made to meet the free edge of the posterior tonsil pillar/palatopharyngeal fold at 90 degrees. The wound is deepened until the nasopharyngeal soft palate mucosa is reached at which time it is incised with a scalpel at the junction of the soft palate and lateral pharyngeal wall.

Hard palate incision: The hard palate mucosal incision is marked to follow the curve of the gingiva and extends from the midline anteriorly to the medial aspect of the ipsilateral maxillary tuberosity posteriorly and then to join the soft palate incision (Figs. 33.1 and 33.2). The incision is made with a scalpel and carried through the periosteum to bone.

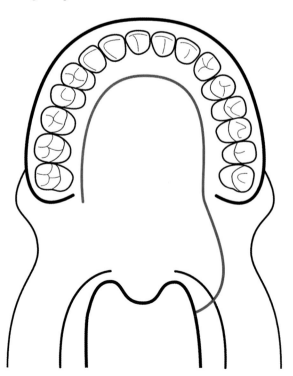

FIGURE 33.1
Hard and soft palate incision for lateral transpalatal access to the nasopharynx.

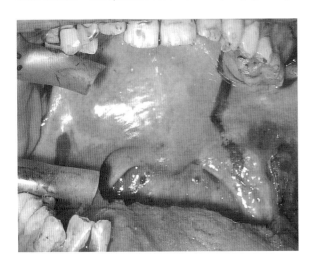

FIGURE 33.2 Hard and soft palate incision marked for lateral transpalatal access.

Palatal Flap

A mucoperiosteal flap based on the contralateral palatine vascular pedicle is elevated in a subperiosteal plane off the underlying bone. The contents of the ipsilateral palatine foramina are ligated and divided. The flap is elevated across the midline while preserving the contents of the incisive canal and the contralateral palatine vascular pedicle. The nasopalatine nerve is preserved as it exits from the incisive foramen in the anterior midline to preserve sensation in the anterior palate. If greater exposure is needed, the anterior hard palate incision can be extended to the contralateral side and the nasopalatine nerve divided as further hard palate mucoperiosteum is elevated. As the palatal flap is elevated, the palatine aponeurosis and inferior choanal mucosa are divided along the posterior free edge of the palatine bone. The palatal flap is retracted in an appropriate manner.

Median Transpalatal Access

The median transpalatal approach can be used for midline lesions involving the posterior wall or roof of the nasopharynx that do not extend into the lateral pharyngeal recesses on either side. This approach is also suitable for midline tumors that extend to the inferior aspect of the nasopharynx or the superior aspect of the oropharynx.

Palatal Incision

Midline palatal incision: A midline incision is marked from the incisive foramen anteriorly to the uvula posteriorly keeping the integrity of the inferior free edge of the soft palate intact. If more exposure is eventually needed, the uvula can be divided in the midline so as to divide the soft palate completely (Figs. 33.3 and 33.4).

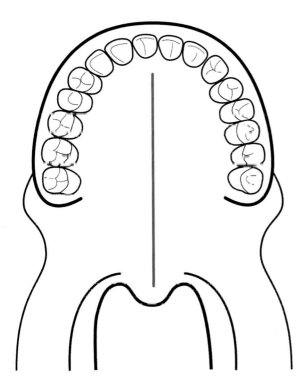

FIGURE 33.3 Midline palatal incision for median transpalatal access to the nasopharynx.

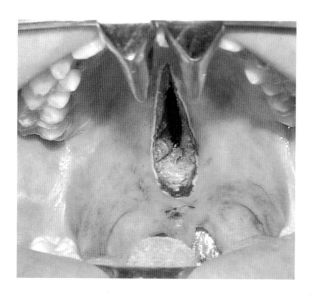

FIGURE 33.4
Midline soft and hard palate incision.

U-shaped palatal incision: A U-shaped incision in the mucosa of the hard palate is marked to follow the curve of the gingiva from the ipsilateral third molar to the contralateral third molar. The incisions are placed anterior to the palatine foramina bilaterally to preserve the palatine vascular pedicles (Fig. 33.5).

Palatal Flap

Midline palatal incision with laterally based flaps: The soft palate is put under tension and the mucosa of the oral surface incised with a scalpel and then the wound deepened, dividing the tissues of the soft palate, until the nasopharyngeal soft palate mucosa is seen, which is also divided with a scalpel. The hard palate mucosal incision is made with a scalpel and carried through the periosteum to the bone. Bilateral mucoperiosteal flaps based on ipsilateral palatine vascular pedicles are elevated in a subperiosteal plane off the bone. The contents of the incisive canal should be preserved. As the palatal flap is elevated, the palatine aponeurosis and inferior choanal mucosa are divided along the posterior free edge of the palatine bone.

U-shaped palatal incision with a posteriorly based flap: A mucoperiosteal flap based on bilateral palatine vascular pedicles is elevated off the bone in a subperiosteal plane. The contents of the palatine foramina are preserved bilaterally. As the palatal flap is elevated posteriorly, the palatine aponeurosis and inferior choanal mucosa are divided along the posterior free edge of the palatine bone.

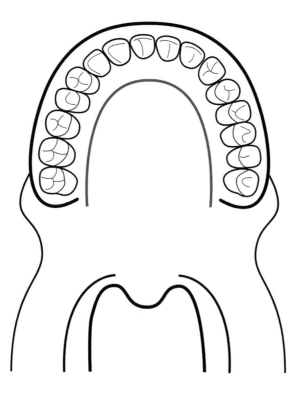

FIGURE 33.5
U-shaped palatal incision for median transpalatal access to the nasopharynx.

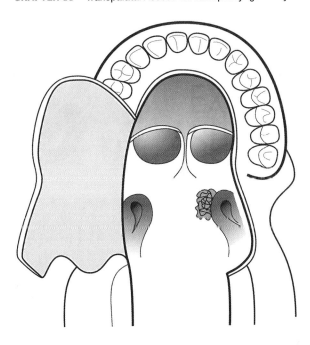

FIGURE 33.6 Exposure of the nasopharynx via a soft palate and hard palate mucoperiosteal flap and removal of the horizontal plate of the palatine bone.

Further Exposure of the Nasopharynx

The mucoperiosteum is elevated off the floor of the posterior nasal cavity, and the horizontal plate of the palatine bone is removed with a bone nibbler or burr to increase exposure of the nasopharynx. Additional exposure is obtained by removing the posterior palatine process of the maxilla after further elevation and preservation of the mucoperiosteum of the floor of the nose, which can be incised along its inferior junction with the nasal septum to further improve exposure. Bilateral mucoperiosteal flaps are elevated off the posterior free edge of the nasal septum, and the vomer removed with a bone nibbler. The posterior ends of the inferior turbinates are removed if necessary (Figs. 33.6 and 33.7).

Nasopharyngectomy

If possible, at least 1-cm margins are marked around the tumor, but as this surgery is usually performed for recurrent nasopharyngeal carcinoma, which may be multifocal, and the original extent of the primary tumor may not be known, a subtotal resection of all nasopharyngeal mucosa including the ipsilateral tubal elevation and auditory tube cartilage is advocated.

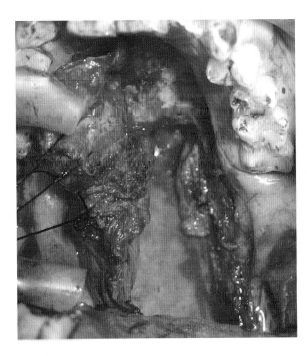

FIGURE 33.7 Soft palate and hard palate mucoperiosteal flap retracted to expose the nasopharynx.

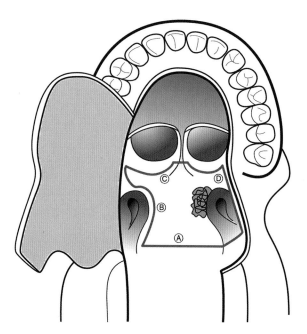

FIGURE 33.8

Nasopharyngectomy incisions: *A*, inferior transverse incision; *B*, vertical posterior wall incision; *C*, superior transverse incision; and *D*, vertical lateral wall incision.

Four incisions are made in the mucosa of the nasopharynx—inferior and superior transverse incisions and ipsilateral and contralateral vertical incisions (Figs. 33.8 and 33.9). If the lateral wall of the nasopharynx including the auditory tube, lateral pharyngeal recess, and lateral nasopharyngeal wall is to be resected, the ipsilateral vertical incision is placed on the lateral wall of the nasopharynx as *the vertical lateral wall incision*; otherwise, the ipsilateral vertical incision is placed on the posterior wall of the nasopharynx as *the vertical posterior wall incision*.

The inferior transverse incision is made transversally across the entire posterior wall of the nasopharynx at the level of the junction of the nasopharynx and oropharynx, approximately at the level of the hard palate, or lower if necessary (Fig. 33.8—Incision A). The incision is carried through the mucosa, pharyngobasilar fascia, constrictor muscle, and buccopharyngeal fascia (together constituting the mucosal space) and then through the alar fascia to reach the prevertebral space. Once the prevertebral space has been entered and the depth of resection appreciated, the tissue of the posterior wall of the nasopharynx, which overlies the longus capitis muscle, is elevated superiorly to the basiocciput. At the basiocciput elevation of nasopharyngeal tissue off the bone of the basiocciput continues in a subperiosteal plane. The midline median or pharyngeal raphé is divided sharply to allow for this elevation, especially where it inserts into the basiocciput. Sharp dissection may also be needed to divide the insertion of the pharyngobasilar, buccopharyngeal, and alar fascia from the basiocciput. Elevation of nasopharyngeal tissue is extended laterally in the plane of the prevertebral space until the fascia of the longus

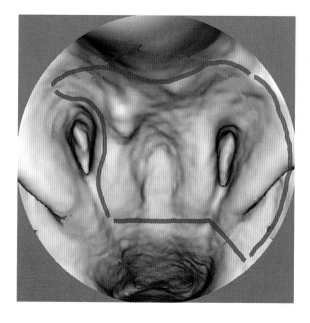

FIGURE 33.9

Nasopharyngectomy incisions superimposed on a virtual endoscopic view of the nasopharynx.

capitis muscle merges with the prevertebral fascia forming the carotid sheath, where the ICA is located and where it should be avoided and not exposed.

The superior transverse incision follows the superior margin of the choana (the junction of the roof of the posterior nasal cavity and the roof of the nasopharynx) bilaterally (Fig. 33.8—Incision C) and is carried through to the sphenoid bone. Medially the incisions reflect around the midpoint of the posterior free edge of the nasal septum if this has not already been removed. Laterally the incisions extend posterior to the posterior ends of the inferior turbinates and onto the lateral margins of the choanae where they are carried through to the underlying medial pterygoid plate. Nasopharyngeal tissue is elevated in a subperiosteal plane off the basisphenoid and basiocciput (the clivus) posteroinferiorly using sharp dissection when necessary.

The vertical posterior wall incision is made at the junction of the posterior wall of the nasopharynx and the medial aspect of the lateral pharyngeal recess (Fig. 33.8—Incision B). The incision continues superiorly and then anterolaterally above the tubal elevation to meet the lateral aspect of the superior transverse incision. Nasopharyngeal tissue is elevated medially from the incision in the plane of the prevertebral space off of the underlying muscle.

The vertical lateral wall incision is made along the lateral margin of the choana between the posterior ends of the inferior and middle turbinates anteriorly and the tubal elevation posteriorly. It is carried through the mucosa to the underlying bone of the medial pterygoid plate. Superiorly the incision meets the lateral end of the superior transverse incision. Inferiorly the *inferior transverse incision* is extended anteriorly in the same transverse plane onto the ipsilateral lateral wall of the nasopharynx to join the *vertical lateral wall incision* at 90 degrees, just superior to the level of the insertion of the soft palate into the lateral pharyngeal wall (Fig. 33.8—Incision D). Since there is no bone underlying the posterior aspect of this anterior extension of the inferior transverse incision, the surgeon must be aware of possible ectatic vessels in the parapharyngeal soft tissue. It is important not to remove the lateral soft palate tissue as this is needed to repair the soft palate at the end of the procedure. Dissection of the nasopharynx starts superior to the remnant of the soft palate. Once the incision is carried through the periosteum, the tissues of the lateral wall of the nasopharynx are elevated posteriorly in the subperiosteal plane. When the posterior free edge of the medial pterygoid plate is reached, the cartilage of the Eustachian tube is divided in the same plane of dissection (in the plane of the medial pterygoid plate). The medial pterygoid plate can be removed with a burr if the medial pterygoid muscle must be removed as an additional margin. Resection of the lateral wall of the nasopharynx must be done with care as mucosa of the lateral pharyngeal recess is closely related to the ICA, which may inadvertently be damaged during resection. Surgical navigation, frequent palpation of the lateral nasopharyngeal tissue, and isolation of the ICA via the neck are some techniques used to protect the integrity of the artery. Once the resection has been accomplished with a combination of sharp and blunt dissection and the specimen delivered en bloc, appropriate frozen section margins are sent from the wound to confirm the adequacy of the resection (Figs. 33.10 and 33.11).

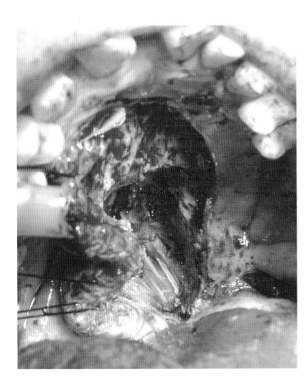

FIGURE 33.10 Postnasopharyngectomy view showing the retracted palatal flap, the posterior free edge of the palatine process of the maxilla, and the longus capitis muscle in the base of the wound.

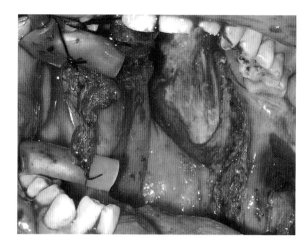

FIGURE 33.11

Postnasopharyngectomy view of the palatal flap retracted to show mucosa of the lower posterior pharyngeal wall and longus capitis muscle in the base of the resection of the posterolateral nasopharynx.

Closure

The wound is irrigated and hemostasis obtained. A fine-bore nasogastric tube is placed for postoperative enteral feeding. The wound may be left to mucosalize or dressed with a split-thickness skin graft taken from the lateral thigh or a mucosal graft taken from the inferior turbinate. Another option is a vascularized septal mucosal flap based on the posterior nasal artery. A 14-Fr 30-mL Foley catheter is inserted into the pharynx via the contralateral nasal cavity, and the balloon, which is inflated with only enough sterile water to prevent the pack from slipping into the oropharynx, is positioned at the inferior margin of the nasopharyngectomy wound and the nasopharynx packed with a length of paraffin gauze to hold the graft in place and aid mucosalization.

It is essential not to put the soft palate wound under tension either from the Foley catheter balloon or from the nasopharyngeal pack. Polyglactin sutures are used to close the palatal wound. All sutures used to close the hard palate mucoperiosteal flap are first preloaded before being tightened and knotted. The soft palate incision is closed in three layers with meticulous attention being paid to the correct repositioning of the mucosal edges. The nasopharyngeal soft palate mucosa is closed through the palatal wound before the soft palate muscular layers, and finally the oral cavity soft palate mucosa is closed (Fig. 33.12). A prefabricated palatal dental splint is securely placed to maintain apposition of the hard palate mucoperiosteal flap against the underlying bone during the healing phase.

POSTOPERATIVE MANAGEMENT

- Perioperative antibiotics are continued for 5 days.
- A chest radiograph is done to confirm the position of the nasogastric tube.
- Chest physiotherapy, tracheostomy care, and suctioning are essential.

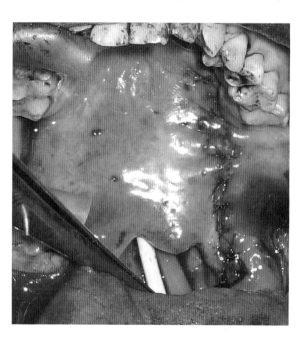

FIGURE 33.12

Closure of the hard and soft palatal wounds prior to application of the prefabricated palatal splint. The fine-bore feeding tube can be seen in the oropharynx as well as a Foley catheter whose bulb will be inflated and carefully retracted into the nasopharynx to maintain the position of the nasopharyngeal pack.

- Antiseptic mouth rinsing and institution-based oral care are given.
- The nasopharyngeal Foley is deflated after 24 hours
- The nasopharyngeal pack is shortened and loosened on day 6.
- The nasopharyngeal pack is totally removed on day 7.
- Rinsing of the nasal cavities and nasopharynx three times a day with normal saline commences on day 7, following removal of the packs.
- The tracheostomy tube is removed on day 8 if there has been no significant bleeding.
- The nasogastric tube is removed and an oral liquid diet begins on day 14.
- A soft diet begins on day 21 if the palatal wounds have healed well.

COMPLICATIONS

The most serious complication is bleeding, and if torrential, then rupture of the ICA must be suspected. This can lead to a stroke or even death. If the ICA is exposed in the nasopharynx, then vascularized muscle should be placed into the nasopharynx to cover and protect the artery. The most common complication is break down of the inferior free edge of the soft palate with eventual palatal insufficiency of varying degrees. Less frequently, the palatal incision breaks down elsewhere with a resultant oronasal or oronasopharyngeal fistula of various sizes. Depending on its position, this can be managed with a palatal dental splint that occludes the fistula. Other delayed complications include otitis media due to auditory tube resection and nasopharyngitis or osteomyelitis due to exposed previously irradiated nasopharyngeal soft tissues or bone.

RESULTS

In a series of 24 patients in whom the transpalatal access was used for nasopharyngectomy, the overall incidence of any palatal wound breakdown leading to varying degrees of dehiscence or palatal fistulas was 54%. Most of the dehiscence occurred at the free edge of the soft palate and was not functionally significant.

The 5-year local relapse-free survival in a series of 97 patients undergoing salvage nasopharyngectomy for residual or recurrent nasopharyngeal carcinoma was 46.7%, while the local control rate at 5 years was 62.8%.

In another series of 246 patients, the 5-year actuarial control of disease in the nasopharynx after the salvage nasopharyngectomy was 74%, and the 5-year disease free survival was 56%.

PEARLS

- The most common indication for a nasopharyngectomy is the management of resectable residual or recurrent NPC.
- Access to the nasopharynx is needed to perform surgery on the nasopharynx.
- There are many surgical approaches to the nasopharynx, of which transpalatal access is one.
- A median transpalatal approach to the nasopharynx is indicated for the surgical excision of resectable midline nasopharyngeal tumors.
- A lateral transpalatal approach to the nasopharynx is indicated for the surgical excision of resectable unilateral nasopharyngeal tumors.

PITFALLS

- Patients with trismus need a mandibular swing approach to access the palate.
- The ICA is at risk of injury during nasopharyngectomy.
- Soft palate wound dehiscence or fibrosis leads to palatal insufficiency.

INSTRUMENTS TO HAVE AVAILABLE

- Dingman mouth gag
- Howarth elevator
- Bone nibbler or rongeur
- Heymann turbinectomy scissors
- Burr

SUGGESTED READING

Morton RP, Liavaag PG, McLean M, et al. Transcervico-mandibulo-palatal approach for surgical salvage of recurrent nasopharyngeal cancer. *Head Neck* 1996;18(4):352.

Fee WE Jr, Moir MS, Choi EC, et al. Nasopharyngectomy for recurrent nasopharyngeal cancer: a 2- to 17-year follow-up. *Arch Otolaryngol Head Neck Surg* 2002;128(3):280.

Brown JJ, Fee WE Jr. Surgical resection of the nasopharynx. *Oper Tech Otolaryngol* 2010;21(1):26.

Vlantis AC, Chan HS, Tong MCF, et al. Surgical salvage nasopharyngectomy for recurrent nasopharyngeal carcinoma: a multivariate analysis of prognostic factors. *Head Neck* 2011;33(8):1126.

Wei WI, Chan JY, Ng RW, et al. Surgical salvage of persistent or recurrent nasopharyngeal carcinoma with maxillary swing approach—critical appraisal after 2 decades. *Head Neck* 2011;33(7):969.

34 ROBOTIC RESECTION OF RECURRENT NASOPHARYNGEAL CANCER

William Ignace Wei

INTRODUCTION

The primary treatment modality for early-stage nasopharyngeal carcinoma (NPC) is radiotherapy and for advanced-stage disease, concomitant chemotherapy and radiation. With the use of intensity-modulated radiotherapy in recent years, the local cancer control rate has improved, while the long-term morbidity has decreased. Despite the better treatment results, there are still a few patients who have residual or recurrent NPC after the initial therapy. Further external radiotherapy in the management of these patients is associated with significant complications especially in the long term and little hope that a modality that failed the first time would succeed the second time. Stereotactic radiation and brachytherapy have been applied with favorable outcomes for some. These types of radiation are only effective when the exact extent of the cancer has been determined accurately with imaging studies so that the cancer could be completely included in the radiation field. This precise determination of the edge of the cancer might be difficult for some patients. The other alternative for management of these residual or recurrent cancer with a curative intention is surgical resection.

Anatomically, the nasopharynx is located in the center of the head; it is over 10 cm from the skin surface from all sides. It is difficult to get adequate exposure for removal of cancer at this site. Various approaches have been described in the literature, and they all require external incisions, and there are associated morbidities. An endoscopic approach for transnasal resection of small tumors in the nasopharynx has been reported. The instruments currently available for endoscopic transnasal surgery when employed for oncologic resection of these tumors have certain limitations. It is difficult to achieve an en bloc resection of the tumor under direct vision especially when the tumor extends to involve the lateral wall of the nasopharynx.

In recent years, the efficacy of transoral robotic surgery in Otolaryngology—Head and Neck Surgery has been established. The da Vinci robot has been used effectively for resection of malignant tumors arising in the oropharynx, supraglottic larynx, and superior hypopharynx. The feasibility of the surgical robot employed for resection of pathologies at the skull base and the nasopharynx has been described. The first successful application for resection of a small recurrent cancer in the nasopharynx has also been reported in recent years.

HISTORY

It is essential to know the stage of the NPC on initial presentation and also the form of therapy such as radiation alone or concomitant chemoradiation. The duration and dosage of radiation should be noted and if chemotherapy was given, the chemotherapeutic agent and the dosages recorded. The time when recurrence was detected should be noted, and any therapy for the management of the recurrence should be documented. This might include further external beam radiotherapy, stereotactic radiation, or brachytherapy. Any medical comorbidities should be recorded.

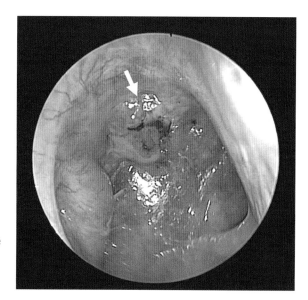

FIGURE 34.1

A small recurrent cancer seen through a 0-degree endoscope located at the superior aspect of right lateral wall of the nasopharynx (*arrow*).

PHYSICAL EXAMINATION

A complete physical examination is essential to exclude metastases to the cervical lymph nodes and to other organs. Palpation of the neck and abdomen should be carried out, and if there is any doubt, an ultrasound examination of these regions should be performed. All suspicious lesions should be investigated further with a fine needle aspiration biopsy or even with positron emission tomography–computed tomography (PET–CT).

Endoscopic Examination

The nasopharynx should be thoroughly examined with both 0-degree- and 30-degree-angled Hopkins rigid endoscopes to ascertain the extent of the tumor (Fig. 34.1). Biopsies around the cancer should be carried out to determine the edges of the tumor and to guide the extent of the resection.

Salvage resection of the primary tumor should only be done when there are no distant metastases. For regional metastasis, a separate surgical salvage procedure such as a neck dissection can be planned either at the same session with the resection of the primary cancer or at a later date.

PREOPERATIVE PLANNING

Imaging Studies

Magnetic resonance imaging (MRI) of the nasopharynx is indicated to see the deep extent of the tumor, its extension in the submucosa of the nasopharynx and paranasopharyngeal space (Fig. 34.2). Its proximity to the

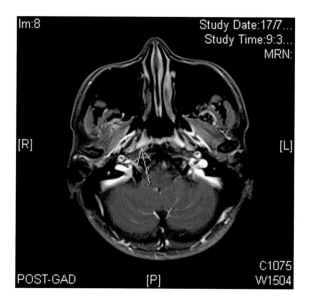

FIGURE 34.2

Magnetic resonance imaging (MRI) of the same cancer (*arrow*) demonstrates that it is only in the fossa of Rosenmüller and has not extended to the paranasopharyngeal space.

internal carotid artery can also be evaluated with the contrast MRI. CT is also indicated if there is any suspicion that the cancer has infiltrated bone, such as the pterygoid plates, the anterior wall of the sphenoid sinus, and the clivus. Either of these imaging studies will demonstrate whether the tumor has involved the paranasal sinuses.

INDICATIONS

The bulk of the recurrent NPC should be at the inferior aspect of either the lateral wall or the posterior wall of the nasopharynx. In general, tumor bulk should be <2 cm in diameter and involve only one Eustachian tube orifice. The tumor should only involve the mucosa or the muscular wall of the nasopharynx. It should not be extending into the paranasopharyngeal space or beyond the pharyngobasilar fascia and not lying close to the internal carotid artery.

CONTRAINDICATIONS

The limitations of employing the robot to carry out resection of the recurrent NPC are those related to the tumor and the clinical condition of the patient. For extensive cancers involving both Eustachian tube orifices and for infiltrative tumors involving the paranasopharyngeal space or close to the internal carotid artery, an anterolateral approach should be carried out to ensure tumor clearance. For those cancers that have extended into the sphenoid sinus or infiltrated the clivus or the pterygoid plates, resection with the robot is unlikely to remove all of the cancer with a clear margin. Robotic resection of the recurrent NPC is done transorally after splitting the palate; thus, the patient should have no trismus and no previous palate surgery. The tongue and intraoral tissue should be pliable and able to stand some stretching. Needless to say, the patient should be well enough medically to tolerate general anesthesia for 3 to 4 hours.

SURGICAL TECHNIQUE

The resection of the cancer is carried out under general anesthesia with the patient in the supine position. The smallest reinforced endotracheal tube suitable for the patient should be used, and it should be a nonkinking one. After proper insertion, the endotracheal tube should be placed over the lower central incisors. A Dingman mouth gag with the longest tongue blade is inserted and opened to its maximum width. A throat pack is inserted, and the palatal incision starts from one side of the base of the uvula (Video 34.1). The incision is extended along the midline of the soft palate onto the mucoperiosteum on the hard palate for three-fourths of the length of the hard palate. The insertion of the soft palate to the posterior edge of the hard palate is detached with electrocautery. All the muscular attachments of the soft palate from the midline to the lateral pharyngeal wall are divided, and the mucoperiosteum of the hard palate is elevated off of the bony surface.

Traction sutures are placed along the incised edge of the soft palate and the mucoperiosteum of the hard palate to facilitate retraction. The suture ends of the traction sutures are inserted into the coils of the spring over the frame of the Dingman retractor to maintain the tension of retraction (Fig. 34.3). After this retraction, the cancer in the nasopharynx comes into view. The handle of the Unitract (Aesculap, Braun), an air pressure–controlled malleable retractor holder, is fixed to the handle of the Dingman retractor, and the body of the Unitract is mounted on the operating table (Fig. 34.4). The head is kept in an extended position that is facilitated by the handle of the Unitract, which was fixed to the Dingman mouth gag in a position that lifts the gag superiorly. Throughout the operation, the retractor holder maintains the position of the Dingman retractor in a fairly rigid status. A plastic catheter is inserted through the nasal cavity to the posterior choana to provide continuous suction of the smoke created by the cautery. This allows an enhanced visualization of the operative field during surgery.

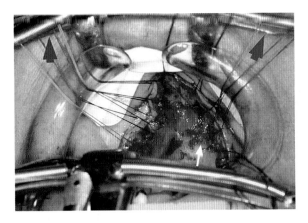

FIGURE 34.3 The Dingman mouth gag is inserted, and the palate is split to expose the cancer (*arrow*) in the left nasopharynx. The traction sutures in the palate are inserted onto the spring over the mouth gag to maintain the traction on the palate (*arrowheads*).

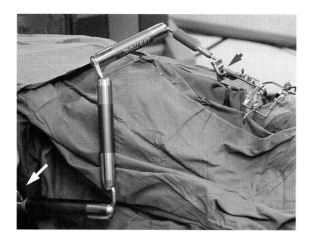

FIGURE 34.4
The Unitract holder is fixed to the side of the operating table (*arrow*) and the handle of the Dingman mouth gag (*arrow head*). This maintains the exposure of the operative field during the resection of tumor with the robot.

The da Vinci surgical robot, model S (Intuitive Surgical Inc., Sunnyvale, CA), is docked from the head end of the table (Fig. 34.5), and the 8-mm diameter 0-degree forward view dual-channel camera is introduced transorally. It is placed just over the tongue blade of the Dingman retractor at the position of the lower incisor. This allows good visualization of the cancer in the nasopharynx and the surrounding tissue. During the operation, an assistant at the operative table provides retraction of soft tissue and suction of smoke and debris to facilitate dissection (Fig. 34.6). The 5-mm Maryland grasping forceps are mounted to the left robotic arm, and the 8-mm scissors with monopolar cautery were mounted to the right robotic arm. The planned incision in the mucosa around the edge of the entire cancer is 1.5 cm, and this is marked with diathermy using the tip of the scissors (Fig. 34.7). The medial crus of the Eustachian tube cushion close to the cancer should be included in the resection. The dissection starts from the inferior aspect of the nasopharynx. The mucosal incision goes from superficial to deep, cutting through mucosa then prevertebral muscle. The cancer and the tissue surrounding it are lifted with the Maryland forceps while at the same time the scissors with the diathermy cut and cauterize the deep aspect of the nasopharyngeal tissue (Fig. 34.8). This was repeated from the lateral aspect of the wall of the nasopharynx. On the side where the Eustachian tube crura are included in the resection, the lateral crus is retracted laterally with the Maryland forceps, and the cautery cuts through the opening of the Eustachian tube going between the two cartilaginous crura. The medial crus is thus included in the specimen. Superiorly, the cautery is used to incise through the mucosa of the nasopharynx down to bone. The scissors in the right robotic arm are then replaced with the 8-mm cautery hook, which also acts as a diathermy tip. The hook lifts the soft tissue of the nasopharynx off the bone and is included in the resection (Fig. 34.9). The cancer and its surrounding tissue are lifted by forceps, and the deep tissue is incised with diathermy, making en bloc resection of the tumor with a margin of soft tissue possible. The internal carotid artery is not exposed or seen during dissection. Following resection of the cancer, the defect in the nasopharynx appears as a slanting trough; the central deep aspect is bone followed by layers of prevertebral muscle, submucosa on the side, and then come back to normal mucosa of the nasopharynx. Mucosal or muscular margins can be taken for frozen section examination to ensure complete tumor resection. A free mucosal graft is taken from the posterior wall of the oropharynx and placed over the raw area in the nasopharynx. A nasogastric tube is inserted through the nasal cavity, and the wound in the nasopharynx and the nasal cavity is packed with Merocel. A hole is drilled on the posterior edge of the hard palate, and a suture passing through this hole and the muscle of the soft palate reattaches the muscle to the bone. The palatal wound is closed in three layers with interrupted absorbable sutures.

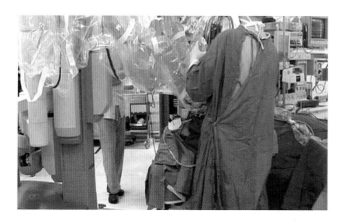

FIGURE 34.5
The da Vinci Robot is docked from the head end of the operating table.

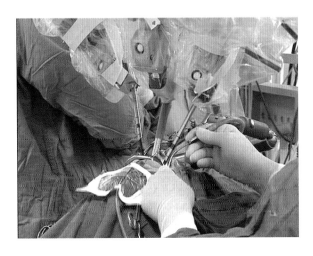

FIGURE 34.6 An assistant is at the operative site removing smoke and debris by suction and preventing trauma of soft tissue by the EndoWrist.

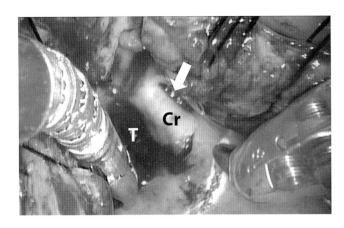

FIGURE 34.7 The diathermy marks the margin of resection; it is 1.5 cm from the cancer (T) that is covered with blood. The left eustachian tube opening can be seen (*arrow*) with the medial crura (Cr), which will be included in the resection.

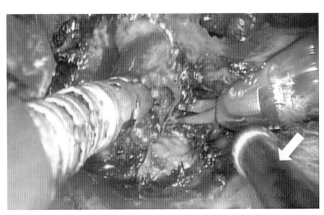

FIGURE 34.8 The cancer with its surrounding tissue is lifted with the Maryland forceps, and the undersurface of the lesion is incised with the scissor with diathermy. The suction (*arrow*) held by the assistant removes smoke and debris.

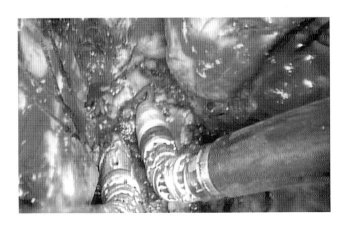

FIGURE 34.9 The monopolar diathermy scissors is changed to a hook that is connected to diathermy; this can flex and scrape all soft tissue from the anterior wall of the sphenoid and clivus.

POSTOPERATIVE CARE

Feeding is started the next day through the nasogastric tube. The nasal packs are removed on the second post-operative day, and oral feeding is started when the palatal wound heals in 2 weeks.

COMPLICATIONS

The immediate complication is bleeding from the wound, but as no major vessels are encountered during the dissection, the bleeding can be managed with packing and pressure.

The other complications are related to the forceful stretching of the tongue. The tongue may swell after releasing the mouth gag, and this could lead to airway obstruction. When this happens, a temporary tracheostomy is indicated. Prolonged rigid stretching of the tongue might lead to temporary palsy of the hypoglossal nerves; these usually recover with time.

One of the late complications is the development of a palatal fistula. As all these tissues were radiated, the healing might not be optimal. The small palatal fistula usually closes spontaneously with conservative management. A larger palatal fistula may need to be closed with a palatal flap.

RESULTS

From January 2010 to March 2012, I have carried out a nasopharyngectomy with the da Vinci Robot on 12 patients. All patients suffered from recurrent cancer of the nasopharynx after radiation or chemoradiation. The median age of these patients was 53 years, and the median duration of the operation was 4 hours. All patients survived the operation. One patient developed angioedema of the tongue, which resulted in brain damage. Another patient had venous bleeding from the nasopharynx that was controlled with nasal packing. A third patient developed temporary hypoglossal nerve palsy due to prolonged retraction of the tongue.

Clear surgical margins of resection were achieved in 10 patients, one patient had a close margin of resection, and the last patient has a positive margin of resection.

With a median follow-up of 19 months, two patients developed local recurrence. One of them had a positive margin of resection, and the other had a clear resection margin. One patient developed a palatal fistula and needed to wear a dental obturator. All patients returned to a normal diet, and no patient developed trismus after the procedure.

PEARLS

- The fundamental difficulty of the operation is the maneuver of instruments in a confined space. The 0-degree endoscope is preferred to a 30-degree endoscope as it gives a panoramic view of the nasopharynx even when it is positioned at the level of the incisor teeth. This gives ample space for the movement of the inserted robotic arms into the nasopharynx. When the 30-degree endoscope is introduced into the oral cavity with the slanting lens toward the roof of the nasopharynx, it takes up some space and limits the movement of the robotic arms:
- The spring over the horizontal bars of the Dingman mouth gag holds securely the stay sutures placed on the split soft palate and hard palate mucoperiosteum, and constant retraction is maintained.
- The assistant at the operating field contributes to suction of blood and smoke and also protects injury of soft tissue in and around the oral cavity from the movements of the robotic arm.
- The EndoWrist of the da Vinci robot cannot remove bone. Thus, when the anterior wall of the sphenoid has to be removed for additional resection margin, it must be done with endoscopic bone instruments transnasally.

PITFALLS

- As the tongue is retracted inferiorly during the whole procedure, edema might occur on releasing the retractor, which might cause airway obstruction. The maintenance of a patent airway should be confirmed before the endotracheal tube is removed at the completion of the operation.
- As all patients who have had previous radiation, the palatal closure might break down at the junction of the hard and soft palate. A hole is drilled at the posterior edge of the hard palate, and the suture passing through this hole and the soft palate musculature will attach soft tissue to the hard palate securely in an effort to reduce this complication.

INSTRUMENTS TO HAVE AVAILABLE

- The da Vinci Robot with the whole range of EndoWrist
- Dingman mouth gag
- A retractor holder to keep the Dingman mouth gag immobilized during the whole surgical procedure. It should be fixed to the side of the operating table to avoid interfering with the movements of the robotic arms.

SUGGESTED READING

O'Malley BW Jr, Weinstein GS. Robotic anterior and midline skull base surgery: preclinical investigations. *Int J Radiat Oncol Biol Phys* 2007;69:S125–S128.

Weinstein GS, O'Malley BW Jr, Snyder W, et al. Transoral robotic surgery: radical tonsillectomy. *Arch Otolaryngol Head Neck Surg* 2007;133:1220–1226.

Ozer E, Waltonen J. Transoral robotic nasopharyngectomy: a novel approach for nasopharyngeal lesions. *Laryngoscope* 2008;118:1613–1616.

Wei WI, Ho WK. Transoral robotic resection of recurrent nasopharyngeal carcinoma. *Laryngoscope* 2010;120:2011–2014.

Yin Tsang RK, Ho WK, Wei WI. Combined transnasal endoscopic and transoral robotic resection of recurrent nasopharyngeal carcinoma. *Head Neck* 2012;34:1190–1193.

35 MAXILLARY SWING

Jimmy Yu-Wai Chan

INTRODUCTION

Nasopharyngeal carcinoma (NPC) is unique among other head and neck malignancies with regard to its epidemiology, pathology, and treatment outcome. It is endemic in southern China and Southeast Asia, with a reported annual incidence of 10 to 50 per 100,000 population. The primary treatment modality for NPC is radiotherapy for early-stage cancers and concomitant chemoradiation for more advanced NPC. Surgical resection is usually reserved for persistent or recurrent cancer after the initial treatment.

Anatomically, the nasopharynx is located at the central skull base in the center of the head, which is over 10 cm from the skin surface in all directions. As a result, adequate exposure for surgical resection of cancers involving this region is often difficult, especially when the cancer has infiltrated the nearby structures.

The maxillary swing approach originated from the observation that during maxillectomy for carcinoma of the maxillary antrum, the nasopharynx was widely exposed when the maxilla was removed. During the maxillary swing operation, the maxillary antrum, including the lateral walls and the floor attached to the anterior cheek flap, is swung laterally as an osteocutaneous flap, in order to expose the pathology in the nasopharynx. After removal of the cancer, the maxillary antrum was returned to its original position and fixed to the rest of the facial skeleton.

HISTORY

A detailed history, physical examination, and imaging studies are crucial for precise preoperative planning in order to achieve the best oncologic and functional outcome. Details of the patient's general health should be sought, including a history of major cardiac or neurologic comorbidities and the need for antiplatelet or anticoagulant consumption. Information such as the initial stage of the cancer on presentation and the subsequent treatment protocol, including the use of induction chemotherapy, concomitant chemoradiation, as well as the type and dosage of external radiation given, is important. The history of recurrent cancer and its subsequent treatment, such as a second course of external radiotherapy, brachytherapy, or surgery, should be obtained. The spectrum of complications from previous treatment, including xerostomia, trismus, hearing problem, loss of smell and taste, velopharyngeal incompetence, and dysphagia, should be thoroughly assessed, as these symptoms may deteriorate further after surgery.

PHYSICAL EXAMINATION

The general status of the patients should be assessed for their fitness for surgery under general anesthesia. Neurologic status, including cranial nerve palsy (such as the abducens nerve), should be noted, as this may signify intracranial tumor extension and, hence, inoperability. The degree of preexisting trismus should be measured, as severe trismus will decrease exposure and increase the difficulty of surgery. The general dental health is assessed, and if necessary, a preoperative dental consultation will be arranged. The neck should be thoroughly examined for cervical lymphadenopathy, and further investigation has to be performed if there is any clinical suspicion of lymph node metastasis. Otoscopy should be carried out since middle ear effusion is a common finding.

INDICATIONS

Pathology of the anterior skull base, including

- Persistent or recurrent NPC after chemoradiation
- Adenocarcinoma or minor salivary gland tumor of the nasopharynx as primary treatment
- Chordoma
- Schwannoma

CONTRAINDICATIONS

- Patients whose medical condition is not fit for general anesthesia
- Persistent or recurrent NPC with significant intracranial extension
- Significant parapharyngeal extension with encasement of the petrosal internal carotid artery
- Patients who have had previous surgery via the midface degloving approach

PREOPERATIVE PLANNING

Routine ultrasound examination of the neck is necessary, and if suspicious lymphadenopathy is evident, ultrasound-guided fine needle aspiration should be performed. Cross-sectional imaging study of the naso-pharynx and the skull base using MRI with intravenous contrast offers the best spatial resolution allowing accurate assessment of the extent of the cancer, the presence of invasion of the parapharyngeal space, retro-pharyngeal lymph node metastasis, as well as the relationship with the petrosal internal carotid artery and the skull base.

The plasma level of Epstein-Barr virus DNA should be measured, and if it is more than 500 copies per milliliter, systemic metastasis should be suspected and whole body [^{18}F]-FDG PET-CT scan should be performed. If necessary, preoperative pulmonary and cardiac optimization should be arranged.

Dental assessment must be performed, and an obturator should be fabricated for each patient before the maxillary swing procedure; this is used to clip onto the teeth on the upper jaw upon return of the swung maxilla, ensuring correct repositioning and precise dental alignment.

Endoscopic examination should be performed before surgery. Biopsy of the lesion of concern is done for histologic confirmation. It also maps the extent of the disease and determines which side of the face to swing during the subsequent surgery.

SURGICAL TECHNIQUE

The operation is carried out under general anesthesia with the patient in the supine position. The head is placed on a soft head ring to allow mobility, and support behind the shoulders should be inserted to extend the neck if a neck dissection or neck exploration is necessary. Endotracheal intubation is carried out through the mouth if possible as this avoids disturbance of the cancer in the nasopharynx. A temporary tracheostomy is then performed, and the endotracheal tube is withdrawn. This avoids the risk of damage to the endotracheal tube during osteotomy, and the tracheostomy protects the airway should postoperative bleeding or edema occur.

Protective eye ointment is used in the contralateral eye, which is draped out of the operative field. The oral cavity and the nasal cavities are irrigated with copious amount of antiseptic solution such as chlorhexidine. Intravenous antibiotics are given on induction of anesthesia, and this usually includes a metronidazole for anaerobic bacteria and a cephalosporin for aerobic bacteria.

 The Weber-Ferguson facial incision is used as it is for maxillectomy; the horizontal limb of the incision is placed at the subciliary region 5 mm below and parallel to the lower eyelid margin (Fig. 35.1; Video 35.1). The incision over the lip is designed to be zigzag to prevent postoperative contracture, and the horizontal limb curves down laterally along the skin crease to stop at about 0.5 cm above the lower edge of the zygomatic arch. Tarsorrhaphy is done for the eye on the side of the swing to avoid inadvertent trauma to the cornea.

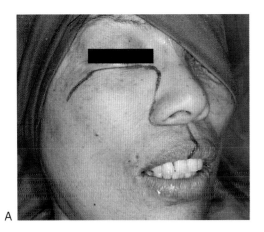

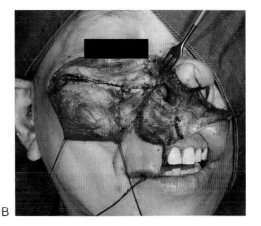

FIGURE 35.1
A: Weber-Ferguson-Longmire incision for right maxillary swing operation. **B:** After skin incision, the underlying osteotomy sites (*blue line*) are exposed. By maintaining the attachment of the maxilla to the overlying soft tissue, the blood supply of the underlying bone is secured.

The lip incision on the lingual surface continues to extend posteriorly to stop between the two central incisors. The palatal wound is created using a curved incision placed at a distance of 0.5 mm from the tooth margin; it is continued posteriorly until the last molar tooth and then continued laterally behind it to stop just before reaching the buccal mucosa. This allows the elevation of soft tissue and mucoperiosteum over the hard palate as a palatal flap with blood supply from the opposite mucoperiosteum of the hard palate and the soft palate.

The incision over the face goes through skin, subcutaneous tissue, and the orbicularis oculi muscle. The thin muscle is lifted together with the facial skin until the orbital rim is reached. The orbital septum should not be cut, or else there will be herniation of the periorbital adipose tissue. The skin incision over the lip is continued, and the orbicularis oris muscle is divided in the line of skin incision.

The horizontal limb of the facial incision goes down to the anterior wall of the maxilla; a limited amount of soft tissue over the anterior wall of the maxilla is elevated to expose a strip of bone for the osteotomy. This osteotomy site is 0.5 cm below the orbital rim and frequently goes through the infraorbital foramen. The infraorbital nerve and vessels are identified and divided. This reduces blood loss when the oscillating saw cuts through the infraorbital foramen. This osteotomy is made to divide only the lower half of the zygoma.

In preparation for the midline osteotomy, soft tissue and mucoperiosteum over the hard plate have to be dissected off of the bony hard palate. The palatal incision goes down to hard palate bone, and the soft tissue together with the mucoperiosteum is lifted with a sharp periosteal elevator. The greater palatine vessels coming through the palatine foramen are seen. These should be divided, and then the palatal flap can be raised further, medially to cross the midline and posterior to the posterior edge of the hard palate. The attachment of the soft palate on the hard palate is divided with diathermy, and the nasal cavity is entered.

A curved osteotome is inserted into the groove between the maxillary tuberosity and the pterygoid plates. The groove lies behind the hamulus, which is lying posteromedial to the molar tooth and can be palpated. The osteotome has to be curved so that when it is placed in the groove and driven by the mallet, it goes vertically upward separating the posterior wall of the maxillary antrum from the pterygoid plates.

Before starting the osteotomy, a 4-hole titanium plate is placed across the osteotomy line on the anterior wall of the maxilla, holes are drilled, and screws are inserted and then removed. These preosteotomy drilled holes will ensure accurate positioning of the maxilla when it is returned to its original site after tumor resection and fixed with the plate and screw. The osteotomy over the anterior wall is carried out by an oscillating saw with a long thin blade. The osteotomy begins in the anterior wall of the maxilla and extends laterally horizontally until the middle portion of the zygomatic arch and then turned downward. Only the inferior part of the zygomatic arch is divided, and thus, after completion of the osteotomy, the inferior orbital rim remains attached to the zygoma.

The soft tissue over the midline is elevated to expose the underlying bone, in preparation for a midline osteotomy. The patient has a high nasal spine; this can be removed with a burr or a rongeur creating a flat bone surface where the titanium plate is placed. Holes are drilled, and screws are inserted and removed similar to the procedure applied on the anterior wall of the maxilla.

An oscillating saw divides the hard palate from anterior to posterior in a straight line. The elevated palatal flap is retracted from the path of the osteotomy and protected. This osteotomy extends through the entire length of the hard palate and inferior part of the nasal septum if there is a septal deviation. The blood loss is minimal with this osteotomy so it is carried out as the first osteotomy. Then the osteotomy of the anterior wall of the maxilla is carried out with the long thin blade; the blade goes through the antrum and divides the lateral wall on its way until it reaches and cuts the post wall. The final osteotomy goes through the medial wall of the antrum and is placed above the inferior turbinate and below the middle turbinate.

After completing the osteotomies, the maxilla drops inferiorly, but remained attached to the anterior cheek flap. The entire osteocutaneous complex is retracted laterally to expose the nasopharynx and the parapharyngeal space (Fig. 35.2). With this exposure, persistent or recurrent cancer in the nasopharynx can be removed together with the Eustachian tube if necessary under direct vision. When present, the retropharyngeal lymph nodes can also be removed.

FIGURE 35.2
A: After the osteotomies, the maxilla (MS) is swung out. The underling cancer (C) in the nasopharynx is exposed. If the parapharyngeal space is involved by the cancer, it is resected en bloc with the pterygoid muscles (PM) down to and including the underlying the pharyngobasilar fascia. **B:** Specimen showing the cancer (C) resected with wide mucosal margins including the ipsilateral eustachian tube (ET).

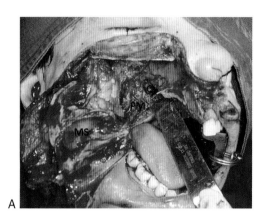
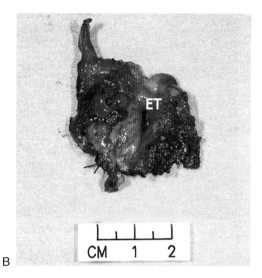

With the osteocutaneous complex including the maxilla swung laterally, the cancer in the nasopharynx with its surrounding tissue is adequately exposed and can be removed with conventional surgical instruments such as scissors and diathermy. The pterygoid plates together with the pterygoid muscle can be removed to improve exposure of the parapharyngeal space on the side of the swing, and any pathologic lymph nodes if present in the region can be removed under direct vision. The internal carotid artery lying outside the pharyngobasilar fascia is situated posteriorly or posterolaterally to the retropharyngeal lymph nodes, and sometimes it could be adherent to the lymph node following radiotherapy. With this wide exposure, the carotid artery can be located with palpation of its pulsation and thus safeguarded during resection of the retropharyngeal lymph nodes.

When the pharyngobasilar fascia has to be resected with the cancer or the retropharyngeal lymph node, the petrosal portion of the internal carotid artery will be exposed. This can be covered with a microvascular free muscle flap to prevent subsequent rupture of the carotid artery.

The frequently employed free muscle flaps include the rectus abdominis or the vastus lateralis muscle. The pedicle is delivered through a tunnel made above the oropharynx to the upper neck. The artery of the flap is joined to the facial or superior thyroid artery, and the venous return is anastomosed to a tributary of the internal jugular vein. The transferred muscle is covered by mucosa within a short period, and this avoids the crusting when skin is used to cover the wound in the nasopharynx.

Increased exposure of the contralateral nasopharynx is achieved following the removal of the posterior part of the nasal septum. Cancers that extend across the midline can be resected up to the medial edge of the Eustachian tube of the opposite side. Following this wide exposure, en bloc resection of the NPC can be carried out including the eustachian tube crura. The inferior turbinate on the side of the swing is removed, and the mucosa covering it is removed. This mucosal sheet is laid onto the raw area in the nasopharynx as a free mucosal graft. This graft frequently survives and facilitates healing, and even if it does not survive, it acts as a temporary dressing for the wound in the nasopharynx.

After excising the cancer and covering the raw area in the nasopharynx, the maxilla is returned to its original position. A few holes are drilled on the posterior edge of the hard palate, and sutures passing through these holes attach the soft palate to the hard palate. A hole is drilled on the base of the nasal bone, a corresponding hole is drilled on the superomedial part of the anterior wall of the maxilla, and a size 26 wire is passed through these holes. The intraoral placement of the prefabricated dental plate ensures accurate repositioning of the maxilla.

While the maxilla is maintained in position with the hand, the two titanium plates are placed over the zygoma and the midline where screw holes were predrilled and the screws inserted (Fig. 35.3). The wire on the superomedial angle of the anterior wall of the maxilla is also tightened to give additional support.

The dental plate is then removed and the palatal flap returned. Two to three sutures are used to fix the posterior part of the flap to the alveolar margin, and the dental plate is reinserted to keep the palatal flap in position.

POSTOPERATIVE MANAGEMENT

After surgery, the patient is nursed in the general ward. It is important to perform frequent suction of the tracheostomy tube to prevent blockage. The cuff of the tracheostomy tube is kept inflated for the first postoperative day in order to protect the airway from blood and secretions from the operative field. Afterward, it should be deflated, and the tracheostomy tube can be removed 3 to 4 days after surgery. Enteral nutrition via the nasogastric tube can be started on postoperative day one until 1 week after surgery when the palatal wound is usually stable enough to allow eating per orally. The nasogastric tube is then removed. Antibiotics are continued

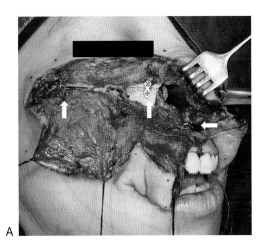 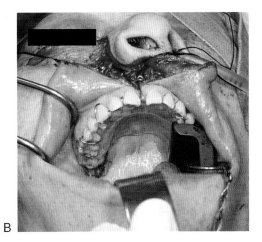

FIGURE 35.3
A: After the cancer is resected, the maxilla is returned to its normal anatomical position and fixed with titanium miniplates and screws (*arrows*). A nasogastric tube is inserted for feeding during the early postoperative period **B:** A prefabricated obturator is inserted to ensure accurate dental approximation.

intravenously, which is then switched to oral administration for a total duration of 1 week. The facial sutures are removed 1 week after surgery, and nasal irrigation using 0.9% sodium chloride solution is started by the patient himself/herself four to six times per day. The patient is then discharged from the hospital.

Mouth-opening exercises starting as early as 8 weeks after surgery effectively prevent trismus. Once developed, it will be more difficult to restore the preoperative degree of mouth opening. The treatment used most commonly is using a stack of tongue depressors between the teeth to push the mouth open over time. Another effective way is to use the TheraBite Jaw Motion Rehabilitation System (Atos Medical, West Allis, WI), which is a patient-operated device for passive stretching of the jaw.

The patients are then followed up regularly in the outpatient clinic, monthly for the first year, and less frequently afterward. Endoscopic examination is performed to ensure satisfactory wound healing and to detect tumor recurrence.

COMPLICATIONS

Most of the potential complications after maxillary swing operation are preventable. Careful patient selection is crucial, and it is important to identify patients with petrosal internal carotid artery encasement and skull base erosion and intracranial extension, as the presence of these signifies inoperability. Early postoperative hemorrhage can be prevented by meticulous hemostasis, and delayed bleeding secondary to carotid artery blowout is avoided by using healthy muscle (such as temporalis muscle flap or free vastus lateralis muscle flap) to cover the exposed artery at the time of surgery. Flap coverage is also indicated in patients with extensive resection resulting in wide area of raw bone exposure. Failure to do so may lead to osteoradionecrosis, which may result in acute bacterial meningitis and death. Careful handling of the palatal mucosal flap is important to prevent palatal fistula formation. Recent modification of the palatal incision so that it no longer overlies on the osteotomy site significantly reduces the incidence of palatal fistulation from 24% to 4.2%.

RESULTS

Between 1989 and 2011, nasopharyngectomy was performed in 312 patients in our institution. Among our patients, 41 (13.1%) had persistent cancer and 271 (86.9%) had recurrent cancer. Resection with negative margins was achieved in 248 (79.5%) patients. All patients survived the operation. The mean hospital stay was 8.6 days. The median follow-up duration was 34 months. The overall 5-year actuarial local tumor control was 74%, and the overall 5-year disease-free survival was 56%. Those with negative resection margins on frozen section and tumor size <1.5 cm in diameter had significantly better local control in the nasopharynx as well as disease-free survival. The majority of the patients had satisfactory healing of the facial wounds (Fig. 35.4).

PEARLS

- Preoperative planning and evaluation of the status of the cancer are essential to achieve good surgical outcome. Those patients with infiltration of the petrosal internal carotid artery and the base of the skull are not surgical candidates.
- Preosteotomy plating using titanium miniplates ensures precise apposition of bone and hence dental occlusal relationships on closure.

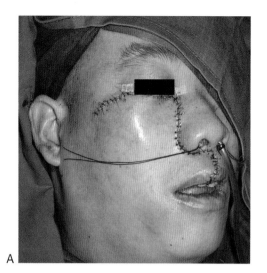
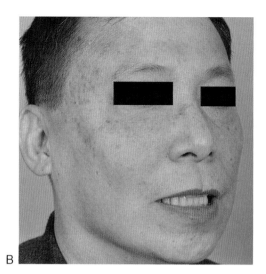

FIGURE 35.4
A: Anatomical closure of the facial wound in layers. **B:** Photo taken 6 months after surgery, showing satisfactory healing of facial wound.

- The contralateral nasopharynx can be approached by removing the posterior portion of the nasal septum.
- For cancers with parapharyngeal extension or when retropharyngeal lymph node metastasis is evident, resection of the tumor en bloc with the pharyngobasilar fascia ensures tumor clearance on the surface of the petrosal internal carotid artery. The resultant exposure of the artery requires healthy tissue coverage, most commonly free vastus lateralis muscle flap, to prevent subsequent fatal carotid artery blowout.

PITFALLS

- Radical resection of a large cancer will result in exposure of a wide area of raw bone at the skull base and cervical spine, increasing the risk of subsequent osteoradionecrosis, especially when a second course of external radiotherapy is required. Prophylactic coverage using microvascular free flap effectively prevents this complication.
- Meticulous handling of the palatal mucosal flap and separating the palatal mucosal incision from the osteotomy line reduce the incidence of palatal fistula formation.
- The majority of the patients experience a variable degree of trismus after surgery. It is essential to starting passive stretching and jaw-opening exercise once wound healing has been completed in order to prevent this complication.

INSTRUMENTS TO HAVE AVAILABLE

- Titanium miniplates and screws and a corresponding drill
- Curved osteotome
- Pneumatic-driven oscillating saw
- Monopolar cautery
- Heavy scissors
- Dental obturator

SUGGESTED READING

Chan JY, Chow VL, Tsang RK, et al. Nasopharyngectomy for locally advanced recurrent nasopharyngeal carcinoma: exploring the limits. *Head Neck* 2012;34(7):923–928.

Chan JY, Chow VL, Mok VW, et al. Prediction of surgical outcome using plasma Epstein-barr virus DNA and (18) F-FDG PET-CT scan in recurrent nasopharyngeal carcinoma. *Head Neck* 2012;34(4):541–545.

Chan JY, Chow VL, Wei WI. Quality of life of patients after salvage nasopharyngectomy for recurrent nasopharyngeal carcinoma. *Cancer* 2012;118(15):3710–3718.

Chan JY, Wei WI. Critical appraisal of maxillary swing approach for nasopharyngeal carcinoma. *Expert Opin Ther Targets* 2012;16(Suppl 1):S111–S117.

Chan JY, Wei WI. Recurrent nasopharyngeal carcinoma after salvage nasopharyngectomy. *Arch Otolaryngol Head Neck Surg* 2012;138(6):572–576.

(Note: Page number in italics denotes figures and those followed by "t" denotes tables.)